The Impact of Sports on Community Health and Development

Mehmet Öçal
https://orcid.org/0000-0001-6973-2611
Burdur Mehmet Akif Ersoy University, Turkey

Mehmet Ata Öztürk
Middle East Technical University, Turkey

IGI Global
Scientific Publishing
Publishing Tomorrow's Research Today

Vice President of Editorial Melissa Wagner
Director of Acquisitions Mikaela Felty
Director of Book Development Jocelynn Hessler
Production Manager Mike Brehm
Cover Design Jose Rosado

Published in the United States of America by
IGI Global Scientific Publishing
701 East Chocolate Avenue
Hershey, PA, 17033, USA
Tel: 717-533-8845 | Fax: 717-533-7115
Website: https://www.igi-global.com E-mail: cust@igi-global.com

Library of Congress Cataloging-in-Publication Data

LCCN: 2026032942 (CIP Data Pending)
ISBN13: 979-8-2600-3174-2
Isbn13Softcover: 979-8-2600-3175-9
EISBN13: 979-8-2600-3176-6
British Cataloguing in Publication Data
A Cataloguing in Publication record for this book is available from the British Library.

Table of Contents

Detailed Table of Contents

Although welfare is a complex concept, its objective is quite clear: to provide a decent life. This objective is pursued through social policies. Social policies are established against social risks and the market to ensure a living standard worthy of human dignity. Through these policies, the market is intervened in to attempt to offer a minimum level of welfare to every individual. At this precise point, sport is regarded as a fundamental field of social policy due to its protective, rehabilitative, and empowering role, as well as its multifaceted and positive effects on human well-being. Comprehensive social policies are implemented to disseminate and expand sport to the grassroots because of these aforementioned effects. Within the scope of this study, the position of sport as a social policy has been evaluated within the framework of welfare regime typologies, and a comprehensive discussion has been conducted on the impact of sport on individual and social welfare.It has been found that spreading sport to the grassroots is a vital factor in making social welfare sustainable.

Sport has multifaceted effects, from breaking down social exclusion to fighting for freedom. This makes sport a fundamental tool of social policy. It positions sport as a core component of social policies that enhance individual well-being and social citizenship. The main objective of this study is to highlight the impact of sport on well-being and to determine which country uses sport more effectively as a social policy. Fort his purpose, chapter is the development of the "Sport-Friendly Country Index," designed to classify 37 countries based on their implementation of sport-related welfare policies. Using "Min-Max Normalization," the index evaluates 14 parameters, including sport-related GDP expenditure, employment, volunteering rates, and bureaucratic structures. The analysis reveals that welfare typologies significantly influence a nation's "sport-friendly" score.

This chapter examines the transformation of sport from a recreational and leisure-time activity into a multidimensional social policy instrument, drawing on both global developments and the Turkish case. The first section scrutinizes the historical evolution of sport as a vehicle of social policy, suggesting its early use in industrial societies as a tool for discipline, its institutionalization within welfare state schemes, and its later reconceptualization within the "Sport for Development and Peace" paradigm. The second section provides a comparative analysis of sport policy development across different countries, including Western and Asian models. The chapter identifies common patterns in sport policy development among differing national contexts: increased state involvement, professionalization, and the tension between elite sport and mass participation.

This study critically examines how sports help combat poverty, particularly in the context of welfare-state changes and social policy. While sports often empower disadvantaged groups and promote well-being, this focus usually obscures deeper causes of poverty, like income inequality and unstable work. The impact of sports policies on poverty depends on welfare regime types. In social democratic regimes, sports complement universal rights. In conservative models, they build local solidarity. In liberal regimes, they are mainly a symbolic, low-cost tool stressing individual responsibility rather than addressing structural roots. The study argues that sports can foster a sense of belonging and provide short-term well-being. However, when used instead of comprehensive social mechanisms, sports make poverty manageable and less visible rather than reducing it. If sports do not align with core welfare responsibilities, they risk becoming a symbolic substitute rather than a structural solution.

This chapter examines the relationship between social welfare levels and sports policies within a socio-economic and structural framework. Sport is considered not merely as a field promoting physical activity, but also as a significant public policy instrument contributing to social integration, equality, public health, and the development of social capital. In this context, the chapter analyzes how sports policies are shaped in high-welfare societies and evaluates their effects on social participation through a comparative perspective with Türkiye.

This study evaluates the distribution and public-interest orientation of sports-related tax incentives in Türkiye, using TÜİK's 2024 Industry and Services Statistics and Revenue Administration tax-expenditure data. In 2024, 13,022 sports enterprises employed 45,097 people. Although sports clubs represented a small share of enterprises, they generated 43.6% of sectoral value added; value added per paid employee was about 9.4 times the annual gross minimum wage. Fitness and bodybuilding centres comprised nearly half of enterprises, yet their corresponding ratio was only 0.84. Türkiye supports national sport through wage exemptions, sponsorship deductions, reduced withholding rates, and income, corporate and value-added tax exemptions. However, insufficient beneficiary-level data prevent reliable evaluation of effectiveness and distributional fairness. The study recommends redirecting support toward community programmes, amateur clubs, young people and persons with disabilities; providing conditional incentives to small fitness centres and sports entrepreneurs; and regularly assessing the cost-effectiveness and distributional impact of all sports-related tax expenditures.

This chapter examines whether government spending on sport truly improves social welfare. While sport is often promoted as a way to enhance health, social inclusion, and community development, evidence shows that its benefits are uneven and sometimes overstated. Public funding frequently supports elite and commercially successful sports rather than community-based activities that benefit wider populations. A key concept discussed is the "subsidy paradox," where funding intended to help disadvantaged groups often benefits already advantaged individuals due to barriers such as cost, access, and social support. The chapter applies theories from economics and social justice to evaluate when sport subsidies are justified. It proposes a capability-based framework that focuses on improving real opportunities for participation, especially for disadvantaged groups. Overall, the chapter calls for fairer distribution, better evaluation, and policy reforms to ensure sport funding genuinely contributes to social welfare.

The intersection of women's sports, social policy, and justice commitments within the global sustainability economy represents an evolving domain of scholarly and policy relevance. This chapter critically examines how gender equity in sports contributes to broader sustainability goals, including social inclusion, economic empowerment, and institutional accountability. It explores structural inequalities that persist in women's sports, such as disparities in funding, media representation, and governance, while situating these challenges within global policy frameworks like the Sustainable Development Goals (SDGs). The chapter further evaluates the role of public policy, corporate engagement, and transnational advocacy in promoting equitable sports ecosystems. By integrating feminist theory, sustainability discourse, and institutional analysis, the study advances a multidimensional understanding of sports as a site of justice. It concludes by proposing policy pathways that align women's sports development with sustainability-driven social transformation

This chapter presents an analysis of sport as a strategic social policy tool, highlighting its potential to advance public health, social inclusion, youth development, and community cohesion. Drawing on theoretical frameworks such as social capital, welfare theory, and the Sport-for-Development and Peace (SDP) approach, this chapter examines how sport can improve physical and mental well-being, empower marginalized populations, foster life skills and education, and strengthen collective identity. Challenges including unequal access, governance issues, commercialization, and ethical concerns are discussed, alongside evidence-based policy recommendations for equitable, inclusive, and sustainable sport-based interventions.

This chapter analyzes sport as a social policy instrument and its impact on the well-being of individuals with disabilities across different welfare state regimes. Rather than treating sport as a neutral or purely recreational activity, it conceptualizes it as a structured policy field shaped by institutional arrangements, state capacity, and ideological orientations. Using a qualitative literature review and a comparative framework based on Esping-Andersen's welfare regime typology, the study examines how liberal, corporatist, and social democratic systems differ in their sport policy approaches. The findings show that participation in sport improves physical, psychological, and social well-being, while fostering self-confidence, social inclusion, and quality of life. However, these benefits are not universal and depend on inclusive infrastructure, public investment, and rights-based policies. The chapter concludes that the effectiveness of sport as a social policy tool is shaped by welfare regime characteristics and broader commitments to equality and inclusion.

Preface

INTRODUCTION

Sport has long been recognized for its contributions to physical fitness, recreation, and entertainment. However, contemporary scholarship increasingly demonstrates that its significance extends well beyond these traditional domains. Across diverse societies and political systems, sport has emerged as a powerful instrument for advancing public health, strengthening social cohesion, promoting inclusion, supporting economic development, and addressing complex social challenges. Governments, international organizations, and civil society actors now view sport as an essential component of broader social policy frameworks capable of enhancing individual well-being while contributing to sustainable community development. This evolving understanding provides the intellectual foundation for *The Impact of Sports on Community Health and Development.*

The primary objective of this volume is to examine sport not merely as an isolated social activity but as an interdisciplinary policy field that intersects with welfare systems, public administration, economics, law, education, health, and social justice. Bringing together contributions from distinguished scholars and practitioners representing multiple countries and disciplinary backgrounds, this edited collection investigates how sport contributes to welfare creation, social protection, equality, community resilience, and inclusive development. While many studies have explored the physiological or economic dimensions of sport, comparatively fewer have examined its role within welfare state institutions and social policy regimes. This volume seeks to address that gap by presenting both theoretical perspectives and evidence-based policy discussions.

A defining characteristic of this book is its comparative and multidisciplinary approach. The contributing authors examine sport through diverse analytical lenses, including welfare regime theory, social capital, capability theory, labor law, public finance, gender studies, disability studies, sustainability, governance, and development policy. Together, these perspectives demonstrate that the social value of sport depends not simply on participation itself but on the institutional arrangements, legal protections, public investments, and policy choices that shape opportunities for equitable access and meaningful participation. Consequently, the chapters encourage readers to move beyond simplistic assumptions regarding the universal benefits of sport and instead critically examine the conditions under which sport contributes to sustainable welfare.

This volume has been prepared for researchers, academics, graduate students, policymakers, public administrators, sport managers, and professionals working within health, education, and community development sectors. We hope that the discussions presented throughout this collection stimulate interdisciplinary dialogue, encourage comparative research, and support evidence-informed policymaking. As societies continue to confront growing inequalities, demographic changes, public health challenges, and sustainability concerns, understanding the role of sport within broader welfare systems has become increasingly important. It is our sincere hope that this book contributes meaningfully to that ongoing conversation.

OVERVIEW OF THE CHAPTERS

The volume opens with Chapter 1, which establishes the conceptual foundation by examining sport as a social policy instrument within different welfare state regimes and discussing its contribution to sustainable social welfare. Building upon this framework, Chapter 2 introduces the innovative *Sport-Friendly Country Index*, providing a comparative assessment of countries according to the effectiveness of their sport-related welfare policies. Chapter 3 traces the historical evolution of sports policies globally and in Türkiye, demonstrating how sport has progressively become an integral component of modern social policy.

The following chapters explore the relationship between sport and welfare from complementary policy perspectives. Chapter 4 critically evaluates whether sport functions as a genuine mechanism for poverty reduction or merely serves as a symbolic substitute for broader welfare interventions. Chapter 5 compares sports policies in Türkiye with those of high-welfare societies, highlighting the connections between public investment, participation, and social inclusion. Chapter 6 examines tax incentives for sport through an international comparative analysis, emphasizing financing models that promote transparency, distributive justice, and public benefit. Chapter 7 addresses the allocation of public sport subsidies, proposing a capability-based framework that prioritizes equitable access and improved social welfare outcomes.

Questions of equality, inclusion, and social justice form the central focus of the next group of chapters. Chapter 8 investigates women's sport within the context of sustainability, justice, and global policy commitments, while Chapter 9 analyzes athletes' social protection through the perspectives of labor law and social security systems. Chapter 10 evaluates Türkiye's state-led sport programs as instruments of social inclusion and welfare policy. Chapter 11 broadens the discussion by examining inclusive sport systems as mechanisms for advancing public health, youth development, and community cohesion. Chapter 12 focuses specifically on individuals with disabilities, demonstrating how welfare regimes influence opportunities for participation and well-being through inclusive sport policies.

The final chapters expand the discussion toward broader questions of governance, social cohesion, and institutional transformation. Chapter 13 explores sport's role in strengthening social cohesion and reducing social risks through community-based programs. Chapter 14 analyzes the relationships among welfare regimes, social justice, and equitable sport policy. Chapter 15 presents the innovative "Samanta Model," illustrating how sports-centered welfare can facilitate indigenous social inclusion through integrated education, healthcare, and sport systems. Chapter 16 critically examines contemporary football as a field shaped by competing forces of financialization and social welfare, while Chapter 17 concludes the volume by discussing the legal, social, and welfare dimensions of modern sport governance and advocating a rights-based approach to athlete protection.

Collectively, these chapters demonstrate the diverse ways in which sport intersects with public policy, legal systems, social institutions, and community development. While each contribution approaches the topic from a distinct disciplinary perspective, together they provide a comprehensive understanding of sport as a strategic instrument for promoting health, equity, inclusion, and sustainable social development.

CONCLUSION

The chapters assembled in this volume collectively illustrate that sport should no longer be viewed solely through the lenses of competition, recreation, or entertainment. Rather, sport has become a multidimensional public policy domain capable of influencing health outcomes, strengthening social capital, promoting equality, enhancing community resilience, and supporting sustainable development. At the same time, the contributors remind us that these positive outcomes are not automatic. The social benefits of sport depend fundamentally upon equitable access, effective governance, inclusive institutions, adequate public investment, and coherent welfare policies.

Another important contribution of this volume lies in its comparative perspective. By examining experiences from different welfare regimes, legal traditions, and national contexts, the book demonstrates that there is no single model for integrating sport into social policy. Instead, successful approaches are shaped by institutional capacity, political priorities, cultural values, and long-term commitments to social justice. The diversity of perspectives presented throughout the volume enriches our understanding of how sport policies can be designed to respond effectively to varying social, economic, and demographic challenges.

We are deeply grateful to all contributing authors whose expertise, commitment, and scholarly rigor have made this collection possible. Their interdisciplinary contributions reflect the richness of contemporary sport policy research and demonstrate the growing importance of collaboration across fields including public policy, economics, sociology, law, health sciences, education, and development studies. We also acknowledge the reviewers and publishing team whose constructive feedback and professional support have strengthened the quality and coherence of this volume.

As editors, we hope this book serves as both a valuable scholarly reference and a practical resource for researchers, educators, policymakers, and practitioners working to harness the transformative potential of sport. We anticipate that the ideas presented here will inspire further research, encourage interdisciplinary collaboration, and contribute to the development of more inclusive, evidence-based, and socially responsive sport policies. Ultimately, if sport is to realize its full potential as a catalyst for healthier, fairer, and more resilient communities, it must continue to be understood and developed as an integral component of broader welfare and social development strategies.

Mehmet Öçal
Burdur Mehmet Akif Ersoy University, Turkey

Mehmet Ata Öztürk
Middle East Technical University, Turkey

Chapter 1
Sport as a Social Policy Tool in Ensuring Welfare

Mehmet Öçal
http://orcid.org/0000-0001-6973-2611
Burdur Mehmet Akif Ersoy University, Turkey

ABSTRACT

Although welfare is a complex concept, its objective is quite clear: to provide a decent life. This objective is pursued through social policies. Social policies are established against social risks and the market to ensure a living standard worthy of human dignity. Through these policies, the market is intervened in to attempt to offer a minimum level of welfare to every individual. At this precise point, sport is regarded as a fundamental field of social policy due to its protective, rehabilitative, and empowering role, as well as its multifaceted and positive effects on human well-being. Comprehensive social policies are implemented to disseminate and expand sport to the grassroots because of these aforementioned effects. Within the scope of this study, the position of sport as a social policy has been evaluated within the framework of welfare regime typologies, and a comprehensive discussion has been conducted on the impact of sport on individual and social welfare.It has been found that spreading sport to the grassroots is a vital factor in making social welfare sustainable.

INTRODUCTION

Social policy, at its core, represents a humanitarian endeavor designed to protect and improve social welfare by addressing the inherent challenges posed by modern economic systems. Often described as the "doctor of capitalism," social policy seeks to repair systemic deficiencies and limit the potential for exploitation through

DOI: 10.4018/979-8-2600-3174-2.ch001

targeted interventions that foster a more equitable society. Within this framework, sport has emerged as a fundamental and multi-dimensional instrument of social policy, evolving from simple physical activity into a systematic social structure deeply integrated into the collective fabric of society. In the contemporary era, the welfare state utilizes sport not merely for physical fitness, but as a flexible tool to achieve broader non-sporting objectives, including social cohesion, economic development, and international relations.

The relationship between sport and social policy is rooted in the recognition of sporting participation as an inherent human right, analogous to the rights to education and health. This perspective positions the provision of sporting opportunities as a primary public service that should be driven by social equity rather than profit motives. As a social phenomenon, sport serves as a vital resource for addressing complex issues such as social exclusion, juvenile delinquency, and public health crises. Specifically, the role of sport in protective and preventive health services is paramount; regular physical activity shields individuals from chronic conditions, thereby enhancing general well-being and providing significant "exchequer benefits" by reducing state health expenditures. Beyond physical health, sport offers essential psychological support, alleviating depression and social isolation by providing a context for social interaction and a sense of belonging.

A cornerstone of effective sports policy is the concept of "spreading sport to the grassroots" (*Tabana Yayılma Politikası*), which is essential for the realization of social justice. By making facilities and activities accessible to all geographical regions—particularly those with low socio-economic development—sport acts as one of the most effective methods to combat social exclusion. For disadvantaged groups, including individuals with disabilities and those from low-income backgrounds, sport provides an indispensable pathway for rehabilitation and social integration based on equal opportunity.

However, the modern commodification of sport poses a significant threat to these humanitarian goals. As fitness is increasingly packaged as a market-driven commodity, material barriers can exclude those living in poverty, risking the transformation of sport into a class-based activity. Furthermore, the influence of neoliberalism has shifted the delivery of sport toward public-private partnerships, which sometimes prioritizes higher-income groups over community objectives. To counter these pressures, state intervention and public investment under the "Sport for All" principle are necessary to ensure that the focus remains on the social, physical, and mental development of every individual

1. SPORT AS A TOOL OF SOCIAL POLICY

Social policy is a humanitarian endeavor. Born as a concession made by capitalism itself during the Industrial Revolution, this approach, which in later years aimed to combat all social problems affecting humanity, fundamentally seeks to protect and improve social welfare. In other words, social policy is essentially the doctor of capitalism. It carries its inherent characteristics and strives to repair its deficiencies. Because the greatest threat to human welfare in post-Industrial Revolution society is capitalism itself, due to its potential for exploiting labor. Social policy, at this point, limits capitalism and implements interventions to improve it in order to protect the system. These interventions take place in the market in a corporatist manner. Various limits and rules are set by laws, and violations of these limits or rules are punished. On the other hand, individuals who fall below the minimum living conditions determined by social policymakers are supported through various social transfers. States that have embraced this humanitarian aim of social policy and intervene in the market at various levels, or are willing to do so, are called welfare states. In other words, a welfare state is a state that implements social policy. Depending on the scope and intensity of social policies, the term welfare state is also used to describe an advanced social state. Due to its rehabilitative, unifying, and protective role, sport is considered one of the fundamental social policy tools within the perspective of both the social and welfare states. Investments made by states to promote and expand participation in sports clearly demonstrate this. The positive effects of sport on the mental and physical health of individuals can also be presented as a justification for this trend (Öçal and Kutlu, 2024; Öçal, et al: 2022; Sütlü and Kutlu, 2025).

Sport throughout human history has evolved from unconscious physical movements into a systematic structure with defined rules that is deeply integrated into individual and social life. In the modern era, sport has transcended being merely a leisure activity or a tool for physical fitness, becoming a flexible, multi-dimensional instrument of social policy used by governments to achieve objectives in social welfare, economic development, and international relations. As a social policy tool, sport serves critical missions including the protection of physical and mental health, ensuring social cohesion, preventing social exclusion, integrating disadvantaged groups into the system, and establishing social justice. The fundamental objective of a social state or welfare regime is to offer citizens a standard, decent living condition worthy of human dignity. Within this framework, the right to participate in sport must be recognized as a fundamental and inherent right, similar to the rights to education and health, and its provision should not be driven by profit motives. The social state is obligated to provide welfare services regardless of language, religion, race, gender, or economic status, and sport acts as a dynamic that expands the multiplier effect of social peace and prosperity (Gençlik & Bakanlığı, 2012; Yerlikaya, 2012; Kasapoğlu and Öçal, 2021; Turaç 2024).

One of the most prominent functions of sport as a social policy tool is observed in the context of protective and preventive health services. Academic research confirms that regular physical activity protects against chronic health issues such as cardiovascular disease, obesity, and diabetes, while enhancing the general well-being of individuals. Building a healthy society reduces state health expenditures while increasing the productivity of working individuals, thereby providing significant economic gains. Consequently, sport serves public health under the philosophy of "active living" as an extension of health policies. However, the benefits of sport are not limited to the physical realm; it also offers psychological support by reducing stress, alleviating depression, and pulling individuals away from social isolation. In modern urban environments, where green spaces are diminishing and sedentary lifestyles are becoming the norm, sport-oriented recreation areas play a vital role in improving public health and strengthening social solidarity (Mumcu et al., 2025; Yerlikaya, 2012; Turaç 2024).

The policy of "spreading sport to the grassroots" (Tabana Yayılma Politikası) plays a vital role in ensuring social justice. If social justice is defined as equal access to services and opportunities provided by public authorities, then making sports facilities and activities accessible across all geographical regions—especially those with low socio-economic development—is one of the most effective methods to combat social exclusion. Encouraging sport among youth is strategically important for reducing crime rates, fighting substance abuse, and directing young people away from harmful habits toward activities compatible with social values. The spirit of togetherness inherent in team sports, which requires individuals to set aside differences to work toward a common goal, transforms sport into a natural mechanism for social integration. Youth centers have become dynamic hubs for this social inclusion, bringing together young people of different ages, nationalities, and beliefs in integrated complexes.

Disadvantaged groups are a primary focus of sport within the scope of social policy. Sport is an indispensable element for the rehabilitation of individuals with disabilities, the development of their physical and mental abilities, and their integration into society. Providing sporting opportunities for the disabled prevents them from feeling excluded and enhances their quality of life, thereby strengthening social equality. Similarly, for children from low-income families, street children, or children under institutional care, sport is a tool for personal development and social attachment based on equal opportunity. However, the commercialization of sport into a massive industry in the modern world can sometimes overshadow these social policy missions. In post-industrial societies, the transformation of sport into a commodity can make it difficult for low-income individuals to access sporting areas, risking the transformation of sport into a class-based activity enjoyed only by a certain elite. At this point, state intervention and public investment under the "sport for all" philosophy act as a balancing element against the commodification of sport (Kasapoğlu et al, 2020).

In the specific case of Turkey, sport policies are built upon a constitutional foundation. Article 59 of the 1982 Constitution defines it as a duty of the state to take measures to improve the physical and mental health of Turkish citizens of all ages and to encourage the spread of sport to the masses. This legal basis is clear evidence that sport is accepted as a social policy tool in the Turkish context. Within the framework of the "Grassroots Policy" implemented in recent years, there has been a significant increase in the geographical distribution of sports investments, with 4,383 sports facilities put into operation between 2005 and 2021. In particular, facility development projects in regions like Southeast and Eastern Anatolia, where socio-economic development needs support, carry great meaning for the fair distribution of welfare services and the establishment of social peace. The number of licensed athletes has also surpassed 10 million following the structural breaks in the early 2000s, reflecting the success of these expansion efforts. The link between education and sport constitutes another cornerstone of social policy. Sport is not just about physical development; it is an educational process where discipline, self-control, teamwork, and ethical values are instilled. Utilizing sport as a primary educational tool in schools allows for the early discovery of talents while fostering a sports culture based on sharing and fun rather than extreme competition. However, the success of sports policies should be measured by how widely these activities spread among the general public rather than just by the number of facilities or medals won by elite athletes. Current statistics indicate that participation rates in sport increase as income and education levels rise; this reality necessitates that the social state provide more incentives and free opportunities to ensure the active participation of low-income groups. The economic dimension of sport is also deeply intertwined with social policy goals. The sports industry has the capacity to create employment, revitalize tourism, and support regional development. It is estimated that millions are employed globally in sport-related sectors such as marketing, management, and media. Large sports organizations allow for the development of infrastructure, increased economic vitality, and the opening of new job fields in the regions where they are held. For example, the 2011 Erzurum Winter Universiade led to massive investments in winter tourism infrastructure and created thousands of temporary and permanent jobs. However, while pursuing these economic growth targets, the "pure" and integrative spirit of sport should not be sacrificed to commercial concerns. The hyper-competitiveness of professional sports and the commodification process driven by star athletes can fuel passive participation, imprisoning the rest of society in the role of mere "spectators". As a social policy tool, sport should aim for an active lifestyle that makes physical activity a part of daily life rather than just a show to be watched (Yerlikaya, 2012).

The globalization of sport since the 1980s has further complicated its role in social policy. While technology and mass media have made sport more accessible to global audiences, they have also subjected it to market pressures that prioritize profit over social value. The “Bosman Rulings” and the rise of multi-national sponsors have turned elite sports into a high-stakes financial sector. In this environment, social policies must work harder to protect the “Sport for All” principle, ensuring that the focus remains on the social, physical, and mental development of every individual regardless of their market value. Effective sports management requires a balance between supporting elite success for national prestige and ensuring that the base of the “sports pyramid”—the general public—has the resources to remain active and healthy. Furthermore, the environmental sustainability of sports facilities and events has become a modern social policy concern. Promoting eco-friendly sports facilities and minimizing the environmental impact of mega-events aligns sport with broader global goals for a sustainable future. Sport can also serve as a tool for “sports diplomacy,” fostering dialogue between nations and enhancing international reputation. These diverse roles underscore why sport cannot be left to the mercy of the free market alone; it requires deliberate, research-based policy making and coordination between ministries of health, education, and sport (Gençlik & Bakanlığı, 2012; Mumcu et al, 2025).

Evaluating sport as a social policy tool is an indispensable element of the modern state's duty to provide social welfare. Sport is a universal language that trains both the body and the soul while reinforcing social justice, eliminating social exclusion, and protecting public health. In Turkey, the constitutionally guaranteed right to participate in sport must be supported by development plans and national policy documents; however, to ensure these goals do not remain merely on paper, they must be strengthened by concrete steps such as the efficient use of facilities, positive discrimination for disadvantaged groups, and the expansion of sports education to all ages. Against the alienation and polarization created by global capitalist systems, sport will continue to be one of the most powerful tools for bringing humanity together on a common ground of ethics and peace. Recognizing sport for its true value as a social policy instrument is the key to both individual happiness and social harmony (Turaç 2024; Kumar et al., 2018; Verdot and Schut, 2012).

2. THE IMPACT OF SPORT ON SOCIAL WELFARE

Sport is no longer viewed merely as a set of physical movements or a simple leisure activity; it has evolved into a systematic social structure that is deeply integrated into both individual lives and the collective fabric of society. In the contemporary era, sport has become a multi-dimensional instrument of social policy, utilized by governments to achieve diverse non-sporting objectives such as enhancing social welfare, fostering economic development, and improving international relations. The malleability of sport allows it to serve as a significant resource for addressing complex social problems, including social exclusion, juvenile delinquency, and public health crises such as childhood obesity. The fundamental purpose of the modern welfare state is to ensure a decent standard of living for its citizens, and in this context, the right to participate in sport is increasingly recognized as an inherent right, akin to the rights to education and health. This perspective positions sport as a primary public service where the provision of opportunities should ideally be driven by social equity rather than profit motives. As a social phenomenon, sport serves as a source for promoting peace, education, and health, aligning with global development goals (Bloyce and Smith, 2010; Donnelly, 2008).

The impact of sport on individual welfare is most clearly seen through its effect on subjective wellbeing (SWB) and life satisfaction. Academic research indicates that engagement in sport is positively and significantly associated with higher levels of life satisfaction. Within the framework of "Wellbeing Valuation," researchers have sought to place a monetary value on these benefits, revealing that participation in sports such as swimming or team activities can generate thousands of pounds in annual "welfare gain" for an individual. For instance, team sports are found to have a particularly strong impact on life satisfaction, often exceeding the perceived value of individual fitness activities. Interestingly, while general physical activity is broadly beneficial, competitive sport carries specific psychosocial benefits derived from social interaction and the formation of social relationships. This "social interaction" nature of sport is a key determinant of the happiness reported by participants. For older adults, the positive effect of individual sports on life satisfaction is even more pronounced, suggesting that sport plays a vital role in maintaining the quality of life during the aging process (Taylor et al., 2014; Fujiwara et al., 2014).

From a physiological and psychological perspective, regular sporting participation serves as a critical component of protective and preventive health services. It is well-documented that physical activity protects against chronic conditions such as cardiovascular disease, type II diabetes, obesity, and osteoporosis. The biological mechanisms activated by sport increase cardiovascular fitness and reduce mortality risk, while physiological mechanisms help regulate stress hormones. Beyond the physical, the mental health benefits of sport are substantial, including a reduced risk of depression, anxiety, and suicidal ideation, particularly among adolescents. Organized sport provides a social context that combats feelings of social isolation, a common symptom of poor mental health, by fostering self-esteem, self-efficacy, and a sense of belonging. Even single bouts of moderate aerobic exercise have been shown to improve neurocognitive function in children with conditions such as ADHD (Kumar et al., 2018; Taylor et al., 2014).

However, the relationship between sport and health is not without its contradictions. Policy-makers often ignore the inherent risks of competitive sport, such as physical injury. In some cases, for younger adults, the medical costs resulting from sports injuries can actually offset the economic benefits of disease prevention. Competitive sport, unlike general physical activity, often involves mock battles where aggression and physical contact are central features, potentially leading to long-term health complications. Furthermore, while sport is often marketed as a universal panacea, it is a social construction whose meaning is given by its participants and defining agents; thus, it can also be used to promote ideological conformity, nationalism, or even inequitable attitudes (Donnelly, 2008; Murphy and Waddington, 1998; Bloyce and Smith, 2010).

The concept of social capital is central to understanding the societal welfare impacts of sport. Sport acts as a form of "social glue," providing bonding capital by increasing social connectedness and a sense of belonging within communities. It can also foster bridging capital by bringing together individuals from different ethnic or socio-economic backgrounds, thereby reducing tensions and promoting cultural understanding. Participation in sport as a voluntary association is a primary source of social interaction that develops trust and civic engagement. For marginalized groups, such as refugees or asylum seekers, sports programs like "Football for Inclusion" serve as a bridge to wider society, helping them acquire local knowledge and build social networks. These programs often utilize "role models" who share common identities with participants to enact proper conduct and guide excluded youth toward social inclusion.

Despite its potential as a tool for social inclusion, sport in its current formalized form is often exclusionary by nature. Significant portions of the population, particularly those living in poverty, face material barriers to participation, including the costs of equipment, facility entry fees, and transportation. Poverty remains the single greatest barrier to participation in sport and physical activity, creating a linear relationship where those with higher incomes participate at much higher rates. This is exacerbated by the commodification of sport, where fitness is packaged as a desirable image and sold as a transaction, often excluding those below the "threshold of social exclusion". Furthermore, social exclusion in sport is a function of cultural norms that have historically defined "legitimate bodies," leading to the under-representation of women, persons with disabilities, and ethnic minorities in both participation and leadership roles (Kumar et al, 2018; Taylor et al, 2014).

The delivery of sport as a welfare tool has undergone significant transformations due to the influence of neoliberalism. In many Western countries, there has been a shift from state-centered provision to public-private partnerships involving social entrepreneurs and non-profit associations. While public sector facilities typically pursue community and social objectives, private sector operators are often driven by profit motives and focus on higher-income groups. However, empirical evidence suggests that from the end-user's perspective, the type of facility—whether public or private—has little direct effect on the perceived health, wellbeing, or social capital outcomes. This implies that individuals may adapt their behavior to maximize their utility regardless of the institutional arrangement, provided they have access to the opportunity (Ekholm, 2016; Kumar et al, 2018).

Economic welfare in the professional team sports industry also presents a unique area of analysis. In professional leagues, social welfare is often defined as the sum of aggregate fan surplus, club profits, and player salaries. Models suggest that leagues where all clubs are profit-maximizers may dominate other structures in terms of social welfare, whereas mixed leagues with different objective functions can lead to inefficiencies. Regulations such as salary caps and revenue sharing have complex effects on welfare, with some evidence suggesting that revenue sharing may actually decrease social welfare in certain competitive environments (Dietl et al, 2009).

The "Sport for All" ideal remains a global challenge, as the policy often fails to reach the most disadvantaged or disabled groups in practice. Tackling social exclusion requires more than just "opening the doors" to existing systems; it necessitates fundamental changes to policies and practices through collaboration with those currently outside the system. Community sports initiatives often aim to address these deficiencies by using flexible, people-centered approaches that lower the threshold for participation. However, critics argue that many sport-based interventions are based on "sport evangelism" or the "great sport myth"—the uncritical belief that sport inherently does good—rather than hard evidence. Evaluation of these programs is often limited, making it difficult to definitively say "what works" in reducing the complex causes of social exclusion (Coalter, 2017; Verdot and Schut, 2012).

In terms of economic impact, the promotion of physical activity through sport is seen as a "best buy" in public health because of its potential to reduce mortality and save on national healthcare costs. In the UK alone, physical inactivity is estimated to cost the economy billions of pounds annually in healthcare expenditures, lost productivity, and sickness absence. Increasing moderate physical activity by just 10% could prevent thousands of premature deaths and save the taxpayer billions. These "exchequer benefits" provide a robust case for government investment in the sport sector, especially in times of economic austerity (Verdot and Schut, 2012; Collins, 2003).

Ultimately, the individual and social welfare impact of sport depends on how it is organized and performed. While sport has the power to unite, create hope, and break down barriers, it is not a universal panacea. The pedagogical rationales of social change embedded in sports programs often focus on shaping active, responsible, and self-governing citizens who are empowered to manage their own risks and inclusion. This shift toward "responsibilization" places the burden of change on the individual rather than addressing structural inequalities. Therefore, while sport remains an essential component of modern welfare provision, its effectiveness as a social policy tool requires research-based policy-making and coordination between various government departments, including health, education, and justice (Ekholm, 2016; Murphy and Waddington, 1998).

IN CONCLUSION: PROMOTING SPORT AT THE GRASSROOTS LEVEL FOR SUSTAINABLE WELL-BEING

The evolution of sport from simple physical movements into a systematic social structure has solidified its role as a deeply integrated component of both individual and collective existence. In the modern era, sport is no longer viewed merely as a leisure activity but has transitioned into a multi-dimensional instrument of social policy, utilized by governments to achieve critical objectives in social welfare, economic development, and international relations. The fundamental premise of the modern welfare state is to ensure a decent standard of living for all citizens, and within this humanitarian endeavor, the right to participate in sport must be recognized as an inherent and fundamental right, equivalent to the rights to education and health. As social policy often acts as the "doctor of capitalism," striving to repair systemic deficiencies and protect human welfare, sport serves as a rehabilitative and unifying tool that limits the potential for social exploitation by fostering a more equitable society.

The importance of sport policies in achieving sustainable welfare is most clearly demonstrated through their impact on both public health and individual life satisfaction. Academic research confirms that regular sporting participation functions as a vital component of protective and preventive health services, shielding individuals from chronic conditions such as cardiovascular disease, obesity, and diabetes. By building a healthier society, these policies not only enhance the general well-being of the population but also provide significant economic "exchequer benefits" by reducing state health expenditures and increasing the productivity of the workforce. Furthermore, engagement in sport is significantly associated with higher levels of subjective well-being, where participation in team activities can generate thousands of pounds in annual "welfare gain" for an individual through the formation of social relationships and increased life satisfaction.

Central to the success of these objectives is the policy of "spreading sport to the grassroots" (Tabana Yayılma Politikası), which is essential for ensuring true social justice. If social justice is defined as equal access to opportunities provided by public authorities, then making sports facilities accessible across all geographical regions—especially those with low socio-economic development—becomes one of the most effective methods to combat social exclusion. By prioritizing the "base of the sports pyramid," governments can ensure that the general public has the resources to remain active and healthy, rather than focusing solely on elite success for national prestige. This grassroots approach is strategically important for youth development, as it provides a natural mechanism for social integration, reduces crime rates, and directs young people away from harmful habits like substance abuse.

Moreover, sport acts as a form of "social glue," providing the bonding and bridging capital necessary for a stable society. It brings together individuals from diverse ethnic or socio-economic backgrounds, fostering trust, civic engagement, and cultural understanding. For disadvantaged groups, such as individuals with disabilities, low-income families, or refugees, sport serves as an indispensable tool for rehabilitation and social attachment based on equal opportunity. However, for these benefits to be sustainable, sport policies must actively resist the commodification of sport. In post-industrial societies, the transformation of fitness into a market-driven commodity can create material barriers for those living in poverty, risking the exclusion of those who fall below the "threshold of social exclusion". Therefore, state intervention and public investment under the "Sport for All" philosophy are required to balance these market pressures and ensure that participation remains inclusive regardless of an individual's market value.

The sustainability of these welfare impacts also depends on modernizing sport policies to include environmental sustainability and social diplomacy. Promoting eco-friendly sports facilities and minimizing the environmental impact of major events aligns the sport sector with broader global goals for a sustainable future. Additionally, the success of sports policies should be measured not by the number of medals won by elite athletes, but by the breadth of participation among the general public. While the professional sports industry contributes to economic welfare through employment and tourism, the "pure" and integrative spirit of sport must be protected from becoming a mere consumer show that encourages passive "spectator" behavior.

In conclusion, evaluating sport as a social policy tool is an indispensable element of the modern state's duty to provide social welfare. Sport is a universal language that trains both the body and the soul while reinforcing social justice and protecting public health. To ensure that the goal of sustainable well-being does not remain merely on paper, it must be supported by concrete steps such as the efficient use of facilities, positive discrimination for disadvantaged groups, and research-based policy-making. Against the alienation and polarization created by global systems, sport remains one of the most powerful tools for bringing humanity together on a common ground of ethics and peace. Ultimately, recognizing sport for its true value as a social policy instrument is the key to achieving both individual happiness and long-term social harmony

REFERENCES

Bloyce, D. ve Smith, A. (2010). *Sport policy and development: An introduction.* Routledge.

Coalter, F. (2017). Sport for social inclusion: Evidence-based policy and practice. *Social Inclusion (Lisboa), 5*(2), 141–149. DOI: 10.17645/si.v5i2.852

Collins, M. F. (2003). *Sport, physical activity and social exclusion.* Routledge. DOI: 10.4324/9780203167267

Dietl, H., Lang, M., & Werner, S. (2009). Social welfare in sports leagues with profit-maximizing and/or win-maximizing clubs. *Southern Economic Journal, 76*(2), 375–396. DOI: 10.4284/sej.2009.76.2.375

Donnelly, P. (2008). Sport and human rights. *Sport in Society, 11*(4), 381–394. DOI: 10.1080/17430430802019326

Ekholm, D. (2016). Sport as a means of responding to social problems: Rationales of governing welfare and social change [Doktora tezi, Linköping Üniversitesi].

Fujiwara, D., & Kudrna, L. ve Dolan, P. (2014). Quantifying and valuing the well-being impacts of culture and sport. Department for Culture, Media & Sport.

Kasapoğlu, M. M., & Öçal, M. (2021). Türkiye'de spor yatırımlarının tabana yayılması politikasının sosyal adalet açısından önemi. *Yönetim ve Ekonomi Araştırmaları Dergisi, 19*(3), 173–191. DOI: 10.11611/yead.991462

Kumar, H., & Downward, P. (2018). Sport participation: From policy, through facilities, to users' health, well-being, and social capital. *Sport Management Review, 21*(5), 549–562. DOI: 10.1016/j.smr.2018.01.002

Mumcu, H. E., Mumcu, N., Kusan, O., ve Öztürk, O. (2025). İki temel politika: Herkes için spor ve elit spor politikası. EFES Spor Bilimleri Dergisi, 1(1), 20-49.

Murphy, P., & Waddington, I. (1998). Sport for all: Some public health policy issues and problems. *Critical Public Health, 8*(3), 193–205. DOI: 10.1080/09581599808402907

Öçal, M., ve Kutlu, Ö. (2024). İstihdamın karanlık yüzü: Ter atölyelerine (sweatshop) insani bir bakış ve ter indeksi ile bir kıyaslama. Çalışma ve Toplum, 2024/4, 1391-1424. https://doi.org/.DOI: 10.54752/ct.1569636

Öçal, M., & Kutlu Dönmez, Ö. (2022). Ruhsal engeli olan bireylerin evsizlik sorununa insani bir bakış ve çözüm önerisi: "Önce konut yaklaşımı". *Mehmet Akif Ersoy Üniversitesi İktisadi ve İdari Bilimler Fakültesi Dergisi*, *9*(3), 2006–2026. DOI: 10.30798/makuiibf.1097609

Sütlü, S., & Kutlu, Ö. (2025). Profile of substance individual with substance use disorders: Community-based project results. *Journal of Substance Use*, *30*(5), 761–766. DOI: 10.1080/14659891.2024.2403079

Taylor, P., Davies, L., Wells, P., & Gilbertson, J. ve Tayleur, W. (2014). A review of the social impacts of culture and sport. Sheffield Hallam University.

T.C. Gençlik ve Spor Bakanlığı. (2012). *Ulusal gençlik ve spor politikası belgesi.* GSB.

Turaç, G. (2024). Spor odaklı rekreasyon alanlarının toplumsal sağlık ve sosyal etkileşim üzerindeki rolü. *Beden Eğitimi ve Spor Bilimleri Dergisi*, *18*(3), 621–636. DOI: 10.61962/bsd.1588768

Verdot, C., & Schut, P.-O. (2012). Sport and social inclusion: The political position vs. practices. *EJSS European Journal for Sport and Society*, *9*(3), 203–227. DOI: 10.1080/16138171.2012.11687897

Yerlikaya, B. (2012). Spor kavramında dönüşüm ve sporun bir sosyal politika aracı olarak kullanımı [Yüksek lisans tezi, Marmara Üniversitesi]

Chapter 2
Welfare Through Sport: A Comparison With the Sport-Friendly Country Index

Mehmet Muharrem Kasapoğlu
http://orcid.org/0009-0009-3943-8556
Turkish Grand National Assembly, Turkey

Mehmet Ata Öztürk
Independent Researcher, Turkey

ABSTRACT

Sport has multifaceted effects, from breaking down social exclusion to fighting for freedom. This makes sport a fundamental tool of social policy. It positions sport as a core component of social policies that enhance individual well-being and social citizenship. The main objective of this study is to highlight the impact of sport on well-being and to determine which country uses sport more effectively as a social policy. Fort his purpose, chapter is the development of the "Sport-Friendly Country Index," designed to classify 37 countries based on their implementation of sport-related welfare policies. Using "Min-Max Normalization," the index evaluates 14 parameters, including sport-related GDP expenditure, employment, volunteering rates, and bureaucratic structures. The analysis reveals that welfare typologies significantly influence a nation's "sport-friendly" score.

INTRODUCTION

The role of sport in contemporary society has undergone a profound transformation, moving beyond the traditional focus on elite performance to become a primary instrument of modern governance. As societies face increasing structural

DOI: 10.4018/979-8-2600-3174-2.ch002

problems such as inequality, exclusion, and public health crises, sport is viewed as a "malleable resource" and a "productive force of governing". This evolution positions sport within "third-generation" social policies, which focus on combating social exclusion, protecting the rights of disadvantaged groups—including women, children, and the handicapped—and ensuring social peace.

At its core, the relationship between sport and welfare rests on the concept of social citizenship, where access to physical activity is treated as a social right that provides the resources necessary for citizens to lead satisfying and productive lives. Sociologically, this is analyzed through diverse perspectives: Structural-Functionalism views sport as a critical subsystem maintaining social order, while Conflict Theory frames it as a compensatory social policy intended to reduce the "bodily capital" gap between classes. Furthermore, New Institutionalism explains a global isomorphism where international organizations like the WHO drive countries to adopt similar "active life" strategies.

This research seeks to address a fundamental question: "Can welfare regimes be subjected to a classification within the framework of the sport policies they implement?". To answer this, a "Sport-Friendly Country Index" was developed, analyzing 37 countries across 14 parameters, including sport investments relative to GDP, employment rates, volunteering, and bureaucratic structures. By utilizing Min-Max Normalization (Feature Scaling), the index standardizes diverse data into a "Sport-Friendly Score" between 0 and 1. This allows for a comprehensive comparative analysis of how different welfare typologies—liberal, social-democratic, conservative, and Southern European—prioritize sport as a social policy tool to enhance collective welfare

1. THE RELATIONSHIP BETWEEN SPORT AND SOCIAL POLICY

The relationship between sport and social policy has undergone a profound transformation, evolving from a secondary concern into a primary instrument of modern governance used to address complex societal challenges. Public authorities increasingly view sport as a "malleable" resource capable of delivering non-sport policy objectives in areas as diverse as public health, crime prevention, social cohesion, and international diplomacy. This expansion reflects a shift from seeing sport as a mere recreational activity to viewing it as a productive force for the governing of society and a solution to social problems arising from increased inequality, segregation, and exclusion. In the contemporary era, sport is recognized as a component of "third-generation" social policies, which focus on combating social exclusion, protecting the rights of disadvantaged groups—including women, children, and the handicapped—and ensuring social peace (Bergsgard, et al., 2007; Yerlikaya and Öcal, 2015; Öçal and Kutlu, 2023a).

In terms of social justice, sport policy serves as a fundamental building block of the social state, aiming to provide all citizens with equal and decent access to welfare services regardless of language, religion, race, or socioeconomic status. This is exemplified in the Turkish context through the "Grassroots Policy" (*Tabana Yayılma Politikası*), which is conceptualized as a turning point for social justice. This policy is anchored in the Turkish Constitution of 1982 (Article 59), which tasks the state with taking measures to develop the physical and mental health of citizens and encouraging the spread of sport to the masses. To achieve regional equity, the Turkish state has prioritized facility investments in historically disadvantaged areas; for instance, between 2005 and 2021, the highest number of new sports facilities were built in the Southeastern and Eastern Anatolia regions. By focusing on low-development regions, social policy aims to eliminate social exclusion and ensure that economically lagging areas benefit more intensely from public welfare services. Sport is also utilized as a critical tool for the social inclusion of disadvantaged groups, particularly children and youth at risk. Projects like the "Social Support Program" (SODES) target individuals in regions under the risk of poverty, using sport to improve their physical and mental status and help them express themselves better. Furthermore, specific protocols between sports ministries and social service agencies ensure that children in state care have free access to sports complexes to promote healthy psycho-social development. The number of "Youth Centers" (*Gençlik Merkezleri*), designed as integrated complexes where youth of different backgrounds can interact under state supervision, has seen a 4000% increase since 2002, growing from 9 to over 360 centers. These centers serve as dynamic hubs for social harmony and the internalization of positive social norms (Kasapoğlu ve Öçal, 2021; Yerlikaya and Öcal, 2015).

Another major dimension of sport as social policy is its use in crime prevention and urban safety. In Sweden, interventions such as "Midnight Football" target youth aged 12–25 on late weekend evenings in socio-economically disadvantaged urban peripheries. This policy is built on the "governmental rationality" that sport can act as a "social vaccine" against gangs, crime, and drug addiction by providing community engagement and resilience. From a governing perspective, these programs function as technologies of discipline. By establishing strict rules of play and utilizing coaches as "moral role models," the state seeks to normalize the conduct of marginalized youth. However, these activities also serve as sites of surveillance, where police and social workers monitor participants beyond the field to ensure social control, framing the management of "at-risk" populations as a form of empowerment (Ekholm and Dahlstedt, 2023).

The relationship between sport and social policy is also defined by the "health problematic," where governments treat physical inactivity as a primary risk factor for obesity and premature death. Participation in sport is promoted as a requirement for a productive population and a cost-effective solution to public health challenges. In Turkey, projects like the "Turkey Healthy Nutrition and Active Life Program" involve collaboration between health and sports ministries to "prescribe" physical activity as a preventative measure for cardiovascular diseases and mental disorders. This approach effectively shifts the responsibility for well-being onto the individual, demanding the physical activation of the population to reduce general health expenditures. Within education policy, sport is conceptualized through the "democratic problematic," emphasizing the "right" to participate in fair and inclusive activities. Sport is viewed as a "school of democracy" where children internalize values such as tolerance and collaboration. However, a tension exists between "association fostering" (*föreningsfostran*), which aims for breadth and equality, and "competition fostering" (*tävlingsfostran*), which prioritizes distinction and exclusion. Critics argue that if sport focuses too heavily on elite performance, it may exclude large groups who do not fit the athletic model, thereby undermining the social policy goal of "sport for all" (Österlind, 2016; Karasu, 2025 (sözlükspor).

At the international level, the Sport, Development, and Peace (SDP) sector has emerged as a distinct global policy field supported by the United Nations and the European Union. This sector utilizes sport to pursue global welfare objectives such as conflict resolution, gender equality, and poverty reduction, often centering on the Millennium Development Goals. The SDP sector is divided into four primary ideological domains (Giulianotti, 2011):

- Corporate/Neo-liberalism: Driven by transnational corporations through Corporate Social Responsibility (CSR) programs that prioritize business returns and market legitimacy while delivering equipment to impoverished areas.
- Developmental Interventionism: Associated with mainstream NGOs focusing on human capacity building in underdeveloped settings.
- Strategic Developmentalism: Led by national and intergovernmental organizations—such as UNICEF, UNESCO, and FIFA—that use top-down management to universalize SDP work.
- Social Justice: Advocated by radical NGOs and social movements to challenge systemic inequalities and protect human rights within the sport industry.

Sport policy also serves as a classic "soft power" resource in foreign policy, allowing states to achieve diplomatic goals through attraction rather than coercion. States utilize Sports Mega-Events (SMEs), such as the FIFA World Cup or the Olympic

Games, to enhance international prestige and improve their national "brand". For example, Germany used the 2006 World Cup and its "Land of Ideas" campaign to overturn negative stereotypes and project an image of hospitality and cultural excellence. Similarly, Qatar utilized its wealth to signal its arrival on the world stage, using the 2022 World Cup to showcase Arab capacity for logistical excellence and innovative state-of-the-art technologies, such as carbon-neutral cooling systems (Grix and Brannagan, 2016; Houlihan, et al.,, 2009).

The modern integration of sport into social policy now includes environmental stewardship and sustainability. The sport industry has recognized its ecological footprint, leading to initiatives like the LEED (Leadership in Energy and Environmental Design) mark for stadium construction. Professional leagues partner with environmental action groups to implement "greening" activities, which are seen as a standard component of an organization's social responsibility. These efforts help sport organizations gain organizational legitimacy, build stronger relationships with stakeholders, and save money through efficient operations (Trendafilova, et al.,, 2014).

Despite the high aspirations of these policies, the literature identifies several "wicked problems" and myths that plague the field. One such challenge is the "inspiration myth," where policy-makers claim that elite success inspires mass participation despite evidence showing little correlation between Olympic medals and public activity levels. There is also a persistent "Great Sport Myth," which assumes that sport is inherently pure and good and that participation automatically leads to positive social changes. Critical scholars warn that sport can inadvertently maintain hierarchies and exclude marginalized groups—based on race, gender, or disability—if not managed through rigorous, evidence-based interventions. Modern sport policy has therefore shifted from a "culture of trust" to a "culture of mistrust," where sport organizations must undergo rigorous audits and evaluations to justify public funding and ensure they perform in line with political objectives (Hoekman and Scheerder, 2021; Houlihan, et al.,, 2009; Kellett, et al.,, 2008; Ekholm and Dahlstedt, 2023; Österlind, 2016).

Ultimately, sport and social policy are now inextricably linked through a machinery of governance that seeks to manage the "conduct" of the population. Whether framed as a tool for social justice in Turkey, a social vaccine in Sweden, or a soft power asset in Qatar, sport has been effectively integrated into the toolbox of the modern social investment state. However, the continued reliance on entrenched "storylines" suggests that for these policies to move beyond mere rhetoric, there must be a shift toward more rigorous practices that prioritize genuine human well-being over political optics (Ekholm and Dahlstedt, 2023; Kasapoğlu and Öçal, 2021; Grix and Brannagan, 2016; Österlind, 2016).

2. THE RATIONALE FOR THE WELFARE STATE'S USE OF SPORT AS A SOCIAL POLICY TOOL: IMPACT ON SOCIAL WELFARE

The multifaceted phenomenon of sport has undergone a profound paradigm shift in contemporary governance, evolving from its traditional focus on elite performance and competition into a primary instrument for promoting individual and collective welfare. In the current understanding of development, sport is no longer viewed merely as a recreational activity but as a "productive force of governing" capable of addressing structural social problems such as inequality, exclusion, and public health crises. This transformation is driven by the realization that sport acts as a horizontal policy area that intersects with education, health, urban planning, and social justice, serving as a "social vaccine" against destructive behaviors and a catalyst for personal and societal growth. At its core, the relationship between sport and welfare rests on the concept of social citizenship, where access to physical activity is treated as a social right providing the resources necessary for citizens to lead satisfying and productive lives. This evolution is analyzed through diverse sociological perspectives, such as Structural-Functionalism, which views sport as a critical subsystem maintaining social order and collective consciousness by fostering healthy citizens. Conversely, Conflict Theory interprets the current emphasis on sport in development plans as a response to neoliberal inequalities, framing sport as a compensatory social policy intended to redistribute resources and reduce the "bodily capital" gap between social classes. New Institutionalism further explains the global isomorphism in sport policy, where international organizations like the WHO and UNESCO drive countries to adopt strikingly similar "active life" strategies as a rationalized myth for solving economic and health crises (Narin, 2025; Ekholm, 2016; Seltman, 2026; Washington and Karen, 2001).

The impact of sport on individual well-being begins with its foundational contribution to physical and mental health. Within the framework of the United Nations' Sustainable Development Goals, particularly SDG 3, sport is recognized as a key ally in reducing mortality from non-communicable diseases, such as cardiovascular issues, diabetes, and obesity. Regular participation in sport can reduce the risk of coronary heart disease and stroke by up to 35%, while also improving insulin sensitivity for the prevention of type 2 diabetes. Beyond these physiological markers, sport serves as a vital support for psychological health, particularly for individuals experiencing stress, low mood, or social isolation. Research indicates that participation in community sport programs is consistently related to higher self-esteem, improved life satisfaction, and reduced levels of depression and anxiety. These psychological benefits are often stronger in team-based or socially structured environments compared to solitary exercise, as the group setting fosters a sense of belonging and identity that mitigates feelings of isolation. The internal mechanisms driving these gains are explained through theories of self-determination and self-efficacy, where sport supports basic human needs for autonomy, competence, and relatedness. As individuals engage in sport voluntarily and bond with teammates, they achieve a sense of mastery that accumulates into meaningful psychological recovery, a process described by the broaden-and-build theory where positive emotions create lasting resilience (Narin, 2025; Im, et al., 2026; Eather, et al., 2023).

On a societal level, sport acts as a powerful vehicle for social inclusion and community cohesion, providing a unique platform that brings together individuals from diverse linguistic, ethnic, and socioeconomic backgrounds under common rules and symbols. In the Turkish context, the adoption of the "Grassroots Policy" (Tabana Yayılma Politikası) exemplifies the use of sport for social justice and regional equity. By prioritizing the construction of sports facilities in historically disadvantaged regions like Southeastern and Eastern Anatolia, the state uses sport to eliminate social exclusion and ensure that economically lagging populations benefit intensely from public welfare services. This policy treats sport as a tool to bridge the gap between marginalized youth and the wider society, providing them with a "school of democracy" where they internalize positive social norms. The role of sport in crime prevention and urban safety is another vital dimension of its social utility. In welfare states like Sweden, interventions such as "Midnight Football" target marginalized youth in segregated urban peripheries during late weekend evenings. These programs operate on a governmental rationality that spontaneous sport participation can foster resilience to gangs, drugs, and antisocial behavior by providing a productive sense of community. Within this regime of practice, sport functions as a technology of discipline and surveillance, seeking to normalize the conduct of youth through the influence of coaches who serve as "authentic role models". By establishing moral bonds, these programs strive to build social capital, defined as a shared feeling of trust and reciprocity that makes local neighborhoods safer (Teke and Karakuş, 2022; Narin, 2025; Ekholm, 2016).

The relationship between sport and welfare also extends to the professional level, where the state's role is dictated by its specific welfare regime. Comparative analysis of European countries reveals distinct models: Social Democratic regimes, such as Norway, view sport as a decommodified right of citizenship with high state funding and universal social protection. In contrast, Liberal regimes reflect a commitment to market solutions with a more passive state role that encourages the commercialization of sport. Post-socialist models, like those in Croatia and Poland, often involve "public employment" schemes, such as enrolling elite athletes in the military or police to provide them with salaries and pensions. For example, in Croatia, athletes are classified based on achievement, and top-tier performers are eligible for national scholarships and inclusion in reserve troops, ensuring a monthly salary while maintaining their athlete status. These institutional variations demonstrate that athlete welfare is not uniform but is deeply embedded in national policy traditions that determine the degree of social protection and income stability for sports professionals (Seltman, 2026).

Economic analysis further reinforces the role of sport as a component of the modern welfare state. Sport is a rapidly growing industry that substantially contributes to the dynamization of regional economies through job creation, sports tourism, and the manufacturing of equipment. From a public policy perspective, sport offers a cost-effective solution to the global "inactivity pandemic". By prescribing physical activity as a preventative measure, governments can significantly reduce the massive systemic costs associated with chronic diseases and healthcare expenditures, as seen in the German "Rezept für Bewegung" (Exercise Prescription) program. Within professional leagues, the objectives of sports clubs—whether profit-maximizing or win-maximizing—significantly impact social welfare. In profit-maximizing leagues, owners prioritize financial returns, which may lead to higher competitive balance but potentially lower overall quality. Win-maximizing clubs, common in European soccer, invest all available revenue into talent, maximizing league quality and fan utility but often leading to a financial "rat-race" (Madden, 2015; Dietl et al., 2009).

The integration of ethics and values into sport is essential for these social benefits to be realized. Ideally, sport promotes fundamental values such as teamwork, discipline, and mutual respect, with Fair Play being the "essence and soul" of the game. Fair Play is defined as a life view based on respect for oneself, opponents, teammates, and referees, explicitly rejecting the "win at all costs" mentality. However, the literature warns of a "breakthrough" or "rupture" in these values caused by the industrialization and commercialization of sport. When winning becomes the highest value, it leads to the justification of immorality, such as doping, match-fixing, and the normalization of unethical behavior. This negative value transfer can harm society if people begin to normalize observed professional misconduct in their own daily lives. Furthermore, a much broader definition of "sports-related violence" (SRV) is now used in research to include not only player and crowd violence but also abusive coaching practices, exploitative labor, and environmental degradation. Sociologists argue that it is necessary to view these varied manifestations as a matrix of interconnected behaviors underpinned by broader social structures such as gender, race, and social class (Abanoz and Soyer, 2018; Young, 2019).

Despite the overwhelming "sport evangelism" and the "Great Sport Myth"—the uncritical assumption that sport is inherently good—critics point out several "wicked problems" and limitations. Sport-based interventions cannot single-handedly solve deep structural issues like poverty or unemployment. Furthermore, if not managed through evidence-based practices, sport can inadvertently maintain social hierarchies or exclude marginalized groups based on race or gender. Modern sport policy has thus shifted from a "culture of trust" to a "culture of mistrust," where organizations must undergo rigorous audits and evaluations to justify their social utility and public funding. The fragmentation of "the social" into particular domains like "the self," "the community," and "the place" shifts the responsibility for welfare from the state to the individual, demanding that subjects become self-governing agents of their own inclusion. For example, sport programs often focus on "subjectification"—shaping citizen subjects who are self-aware, active, and capable of taking responsibility for their own health and social integration. This responsibilization of individuals and communities is a hallmark of advanced liberal governance, where the state governs "at a distance" by mobilizing the "will to empower" within citizens (Young, 2019).

Ultimately, sport has been effectively integrated into the toolbox of the modern social investment state. By activating the self, mobilizing the community, and disciplining the place, sport-based social policy strives to produce a healthier, more compliant, and more cohesive population. Whether through the Swedish model of risk management in the urban periphery, the Turkish strategy for regional social justice, or the global Sport, Development, and Peace (SDP) sector, sport is conceptualized as a vital means of responding to social problems because it aligns individual activity with the macro goals of an "active society". However, for these policies to move beyond mere rhetoric, there must be a shift toward more rigorous, evidence-based practices that prioritize genuine human well-being over political optics. The continued reliance on entrenched "storylines" and myths suggests that sport's social potential remains a contested terrain, requiring constant critical scrutiny to ensure that its benefits are equitably distributed across all strata of society. In this context, sport is not just a game; it is a complex field of social interaction, a site of governance, and a laboratory for understanding the evolving nature of the welfare state and its citizens (Kasapoğlu & Öçal,, 2020).

3. WHICH COUNTRY IS MORE SPORTS-FRIENDLY? A COMPARISON USING THE SPORTS-FRIENDLY COUNTRY INDEX

The main problem statement of the research is formed by the question: "Can welfare regimes be subjected to a classification within the framework of the sport policies they implement?". To seek an answer to this problem statement, a Sport-Friendly Country Index has been developed within the scope of the research. The promotion of sport by spreading it to the grassroots as a welfare policy is a process brought about by many factors. In a spectrum ranging from the state's sport investments to the presence of sport within the education system, sport constitutes one of the basic policy areas in the realization of a humane life, which welfare regimes commit to those living under their auspices by increasing social welfare.

On the contrary, the social state and social policy, which is its foundation, is the only philosophy that humanizes capitalism's perspective on people. The social state, based on social policy described as a human pursuit, becomes a guarantor for all individuals for a life worthy of human dignity. In fact, the social state is a shield that protects individuals from the market. It is attempted to limit the negative impact of the capitalist market on human welfare through the social policies put forward by the social state. The social state draws "red lines" for the market and tries to prevent these lines from being crossed with a corporatist style of action. These red lines appear as prohibitions, obligations, and incentives in every field concerning human welfare (Öçal and Kutlu, 2023b; Alcock, et al.,, 2002).

One of the most important social policy actions of states that define themselves as a social state and have accepted making sacrifices for the goodness, well-being, and welfare of individuals has been the protection and development of welfare through sport. Sport and the spreading of sport to the grassroots, which have a very important impact on social welfare, are defined today as a fundamental duty of the social state. However, even though it is defined as a fundamental social state duty, differences arising from welfare regime typologies cause the social policies implemented by states for the grassroots spread and promotion of sport to differentiate in terms of degree, intensity, and scope, as is the case in all social policy applications.

Differences in the political, economic, and socio-cultural values and traditions of states differentiate the social policies they implement. Although the implemented actions are essentially carried out for human welfare and characterized as social policy, the levels of these social policies vary due to the variables emphasized. In short, the social policies implemented by states regarding sport differ. There is no clear indicator regarding the degree of importance each state gives to sport and its dissemination, and at what level it provides social policy to individuals (Esping-Andersen, 1990; Titmuss, 1968; Özdemir, 2005).

Within the scope of this study, an index has been developed regarding the grassroots spread and promotion of sport as a welfare policy. With this index, different values that can be accepted as indicators for the grassroots spread and promotion of sport have been analyzed by correlating them with each other. A "sport-friendly score" has been calculated for each country, and in line with this score, it has been determined which country is more "sport-friendly." Within the scope of the developed index, "Min-Max Normalization," also known as "Feature Scaling," has been used.

3.1. Construction of the Sports-Friendly Country Index

The parameters to be analyzed within the scope of the index in question have been determined as a result of academic studies conducted on the subject. In other words, the parameters to be analyzed in measuring the sport-friendly scores of countries were identified as a result of research pointing to the elements of the concepts of grassroots spread and promotion of sport. In other words, the measurement parameters of the index study were created with inferences obtained from research on how welfare regimes can be characterized as sport-friendly. According to these researches, the most prominent features observed in sport-friendly countries are indicated as: the high ratio of sport investments within the gross domestic product, the promotion of sport and athletes, the rate of volunteering, the legal and political organizational potential of sport, and employment in the sport sector.

There are undoubtedly many factors and variables of being a sport-friendly welfare regime. However, data regarding these variables are not accessible for every country. Within the scope of this study, a Sport-Friendly Country Index has been developed based on the parameters given above in order to determine which country is more "sport-friendly." In this context, parameters regarding being a sport-friendly country have been divided into three: social policies, individual factors, and sport in terms of bureaucratic priority. Social policies have been examined under three main and three sub-headings. While individual factors include data on satisfaction and orientation towards sport pointing to the effectiveness of incentives and grassroots spread provided by the welfare regime, sport in terms of bureaucratic priority grades the legal and bureaucratic structuring of the welfare regime regarding sport.

The purpose of the developed index is to determine how sport-friendly which welfare regimes are. At this point, it is aimed to develop measurement tools for this purpose and to make inter-country data comparable. The developed "sport-friendly country index" has measured by standardizing the social policies that states have implemented for the grassroots spread and promotion of sport. Following the analyses performed, it has been statistically demonstrated which country is more "sport-friendly." The index reveals the Sport-Friendly Country Score based on the scope and intensities of the social policies applied by welfare regimes towards sport. With this score, countries are put into a "sport-friendly" ranking. On the other hand, the effectiveness of the sport policies of today's welfare regimes gains further clarity with the developed index.

3.2. Statistical Analyses

The normalization method was used in order for very different data to be correlated with each other and for evaluations to be made within the scope of the

Sport-Friendly Country Index. Within the scope of the developed index, "Min-Max Normalization," also known as "Feature Scaling," was used. "Feature Scaling" is a statistical formula that is used and accepted for validity, especially in classifying data of different quality and quantity by reducing them into a single piece of data; in other words, in distinguishing the data class called the target set from all other possible objects called outliers. The method, in its most commonly used definition, is a scaling process also called standardize and normalize. This standardization process transforms different data into a value between 0 and 1. In this way, the comparability of different data is ensured (Yıldırım, 2014; Anorim, et al., 2023; Juszczak, et al., 2002).

"Feature Scaling" can be used with two different equations in terms of the quality of the data to be analyzed. These are the benefit and cost equations. While the benefit equation is $x'=(x-min(x))/(max(x)-min(x))$, the cost equation is $x'=(min(x)-x)/(max(x)-min(x))$. Two different equations are used by preference in line with the direction of the data's impact on the analysis (Han, et al., 2012).

The "Sport-Friendly Country Index" sets out from the social policies that welfare regimes apply to individuals, which affect them directly and indirectly, and the impact of these policies on individuals' orientation towards sport. At this point, the index components are listed below:

A1= Ratio of State's Sport Expenditure to GDP (%)
A2= Household's Average Annual Sport and Sport Equipment Expenditure (Dollar) (PPS)
A3= Ratio of Those Who Did Not Participate in Sport in the Last 1 Year to Total Population (%) (Cost Equation)
A4= Ratio of Employment in the Sport Sector to Total Employment (%)
A5= Ratio of Those Engaged in Sport Activities at Least Four Times in the Last 1 Year to Population (%)
A6= Average Time Spent in Sport in the Last 1 Year (Minutes)
A7= Volunteering Participation Rate (%)
A8= Ratio of Those Spending 150 Minutes and Above in Health-Enhancing Aerobic Activities to Population (%)
A9= Ratio of Those Satisfied with Provided Sport Opportunities to Population (%)
A10= Award Given to Successful Athletes (For Gold Medal in Olympics) (Dollar)
A11= Employment Opportunity as an Athlete in the Public Sector for Successful Athletes
A12= Status of Physical Education or Sport Lesson Inclusion in the Curriculum in ISCED-I and ISCED-II

A13= Existence of Independent Sport Law
A14= Existence of Independent Ministry of Sport
Sport-Friendly Country Index= $(A1+A2+A3+A4+A5+A6+A7+A8+A9+A10+A11+A12+A13+A14)/14$

The benefit equation of the relevant normalization was used for A1, A2, A4, A5, A6, A7, A8, A9, A10, A11, A12, A13, and A14, while the cost equation was utilized for A3. Unlike other parameters, the increase in the A3 value, expressed as individuals' non-participation in sport, produces a cost-oriented rather than a benefit-oriented effect on the individual and society.

CONCLUSION AND DISCUSSION

The Sport-Friendly Country Index determined the degree of a "sport-friendly" country by classifying countries and welfare regimes according to the content and type of social policies they implement for the promotion and grassroots spread of sport. The scope of the index includes European Union countries and countries in the position of candidate for membership. Furthermore, the United Kingdom, which left the union through the Brexit process, and selected Balkan countries were also included in the study. Within this scope, the panel data set used in the analysis was accessed through EUROSTAT, the Olympic Data Bank, and various EU publications, and the accessed data were subjected to normalization analysis using the SPSS program.

Considering that many of the countries within the scope of the index are classified within different welfare regime typologies, it is thought that sufficient coverage has been reached for classification. As a result of the analyses performed by subjecting the data regarding the grassroots spread and promotion of sport in selected countries to normalization, a sport-friendly country score between 0 and 1 has been obtained for each country. Subsequently, the values in question were classified, and a "sport-friendly country" ranking was established.

Table 1. Analysis of Grassroots Spread and Promotion of Sport Practices of Selected Countries According to the Sport-Friendly Country Index

Ülke	A1	A2	A3	A4	A5	A6	A7	A8	A9	A10	A11	A12	A13	A14	Spor Dostu Skoru
Belgium	0,214286	0,53667	0,978673	0,169231	0,56682	0,849462	0,530303	0,39685	0,900763	0,049091	1	1	0	1	0,744740867
Bulgaria	0	0,095563	0,933649	0,088462	0,041475	0,387097	0,262626	0,113386	0,251908	0,126364	1	1	1	1	0,57277538
Czechia	0,214286	0,193888	0	0,1	0,447005	0,612903	0,704545	0,330709	0,770992	0,090909	1	1	1	1	0,678657917
Denmark	0,142857	0,521191	0,938389	0,446154	0,576037	0,27957	0,805556	0,807874	0,267176	0,014455	0	1	1	0	0,618114238
Germany	0,142857	0,566782	0,981043	0,15	0,391705	0,72043	0,608586	0,707087	0,816794	0,02	1	1	0	0	0,645934847
Estonia	0,357143	0,2076	0,969194	0,311538	0,281106	0,591398	0,247475	0,341732	0,751908	0,106364	0	1	1	0	0,560496251
Ireland	0	0,60115	0,966825	0,311538	0,714286	0,483871	1	0,522835	0,648855	0	0	1	1	1	0,74994174
Greece	0,357143	0,328223	0,945498	0,180769	0,16129	0,752688	0,426768	0,244094	0,30916	0,090909	0	1	1	1	0,617867559
Spain	0,285714	0,456462	0,93128	0,369231	0,506912	0,709677	0,204545	0,492913	0,70229	0,100909	0	1	1	1	0,705448567
France	0,357143	0,488266	0,945498	0,330769	0,281106	1	0,674242	0,366929	0,820611	0,078182	1	1	1	0	0,75843145
Croatia	0,214286	0,312595	0,978673	0,161538	0,419355	0,129032	0,373737	0,248819	0,564885	0,042727	1	1	1	1	0,676877107
Italy	0,142857	0,446507	0,954976	0,203846	0,152074	0,763441	0,136364	0,245669	0,51145	0,193636	1	1	1	1	0,7046201
Cyprus	0,071429	0,618072	1	0,2	0,373272	0	0,068182	0,288189	0,347328	0,156364	0	1	1	1	0,556621405
Latvia	0,071429	0,180051	0,938389	0,115385	0,073733	0,354839	0,169192	0,253543	0,576336	0,140909	1	1	1	0	0,533982246
Lithuania	0,142857	0,201752	0,938389	0,134615	0,073733	0,55914	0	0,264567	0,541985	0,166364	1	1	1	1	0,638490995
Luxembourg	0,357143	1	0,900474	0,176923	0,37788	0,784946	0,618687	0,64252	0,805344	0	1	1	1	1	0,87853785
Hungary	0,428571	0,313466	0,938389	0,169231	0,170507	0,731183	0,209596	0,444094	0,652672	0,136364	0	1	1	0	0,563097479
Malta	0,142857	0,427718	0,992891	0,130769	0,156682	0,258065	0,179293	0,127559	0,076336	0,01	0	1	1	1	0,500197269
Netherlands	0,285714	0,592116	0,921801	0,307692	1	0,741935	0,691919	0,911811	0,69084	0,029091	0	1	0	1	0,742992719

continued on following page

Table 1. Continued

Ülke	A1	A2	A3	A4	A5	A6	A7	A8	A9	A10	A11	A12	A13	A14	Spor Dostu Skoru
Austria	0,142857	0,631809	1	0,165385	0,313364	0,806452	0,505051	0,625197	0,671756	0,019091	1	1	1	1	0,807360081
Poland	0,285714	0,195033	0,914692	0,103846	0,152074	0,634409	0,482323	0,255118	0,90458	0,046364	1	1	1	1	0,724922961
Portugal	0,142857	0,377224	0,938389	0,303846	0,460829	0,634409	0,169192	0,201575	0,973282	0,083636	0	1	1	0	0,571385431
Romania	0,142857	0,131498	0,862559	0	0,013825	0,795699	0,138889	0,061417	0,507634	0,131818	1	1	1	0	0,52601787
Slovenia	0,214286	0,418386	0,969194	0,211538	0,322581	0,473118	0,333333	0,448819	0,660305	0,020909	1	1	1	1	0,733860906
Slovakia	0,142857	0,158052	0,976303	0,107692	0,271889	0,494624	0,469697	0,415748	0,541985	0,053636	1	1	1	1	0,693862167
Finland	0,428571	0,484508	0,85782	0,369231	0,460829	0,634409	0,770202	0,499213	1	0,053636	1	1	1	0	0,778038141
Sweden	0,428571	0,519025	0,940758	0,496154	0,576037	0,72043	0,871212	0,823622	0,679389	0	0	1	1	0	0,732290862
Iceland	1	0,303984	0,92891	1	0,299539	0,645161	0,20202	0,815748	0,854962	0	0	1	1	0	0,731847705
Norway	0,214286	0,623697	0,864929	0,392308	0,788018	0,731183	0,633838	1	0,694656	0	0	1	1	0	0,722083182
Switzerland	0,142857	0,724436	0,921801	0,311538	0,797235	0,731183	0,727273	0,815748	0,706107	0,04	0	1	0	1	0,719834337
United Kingdom1	0,214286	0,532837	0,957346	0,419231	0,345622	0,645161	0,335859	0,314961	0,530534	0	1	1	0	1	0,663257882
Bosnia and Herzegovina	0	0,041236	0,78673	0,1	0,069124	0,290323	0,103535	0,001575	0,026718	0	0	1	1	0	0,310840084
Montenegro	0	0,139064	0,739336	0,2	0,230415	0,16129	0,436869	0,034646	0,522901	0,036364	0	1	1	1	0,500080373
North Macedonia2	0,071429	0,018938	0,71564	0,023077	0,115207	0,354839	0,128788	0,022047	0,236641	0	0	1	1	0	0,335146008

Ülke	A1	A2	A3	A4	A5	A6	A7	A8	A9	A10	A11	A12	A13	A14	Spor Dostu Skoru
Albania	0,071429	0	0,78673	0,038462	0	0,430108	0,318182	0	0,103053	1	0	1	1	1	0,522542068
Serbia	0,071429	0,123037	0,957346	0,176923	0,152074	0,709677	0,300505	0,2	0	0,205455	0	1	1	1	0,536040498
Turkey	0,2	0,239181	0,933649	0,05	0,032258	0,655914	0,29798	0,020472	0,301527	0,481818	1	1	1	1	0,65570902

Referance: Eurostat, General government expenditure by function (COFOG), https://ec.europa.eu/eurostat/databrowser/view/gov_10a_exp$dv_584/default/table?lang=en&category=sprt.sprt_gov., Eurostat, Mean consumption expenditure of private households on sporting goods and services by COICOP consumption purpose, https://ec.europa.eu/eurostat/databrowser/view/sprt_pcs_hbs/default/table?lang=en&category=sprt.sprt_exp., Eurostat, Persons not participating in cultural or sport activities in the last 12 months, https://ec.europa.eu/eurostat/databrowser/view/ilc_scp06$dv_2402/default/table?lang=en&category=sprt.sprt_pcs.sprt_pcs_ilc., Eurostat, Employed persons in sport, https://ec.europa.eu/eurostat/databrowser/view/sprt_emp_sex/default/table?lang=en&category=sprt.sprt_emp., Eurostat, Persons participating in cultural or sport activities in the last 12 months, https://ec.europa.eu/eurostat/databrowser/view/ilc_scp03$dv_551/default/table?lang=en&category=sprt.sprt_pcs.sprt_pcs_ilc., Eurostat, Time spent, participation time and participation rate in the main, https://ec.europa.eu/eurostat/databrowser/view/tus_00age$dv_167/default/table?lang=en&category=sprt.sprt_pcs.sprt_pcs_tus., Eurostat, Persons participating in formal voluntary activities, https://ec.europa.eu/eurostat/databrowser/view/ilc_scp23$dv_2403/default/table?lang=en&category=sprt.sprt_pcs.sprt_pcs_ilc., Eurostat, Time spent on health-enhancing (non-work-related) aerobic physical activity, https://ec.europa.eu/eurostat/databrowser/view/hlth_ehis_pe2e$dv_300/default/table?lang=en&category=sprt.sprt_pcs.sprt_pcs_pha., Eurostat, Perception survey results, https://ec.europa.eu/eurostat/databrowser/view/urb_percep$dv_283/default/table?lang=en&category=sprt.sprt_pcs.sprt_pcs_urb., Olimpics, Winner Reward, https://www.olympics.com/ioc/ioc-overview/ioc-history/ancient-olympic-games/rewards., Jürgen, M, vd, Good Governance in the Employment Relations of Athletes in Olympic Sports in Europe: Understanding Evaluating – Improving, 2022, European Commission, Physical Education and Sport at School in Europe Eurydice Report, 2013; European Institute for Gender Equality, National ministries with responsibility for sports, chrome-extension://efaidnbmnnnibpcajpcglclefindmkaj/https://eige.europa.eu/sites/default/files/wmid_mapping_sp_natmin_1.pdf.,

In Table 1, where the Sport-Friendly Country Index is shown, the minimum value of the index was identified as 0.3108 for Bosnia and Herzegovina, while the highest value was identified as 0.8785 for Luxembourg. The average "Sport-Friendly Score" of 37 countries was calculated as 0.6409. Turkey's index value is 0.6557. The distinctions of welfare typologies also emerge in the analysis performed. Truly looking at it, the countries where the analysis was carried out are divided into at least four as liberal, social-democratic, conservative, and Southern European typologies according to the classifications performed by Esping-Andersen (1991) and Leibfried (1993). This distinction is clearly striking when the range of the index is examined. Especially the ratio of sport investments to GDP, the awarding of successful athletes, employment guarantees, and the existence of an independent ministry have been decisive in how sport-friendly the analyzed countries are. All countries examined within the scope of the index are countries that implement social policies that promote and encourage sport in individuals. At this point, although all the countries evaluated are "sport-friendly," four degrees were revealed when they were classified according to the intensity levels of the policies they implemented. Social transfers to be evaluated in the index developed by us, the importance degrees of social transfers, or new countries to be added may reveal differences in the said grading (Esping-Andersen, 1990; Leibfried, 1993)

Figure 1. Ranking of Sport-Friendly Countries According to the Sport-Friendly Score

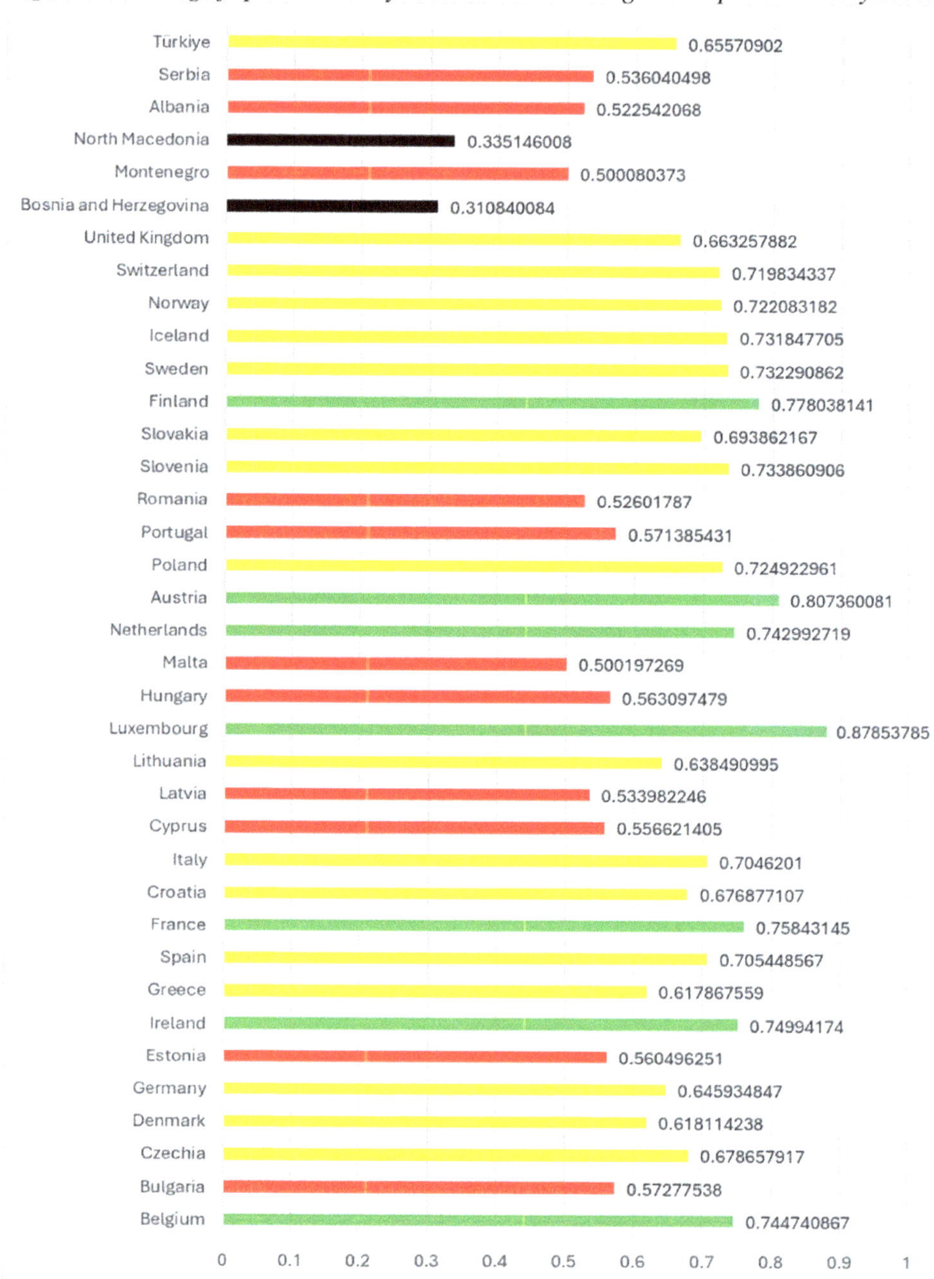

According to the developed Sport-Friendly Country Index, Finland, Austria, Belgium, Ireland, France, Luxembourg, and the Netherlands can be evaluated as a "Sport Regime" located in the green category. While 17 countries, including Turkey, are positioned as "sport-friendly countries," 11 countries can be expressed as "medium-degree sport-friendly countries" and two countries as "low-degree sport-friendly countries." At this point, it can be said that Turkey has a sport-friendly score in a course close to the performance of conservative welfare regimes. It is observed that the distribution of sport-friendly countries also shows similarities with welfare regime typologies. Accordingly, it has been seen that the welfare regimes defined as sport regime countries in the green category are strong social states classified as conservative and social-democratic welfare regimes. On the other hand, it is striking that the medium and low-degree sport-friendly countries are countries expressed as the Southern European welfare regime type, which, although they define themselves as a social state, can implement palliative social policies. The classification of sport-friendly countries, created based on the Sport-Friendly Country Score, has provided an opportunity to make an inter-country comparison based on the social policies that selected countries implement for individuals.

REFERENCES

Abanoz, E. I., & Soyer, F. (2018). Sporun toplumsal değerler üzerindeki etkisi hakkında bir çalışma. *Uluslararas Insan Bilimleri Dergisi, 15*(1), 309–318. DOI: 10.14687/jhs.v15i1.4951

Alcock, P., & Erskine, A. May, May, M. (2002). The Blackwell Dictionary of Social Policy, Oxford: Blackwell Publishing.

Anorim, L., Cavalcanti, G., & Cruz, R. (2023). The choice of scaling technique matters for classification performance. *Applied Soft Computing, 133.* Advance online publication. DOI: 10.1016/j.asoc.2022.109924

Bergsgard, N. A., Houlihan, B., Mangset, P., Nødland, S. I., & Rommetvedt, H. (2007). *Sport policy: A comparative analysis of stability and change*. Elsevier.

Dietl, H. M., Lang, M., & Werner, S. (2009). Social welfare in sports leagues with profit-maximizing and/or win-maximizing clubs. *Southern Economic Journal, 76*(2), 375–396.

Eather, N., Wade, L., Pankowiak, A., & Eime, R. (2023). The impact of sports participation on mental health and social outcomes in adults: A systematic review and the 'Mental Health through Sport' conceptual model. *Systematic Reviews, 12*, 102. DOI: 10.1186/s13643-023-02264-8

Ekholm, D. (2016). *Sport as a means of responding to social problems: Rationales of government, welfare and social change* (Linköping Studies in Arts and Science No. 687). Linköping University.

Ekholm, D., & Dahlstedt, M. (2023). *Sport as social policy: Midnight football and the governing of society*. Routledge.

Esping-Andersen, G. (1990). *The Three Worlds of Welfare Capitalism*. Polity Press.

European Institute for Gender Equality. National ministries with responsibility for sports, chromeextension://efaidnbmnnnibpcajpcglclefindmkaj/https://eige.europa.eu/sites/default/files/wmid_mapping_sp_natmin_1.pdf

Eurostat, Mean consumption expenditure of private households on sporting goods and services by COICOP consumption purpose, https://ec.europa.eu/eurostat/databrowser/view/sprt_pcs_hbs/default/table?lang=en&category=sprt.sprt_exp

Eurostat, Employed persons in sport, https://ec.europa.eu/eurostat/databrowser/view/sprt_emp_sex/default/table?lang=en&category=sprt.sprt_emp

Eurostat, General government expenditure by function (COFOG), https://ec.europa.eu/eurostat/databrowser/view/gov_10a_exp$dv_584/default/table?lang=en&category=sprt.sprt_gov

Eurostat, Perception survey results, https://ec.europa.eu/eurostat/databrowser/view/urb_percep$dv_283/default/table?lang=en&category=sprt.sprt_pcs.sprt_pcs_urb

Eurostat, Persons not participating in cultural or sport activities in the last 12 months, https://ec.europa.eu/eurostat/databrowser/view/ilc_scp06$dv_2402/default/table?lang=en&category=sprt.sprt_pcs.sprt_pcs_ilc

Eurostat, Persons participating in cultural or sport activities in the last 12 months, https://ec.europa.eu/eurostat/databrowser/view/ilc_scp03$dv_551/default/table?lang=en&category=sprt.sprt_pcs.sprt_pcs_ilc

Eurostat, Persons participating in formal voluntary activities, https://ec.europa.eu/eurostat/databrowser/view/ilc_scp23$dv_2403/default/table?lang=en&category=sprt.sprt_pcs.sprt_pcs_ilc

Eurostat, Time spent on health-enhancing (non-work-related) aerobic physical activity, https://ec.europa.eu/eurostat/databrowser/view/hlth_ehis_pe2e$dv_300/default/table?lang=en&category=sprt.sprt_pcs.sprt_pcs_pha

Eurostat, Time spent, participation time and participation rate in the main, https://ec.europa.eu/eurostat/databrowser/view/tus_00age$dv_167/default/table?lang=en&category=sprt.sprt_pcs.sprt_pcs_tus

Giulianotti, R. (2011). The sport, development and peace sector: A model of four social policy domains. *Journal of Social Policy*, *40*(4), 757–776. DOI: 10.1017/S0047279410000930

Grix, J., & Brannagan, P. M. (2016). Of mechanisms and myths: Conceptualising states' "soft power" strategies through sports mega-events. *Diplomacy and Statecraft*, *27*(2), 251–272. DOI: 10.1080/09592296.2016.1169791

Han, J., Kamber, M., & Pei, J. (2012). *Data minin: concepts and techniques*. Morgan Kaufman Press.

Hoekman, R., & Scheerder, J. (2021). Sport policy practice and outcome: Theoretical and empirical approaches. *European Journal of Sport Science*, *18*(2), 103–113. DOI: 10.1080/16138171.2021.1926772

Houlihan, B., Bloyce, D., & Smith, A. (2009). Developing the research agenda in sport policy. *International Journal of Sport Policy and Politics*, *1*(1), 1–12. DOI: 10.1080/19406940802681186

Im, Y.-J., Jung, H.-Y., & Kim, S.-G. (2026). The effects of public sports welfare programs on participants' psychological well-being recovery. *Journal of Sport and Applied Science*, *10*(1), 17–23. DOI: 10.13106/jsas.2026.vol10.no1.17

Juszczak, P., Tax, D., & Duin, R. (2002). Feature scaling in support vector data description. *8th Annual Conf. Of The Advanced School For Computing And Imaging.*

Jürgen, M (2022), Good Governance in the Employment Relations of Athletes in Olympic Sports in Europe: Understanding Evaluating – Improving, European Commission, Physical Education and Sport at School in Europe Eurydice Report.

Kasapoğlu, M. M., & Öçal, M. (2021). Türkiye'de spor yatırımlarının tabana yayılması politikasının sosyal adalet açısından önemi. *Yönetim ve Ekonomi Araştırmaları Dergisi*, *19*(3), 173–191. DOI: 10.11611/yead.991462

Kellett, P., Hede, A.-M., & Chalip, L. (2008). Social policy for sport events: Leveraging (relationships with) teams from other nations for community benefit. *European Sport Management Quarterly*, *8*(2), 101–121. DOI: 10.1080/16184740802024344

Leibfried, S. (1993). Towards a European welfare state? In Jones, P. (Ed.), *New Perspectives on the Welfare State in Europe* (pp. 135–156). Routledge.

Madden, P. (2015). Welfare economics of "financial fair play" in a sports league with benefactor owners. *Journal of Sports Economics*, *16*(2), 159–184. DOI: 10.1177/1527002512465759

Narin, M. (2025). Sekiz ülke politikasında sporun performanstan toplumsal refaha evriminde sosyolojik analiz. *Fenerbahçe Üniversitesi Spor Bilimleri Dergisi*, *5*(2), 3–13.

Olimpics, Winner Reward, https://www.olympics.com/ioc/ioc-overview/ioc-history/ancient-olympic-games/rewards

Öçal, M., & Kutlu, Ö. (2023a). A Study On Welfare And Lıvıng Condıtıons Of Dısadvantaged Groups: The Case Of Burdur Provınce. *Journal of Management and Economics Research*, *21*(3), 410–425. DOI: 10.11611/yead.1333231

Öçal, M., & Kutlu, Ö. (2023b). Two Sides of the Coin in Ageing in Place: Neighbourhood Safety and Elder Abuse. In Asiamah, N. (Eds.), *Sustainable Neighbourhoods for Ageing in Place*. Springer., DOI: 10.1007/978-3-031-41594-4_5

Österlind, M. (2016). Sport policy evaluation and governing participation in sport: Governmental problematics of democracy and health. *International Journal of Sport Policy and Politics*, *8*(3), 347–362. DOI: 10.1080/19406940.2015.1123755

Özdemir, S. (2005). Sosyal Gelişim Düzeyleri Farklı Refah Devletlerinin Sınıflandırılması Üzerine Bir İnceleme. *Sosyal Siyaset Konferansları, 49*, 231–266.

Teke, M. S., & Karakuş, S. (2022). Sporun sosyal gelişim sürecine etkisi. *Journal of Social. Humanities and Administrative Sciences, 8*(53), 733–736. DOI: 10.29228/JOSHAS.62508

Titmuss, R. M. (1968). *Commıtment to Welfare*. Pantheon Books. DOI: 10.1111/j.1467-9515.1968.tb00093.x

Trendafilova, S., McCullough, B., Pfahl, M., Nguyen, S. N., Casper, J., & Picariello, M. (2014). Environmental sustainability in sport: Current state and future trends. *Global Journal on Advances in Pure & Applied Sciences, 3*, 9–14.

Washington, R. E., & Karen, D. (2001). Sport and society. *Annual Review of Sociology, 27*(1), 187–212. DOI: 10.1146/annurev.soc.27.1.187

Yerlikaya, B., & Öcal, A. T. (2015). Sports as a social policy tool in Turkey. *British Journal of Arts and Social Sciences, 20*(1), 38–52.

Yıldırım, F. (2014). *Gri ilişkisel analiz*. Dora Publising.

Young, K. (2019). *Sport, violence and society* (2nd ed.). Routledge. DOI: 10.4324/9781315737089

ENDNOTES

1 Due to the Brexit process, the compiled data for the United Kingdom are dated 2019

2 In the EUROSTAT database, the latest updated data for North Macedonia is dated 2017.

Chapter 3

A Look at the Development of Sports Policies in the World and in Türkiye From a Social Policy Perspective

Mehmet Muharrem Kasapoğlu
http://orcid.org/0009-0009-3943-8556
Turkish Grand National Assembly, Turkey

Nice Şenolan
Turkish Grand National Assembly, Turkey

ABSTRACT

This chapter examines the transformation of sport from a recreational and leisure-time activity into a multidimensional social policy instrument, drawing on both global developments and the Turkish case. The first section scrutinizes the historical evolution of sport as a vehicle of social policy, suggesting its early use in industrial societies as a tool for discipline, its institutionalization within welfare state schemes, and its later reconceptualization within the "Sport for Development and Peace" paradigm. The second section provides a comparative analysis of sport policy development across different countries, including Western and Asian models. The chapter identifies common patterns in sport policy development among differing national contexts: increased state involvement, professionalization, and the tension between elite sport and mass participation.

DOI: 10.4018/979-8-2600-3174-2.ch003

INTRODUCTION

Traditionally viewed as a recreational pastime or a form of entertainment, sport has undergone a profound transformation, evolving into a multidimensional instrument of social policy. In the contemporary era, modern states increasingly utilize sport to address complex societal challenges, moving beyond its intrinsic value to leverage its capacity for "development through sport". This paradigm shift positions sport as a mechanism of social engineering designed to improve the social fabric by fostering better social behavior, moral well-being, and economic efficiency. As a guarantor of human well-being, social policy involves state intervention in the market to ensure a minimum quality of life, and sport has emerged as a primary tool within this framework, operating on the philosophy that "prevention is cheaper than cure".

The systematic application of sport for social objectives dates back to the late nineteenth century in industrializing European societies. During this period, characterized by urban overcrowding and social fragmentation, institutions like British public schools adopted sport to instill discipline, teamwork, and social order among youth. Similarly, in Germany and Sweden, physical education was employed to rebuild national populations and restore social cohesion. Following the Second World War, the rise of welfare states marked the formal institutionalization of sport within public policy. During this "golden age," sport was explicitly linked to health, education, and social welfare, supported by influential frameworks such as the Council of Europe's 1975 "Sport for All" Charter, which established access to sport as a fundamental citizenship right.

By the late twentieth century, the challenges of globalization, such as marginalization and community disintegration, prompted a further redefinition of sport's role. This era witnessed a transition from "Sport for All"—focused on universal rights—to "Sport for Good," which conceptualizes sport as an instrumental tool to achieve measurable outcomes in areas like crime reduction, social inclusion, and community regeneration. This perspective was globally solidified in 2001 when the United Nations officially recognized sport as a means to achieve non-sport-related objectives, including poverty reduction and gender equality, leading to the institutionalization of the "Sport for Development and Peace" (SDP) paradigm.

The Turkish trajectory offers a compelling case of this evolution, shifting from a centralized, state-led model toward a strategic, rights-based approach. In the early years of the Republic, sport was primarily a vehicle for nation-building and cultivating a disciplined, physically strong citizenry, a mission codified in the 1938 Physical Education Law. The post-1960s planned development era shifted the focus toward mass participation and public health, eventually leading to the 1982 Constitution, which established the promotion of sport as a duty of the state. In the post-2002 period, Türkiye entered an advanced phase characterized by unprecedented infrastructure expansion and a 1000% increase in licensed athletes. Current policies prioritize protecting youth from social risks and utilizing sport as a vital mechanism for social integration and public welfare.

In the neoliberal era, the role of sport has expanded further to include its function as a strategic investment tool for both public and private sectors. Governments now view sports infrastructure not only as a public good but as a catalyst for urban regeneration and economic activity, often utilizing public-private partnerships (PPP) to optimize efficiency. Furthermore, mega-sporting events like the Olympic Games have become essential platforms for soft power, enabling states to enhance national branding and international prestige. Simultaneously, the private sector has embraced sport through club acquisitions and global sponsorships, seeking to capitalize on "meaning transfer"—the process of associating brand identity with the loyalty and emotional attachment found in sporting communities. This study examines these global and national transformations, analyzing the complex interplay between sport, social policy, and economic strategy.

1. SPORT AS A VEHICLE OF SOCIAL POLICY: A HISTORICAL OUTLOOK ON THE GLOBAL AND TURKISH CASES

Social policy is one of the fundamental guarantors of a humane life. Social policy, which refers to state intervention in the market to protect and improve human well-being, essentially sets a boundary for a minimum quality of life in this regard. It strives to protect the boundary it sets through laws. After the 1980s, when efforts to provide welfare through social transfers began to be debated, the preference for social policies in protective and rehabilitative areas has increased. Sport constitutes one of the most important pillars of these social policies based on the philosophy that "preventing is cheaper than paying". Sport embodies protective factors against social risks and rehabilitative factors against negative occurrences. Sport, which has positive effects on individual and social levels ranging from health to psychological well-being and even social inclusion, is for these reasons primarily preferred as an effective social policy tool by most welfare regimes, especially in recent years. Spreading sport to the grassroots and encouraging the athlete constitute the basic starting points of these social policies. At this point, the construction of sports facilities from a local development perspective, the reinforcement of sport culture across all segments of society, and the encouragement of successful athletes through various social policies or cash transfers stimulate the sub-breakdowns of these two fundamental starting points (Kasapoğlu and Öçal, 2021; Öçal and Kutlu, 2024; Öçal and Kutlu, 2023; Öçal, et al., 2022).

Sport has increasingly transcended its traditional role as a leisure-time activity, a form of entertainment, or a purely recreational pursuit, evolving into an instrument through which modern states seek to address a wide range of societal challenges. In this sense, sport can be understood as a mechanism of social engineering, employed to shape and improve the social fabric of society. Governments and public agencies have demonstrated a growing interest in utilizing sport to achieve non-sport-related objectives—what has been conceptualized as "development through sport"—prioritizing outcomes such as improved social behaviour, moral well-being, and economic efficiency (Houlihan et al., 2009). Understanding how sport has evolved from an activity primarily associated with individual physical and mental well-being into a structured instrument of social policy is therefore essential.

The roots of the systematic use of sport for social purposes can be traced back to the late nineteenth century, particularly within industrializing European societies. Rapid industrialization brought about significant social disruptions, including poverty, unemployment, urban overcrowding, and social fragmentation. In response to these transformations, British public schools increasingly incorporated sport into their curricula as a means of instilling discipline, moral values, and social order among youth. Sport was believed to cultivate essential qualities such as leadership, teamwork, loyalty, and self-restraint. Importantly, this integration also emerged as a response to widespread disorder and unrest within schools during that period. Heggie (2016) argues that the processes of industrialization and urbanization throughout the nineteenth century weakened traditional forms of citizenship identity, indirectly contributing to the deterioration of cultural and social institutions. In this context, competitive sports and physical education—centered on improving bodily capacity and discipline—came to be viewed as instruments for restoring social cohesion and civic identity. Historical examples from Germany and Sweden, discussed by Heggie (2016), further illustrate how physical education and sport were utilized by states as mechanisms for strengthening and "rebuilding" populations perceived to be socially or physically degenerate. Thus, even before the formal institutionalization of social policy, sport had already begun to function as an informal policy instrument through which states sought to promote social cohesion, civic consciousness, and social stability.

Following the Second World War, the rise of welfare states marked a turning point in the institutionalization of sport within public policy. Governments began to approach sport more systematically, explicitly linking it to policy domains such as health, education, and social welfare due to its perceived social benefits. The post-World War II era, often referred to as the "golden age" of welfare policy, also represented the period in which sport became increasingly institutionalized within public policy frameworks (Houlihan & White, 2003). The period between the 1950s and the mid-1970s was characterized by the emergence of the activist state model across Europe, whereby governments expanded their commitment to publicly funded welfare services. During this era, the scope of public services extended beyond traditional sectors such as housing and healthcare to include non-traditional areas, including sport. Beginning in the 1960s, expenditures related to sport—particularly investments in sports facilities and public infrastructure—came to be regarded as legitimate forms of government spending. The rationale behind the institutionalization of sport can be observed in influential reports such as the Albemarle Report (1960) and the Wolfenden Report (1960) in the United Kingdom, both of which emphasized the instrumental value of sport in addressing post-war social challenges. These reports highlighted the role of physical activity and organized sport in promoting bodily fitness, fostering social integration, and addressing issues related to youth delinquency and social disorder. Moreover, sport was portrayed as a means of bringing young people into constructive and healthy contact with their peers, reducing tendencies toward criminal behaviour, and contributing to character formation. A major milestone in this process was the Council of Europe's "Sport for All" Charter of 1975, which framed access to sport as a fundamental component of citizenship rights. The Charter represented a significant step in integrating sport into the broader realm of social policy by advocating the extension of the social, educational, and health-related benefits of sport to wider segments of society (Hartmann-Tews, 2006).

By the late twentieth century, the emergence of new societal challenges—particularly those associated with globalization, such as social exclusion, marginalization, and community disintegration—necessitated a redefinition of sport's role within public policy. As policymakers searched for more diverse and innovative instruments to address these issues, sport gained renewed prominence within policy agendas. In particular, this period witnessed the growing recognition of social exclusion as one of the most pressing contemporary challenges, encompassing economic, social, cultural, and political dimensions (Spaaij et al., 2014). In the United Kingdom, for example, the urban riots of the 1980s prompted the Conservative government to increasingly utilize sport as a mechanism for addressing social unrest and promoting community cohesion (Green, 2006). As Coalter (2007) argues, this period marked a significant transformation in the way sport was conceptualized within policy frameworks. Rather than being supported primarily for its intrinsic value, sport came to be justified increasingly in terms of its measurable contributions to broader social and political objectives. The general assumption that "sport is beneficial" was no longer considered sufficient; instead, sport was expected to demonstrate tangible outcomes in areas such as crime reduction, social inclusion, youth development, and community regeneration. This transformation is commonly characterized as a shift from "Sport for All" to "Sport for Good." The former reflected a rights-based understanding of sport, emphasizing universal access as a component of citizenship and social welfare. The latter, by contrast, conceptualized sport as an instrumental policy tool designed to address specific societal problems. Within this framework, public investment in sport was increasingly expected to contribute to strategic policy goals, particularly those related to social inclusion, social cohesion, and community development.

From the 1990s onward, national governments' emphasis on the role of sport in combating social exclusion and promoting social inclusion was increasingly shaped by the influence of supranational and international organizations and their respective policy frameworks. This trend intensified during the 2000s with the formal recognition of sport as a development instrument by major global institutions. Such developments reflected the broader transition of sport from a primarily recreational activity into what became known as the Sport for Development and Peace (SDP) sector, which is grounded in the belief that sport can generate a wide range of positive social outcomes (Spaaij et al., 2014; Ekholm, 2016). As Beutler (2008) highlights, it was only in 2001 that the United Nations officially recognized sport as a means of achieving non-sport-related objectives, including poverty reduction, gender equality, and environmental sustainability. The establishment of the United Nations Office on Sport for Development and Peace, together with the appointment of the first UN Special Adviser on Sport for Development and Peace in the same year, further institutionalized this perspective. This shift was also reflected in the United Nations' 2003 report *Sport for Development and Peace*, which described sport as a versatile and cost-effective instrument for achieving broader development goals. Although sport had previously been utilized informally within various UN initiatives, its systematic integration into international development strategies accelerated following the publication of the 2003 report and subsequent UN resolutions. Importantly, the United Nations did not promote sport for its own sake; rather, it emphasized sport's utility within wider development and peace-building agendas. As outlined in the 2003 report, sport was regarded as a "school for life," capable of fostering values and skills such as self-confidence, leadership, cooperation, discipline, and mutual respect—qualities considered essential for social cohesion. Furthermore, sport was recognized for its capacity to bring together individuals from diverse social, cultural, and ethnic backgrounds, thereby functioning as an effective mechanism for social integration. Its preventative effects on public health, its potential contribution to reducing healthcare expenditures, and its role in enhancing employability through transferable skills such as teamwork, communication, and discipline further reinforced its legitimacy as a social policy instrument. In addition, sport was increasingly viewed as a platform for dialogue and reconciliation between opposing groups, capable of transcending social, cultural, and political divisions. Two years after the publication of the United Nations' 2003 report, 2005 was declared the International

Year of Sport and Physical Education. From this period onward, UN member states increasingly incorporated sport into their national policy agendas. Despite variations in welfare regimes and state capacities, governments across different contexts came to view sport as a relatively low-cost and legitimate means of addressing structural social challenges, including social isolation, youth delinquency, and community fragmentation (Narin, 2025; Ekholm, 2016). Consequently, the historical evolution of sport as a social policy instrument demonstrates that its role has been closely intertwined with broader global governance practices and continuously reshaped in response to evolving societal challenges.

In the Turkish case, the integration of sport into the country's social policy framework did not occur overnight, as was similarly the case at the international level. Rather, sport gradually evolved from being perceived primarily as a form of physical activity into a strategic and multifunctional instrument of social policy through a long process of institutional transformation. The changing role of sport within government agendas reflected broader shifts in national priorities and state-building strategies. In the early years of the Turkish Republic, and particularly until the introduction of planned development policies in the 1960s, sport was primarily promoted as a means of cultivating a healthy, physically strong, and disciplined society. The first Bayar Government (1937–1938) was the first government in Republican history to explicitly include sport in its official programme (Aykın & Bilir, 2013). The government's emphasis on sport was closely linked to the belief that physical activity constituted an essential component of national strength and moral education. In this sense, sport during the early Republican period can be understood as an important element of the new Republic's nation-building and modernization project. This perspective was institutionalized through the Physical Education Law of 1938, enacted during the Bayar Government era, which defined sport as a means of ensuring that citizens acquired physical and moral capacities in accordance with national and revolutionary ideals (Uçar, 2016). The law also established the General Directorate of Physical Education, thereby transforming sport into a centralized and statutory public service. The state's interest in sport during this period was rooted largely in the objective of cultivating a population capable of defending the nation while simultaneously instilling values such as discipline, collective consciousness, and national solidarity (Ayvaz, 2022; Tokatlıoğlu, 2021). From the 1960s onward, with the adoption of planned development strategies, sport began to be addressed more systematically within state policy. A significant milestone in this regard was Article 49 of the 1961 Constitution, which assigned the state responsibility for protecting the physical and mental well-being of citizens. Subsequently, the Second Five-Year Development Plan (1968–1972) identified sport, for the first time, as an educational instrument for raising healthy and strong generations. During the planned development era, the primary focus of state policy was on expanding mass participation in sport and increasing public access to physical activity. From the 1980s onward, sport gained further constitutional significance through Article 59 of the 1982 Constitution, which established the promotion of sport as a duty of the state. In parallel with broader global trends of the period, sport in Türkiye increasingly came to be viewed as a mechanism of social control and social integration, capable of preventing social disintegration and steering young people away from various forms of social risk and delinquency. Beginning in the late 1990s, again in line with international developments, sport became integrated into a broader social inclusion agenda. The Eighth Five-Year Development Plan (2001–2005) represented a particularly important turning point, as it explicitly addressed the barriers faced by marginalized groups in accessing sporting opportunities. From this period onward, sport increasingly came to be conceptualized as a tool for combating social exclusion and discrimination. The establishment of the Turkish National Paralympic Committee in 2002 further demonstrated the state's commitment to utilizing sport as a mechanism for social integration and equal participation.

2. THE EVOLUTION OF SPORT POLICY: AN ANALYSIS OF GLOBAL AND TURKISH DEVELOPMENTS

The evolution and development of sport policy across the globe has followed a broadly similar trajectory in many countries, moving from fragmented and volunteer-led structures toward increasingly institutionalized and state-supported systems (Begović, 2020; Antonie et al., 2024). Despite these common patterns in the development of sport policy, the extent and nature of state intervention have varied significantly across national contexts. Although each country has followed its own historical trajectory, several recurring themes can nevertheless be identified: the professionalization of sport management, the tension between elite sport development and mass participation, and the growing importance of sport within international diplomacy and national image-building efforts (Houlihan & Green, 2011; Coalter, 2017; Grix & Lee, 2013). This chapter examines the evolution of sport policy in various countries through these broader transformations.

With regard to Commonwealth countries and Western models, sport policy in states such as Australia, Canada, and Scotland demonstrates a gradual transition from volunteer-based activities to state-backed systems in which sport is utilized to achieve a variety of national objectives, including the promotion of public health, social cohesion, and international prestige. As Stewart et al. (2004) suggests, the Australian sport policy trajectory can be divided into four distinct stages. The first phase, spanning from 1920 to 1971, is characterized as a period of "benign indifference," during which the organization and financing of sport were largely left to voluntary associations and civil society actors.

The second phase, between 1972 and 1982, marked the beginning of direct federal intervention in sport policy under the Whitlam Labor administration. This period witnessed the establishment of the Australian Institute of Sport, signaling the state's growing recognition of sport as an area of strategic public interest (Stewart et al., 2004). The third phase, covering the years from 1983 to 1996, was characterized by substantial budgetary expansion and institutional development, including the creation of the Australian Sports Commission (Stewart et al., 2004). Finally, the period from 1996 onward is described as the "integration phase," during which efforts were made to balance elite sport success with broader community participation programmes and public health objectives (Stewart et al., 2004).

A similar trajectory can be observed in Canada. During the first half of the twentieth century, the federal government played only a limited role in sport policy, as sport was generally considered to fall within the domains of education and local community activity rather than constituting a distinct policy field (Comeau, 2013). This situation changed significantly with the adoption of the *Fitness and Amateur Sport Act* in 1961, which paved the way for federal involvement in the governance and financing of sport. Throughout the 1970s, high-performance sport increasingly became associated with national pride and national unity within the Canadian context (Comeau, 2013). This period also witnessed the growing professionalization of sport organizations, which gradually evolved into institutional mechanisms through which the state implemented its sport policies.

More recently, the *Canadian Sport Policy* of 2002 and the *Physical Activity and Sport Act* of 2003 marked the beginning of a new phase in Canadian sport policy, one in which sport came to be understood as extending beyond competition and athletic achievement alone. These policy frameworks formalized what has been described as a "social investment approach" (Thibault & Harvey, 2013; Comeau, 2013), whereby sport increasingly became a tool for achieving broader societal objectives, including the improvement of public health, the strengthening of marginalized communities, and the promotion of social inclusion.

In Scotland, the governance of sport functioned for centuries with relatively limited state intervention, relying primarily on local clubs and voluntary associations to organize and maintain traditional sporting practices such as golf and archery (Meir et al., 2024). The transition toward greater state involvement began in the late 1950s, when the government gradually started to finance sports infrastructure and public sporting facilities (Meir et al., 2024). During the 1980s, the policy landscape became increasingly complex as the UK government began to utilize sport as a mechanism for promoting community cohesion and addressing urban unrest (Meir et al., 2024).

Following the re-establishment of the Scottish Parliament in 1998, Scotland developed a more distinctive and autonomous sport policy identity. Since the beginning of the twenty-first century, Scottish sport policy has largely rested on two central pillars: the promotion of health and well-being through sport, and the strategic use of mega sporting events (Jarvie, 2023). In this regard, the Scottish government has increasingly utilized international sporting events such as the 2014 Commonwealth Games and the 2023 UCI Cycling World Championships to stimulate economic activity, enhance tourism, and strengthen Scotland's international visibility and soft power (Meir et al., 2024; Jarvie, 2023).

In contrast, the evolution of sport policy in China closely reflects the country's broader political and economic transformations. Over time, sport evolved from being primarily a mechanism for military preparedness into a sophisticated instrument of international prestige, economic modernization, and soft power projection. Following the establishment of the People's Republic of China in 1949, sport policy was largely centered on improving the physical condition of the population in order to build a strong and militarily prepared nation. Consequently, between 1949 and 1957, sport policies primarily targeted urban workers, rural populations, and military personnel.

According to Zhang and Saunders (2019), after a period of major disruption between 1958 and 1976, China began to modernize its sport system from 1977 onward by moving away from rigid ideological control mechanisms toward a more strategic and institutionalized approach. It was also during this period that participation in sport was formally recognized within the Chinese Constitution, transforming access to sport from a policy preference into a legal entitlement.

Between 1995 and 2008, two principal themes dominated Chinese sport policy: achieving international sporting success and expanding public participation in sport. During this era, China simultaneously pursued elite sport development and mass participation objectives. Through substantial investments in elite sport programmes, the state sought to increase medal success and enhance international prestige, as reflected in initiatives such as the Olympic Glory Plan. At the same time, investments in grassroots and mass sport programmes aimed to improve public health and encourage wider participation. This period also witnessed the introduction of China's first comprehensive legal framework governing sport policy, further institutionalizing the sector.

Since 2009, Chinese sport policy has entered a new phase combining social welfare objectives, economic development strategies, and global competitiveness. Policies such as the Thirteenth Five-Year Plan increasingly addressed complex social issues—including childhood obesity and the declining physical condition of the workforce—thereby demonstrating how sport policy became progressively oriented toward addressing broader societal and economic challenges.

Similarly, the development of sport policy in South Korea closely paralleled the country's broader socio-economic transformation, evolving from a highly state-controlled system into a more people-centered and rights-based framework (Kang & Kwon, 2024). According to Kang and Swon (2024), during the 1960s and 1970s South Korea viewed sport primarily as a tool for enhancing national prestige and competing symbolically with North Korea. Consequently, the government focused heavily on elite athlete development, leading to the establishment of specialized national training centres (Kang & Kwon, 2024). Furthermore, the National Sports Promotion Act of 1961 formally established sport as a responsibility of the state, thereby institutionalizing government involvement in the sector. During this period, sport policy was largely oriented toward achieving success in international competitions, which were perceived as symbolic arenas of political rivalry and national legitimacy.

A major transformation occurred during the 1980s, when South Korea gradually shifted from an exclusive emphasis on elite sport toward a broader mass participation approach. The successful hosting of the 1988 Seoul Olympic Games acted as a major catalyst for this transition (Choi et al., 2019). Following the achievement of international recognition through elite sporting success, the government increasingly began to promote sport as a component of everyday life rather than solely as a domain of international competition. Simultaneously, rising economic prosperity and improvements in living standards generated growing public demand for leisure opportunities and higher quality of life, further reinforcing the role of sport within society (Kang & Kwon, 2024).

The Hodori Plan of 1989 represented a major milestone in this transformation, as it introduced a nationwide strategy for promoting mass participation in sport through investments in sports facilities and community-based programmes (Choi et al., 2019). In this way, the South Korean state actively sought to make sport more accessible to broader segments of society. In recent years, South Korean sport policy has increasingly shifted toward a welfare- and rights-based perspective (Choi et al., 2019). Accordingly, contemporary sport policy in South Korea is no longer concerned solely with medal success or general participation rates; rather, sport is increasingly regarded as an integral component of the broader social welfare system. Current policy frameworks, including initiatives such as *Sport Vision 2018*, specifically target groups such as women, older adults, and low-income populations, reflecting a stronger emphasis on equality, accessibility, and social inclusion (Choi et al., 2019).

In the Turkish case, the development of sport policy has evolved from an elite-centered activity during the late Ottoman period into a centralized state mission aimed increasingly at enhancing social welfare and public well-being. Modern sport first emerged during the Tanzimat era beginning in the 1830s, as part of the broader modernization process intended to align Ottoman society with Western norms. During this period, sport was introduced and largely dominated by non-Muslim minorities and elite social groups, while the broader population remained relatively excluded from sporting activities (Saydam, 2024; Akın, 2005).

During the Second Constitutional Era (1908–1922), however, the role and function of sport underwent a significant transformation. Sport increasingly shifted from being an elite leisure activity into a mechanism for nation-building, military preparedness, and social discipline (Ayvaz, 2022). Physical education and sporting activities were utilized to prepare young people for military service and to instill values associated with patriotism, discipline, and national defence. The emergence of paramilitary youth organizations such as *Türk Gücü Derneği* (1914) and *Osmanlı Genç Dernekleri* (1916) illustrates the extent to which sport became integrated into broader state-building and militarization efforts during the late Ottoman period (Akın, 2005; Ayvaz, 2022). These developments subsequently laid the institutional and ideological foundations for sport policy in the early Republican era.

Between 1922 and 1939, Turkish sport policy evolved through three major institutional phases: *Türkiye İdman Cemiyetleri İttifakı* (1922–1936), *Türk Spor Kurumu* (1936–1938), and finally the enactment of the *Beden Terbiyesi Kanunu* (Law No. 3530) in 1938. During the early Republican period, sport increasingly became a state-directed mission closely aligned with national defence objectives and the creation of a disciplined, modern citizenry. The *Beden Terbiyesi Kanunu,* which established the *Beden Terbiyesi Genel Müdürlüğü* (General Directorate of Physical Education), represented the peak of this centralization process, transforming sport into a top-down policy instrument rather than merely a voluntary civil society activity (Öğüt, 2014; Alev et al., 2021). Under this framework, participation in physical training activities became compulsory for young people, reflecting the state's emphasis on discipline, collective mobilization, and physical preparedness.

Following the Second World War, Turkish sport policy gradually shifted away from its strict militaristic orientation toward a more welfare-oriented and rights-based framework. The primary policy objectives increasingly became improving public health, expanding mass participation, and achieving international sporting success. Although the 1961 Constitution did not contain a specific provision regarding sport, it emphasized the protection of citizens' physical and mental well-being through the recognition of the right to health (Aydın et al., 2007). A particularly important development occurred in 1964, when the Constitutional Court abolished compulsory participation in sport activities (Akın, 2005). As a result, sport ceased to be regarded as an obligation imposed by the state and instead became an area that the state was expected to support in order to promote public well-being.

The 1982 Constitution marked another important turning point by incorporating sport directly into the constitutional framework for the first time. Through Article 59, the promotion of sport became explicitly defined as a public responsibility, obliging the state to encourage participation and develop sporting infrastructure (Sivrikaya & Demir, 2019; Sunay, 2024). Moreover, beginning particularly with the Second Five-Year Development Plan (1968–1972), the state increasingly prioritized "Sport for All" policies over spectator-oriented sporting activities (Sunay, 2024; Saydam, 2024). In this context, public policy aimed to expand access to physical activity and encourage broader participation among citizens.

Between 1982 and 2002, Turkish sport policy entered a phase characterized by stronger legal institutionalization and increasing adaptation to global trends in sport governance and commercialization. A major administrative restructuring took place in 1986 with the enactment of Law No. 3289, which established the General Directorate of Youth and Sports. This reform enabled sport governance to become more centralized, coordinated, and institutionally organized at the national level. Simultaneously, from the 1980s onward, Turkish sport increasingly aligned with global economic and organizational transformations, particularly through the commercialization of football, which evolved into a major entertainment industry attracting investment and commercial activity (Öğüt, 2014; Akın, 2005). A further milestone occurred in 1992, when the Turkish Football Federation gained financial and administrative autonomy, enabling a more professionalized governance structure aligned with international organizations such as UEFA and FIFA (Alev et al., 2021; Öğüt, 2014; Akın, 2005).

Since 2002, Türkiye has entered a more advanced phase in the evolution of sport policy, during which sport has increasingly become a multidimensional national priority and a central pillar of broader public policy strategies. This transformation has been characterized by extensive state investment, institutional modernization, and a growing recognition of sport as a strategic instrument for public health, social cohesion, and national prestige (Güler & Yaman, 2023; Sunay, 2024). The re-establishment of the Ministry of Youth and Sports constituted an important institutional milestone that enabled the delivery of more comprehensive and coordinated services in the field of sport (Alev et al., 2021; Sunay, 2024).

One of the defining characteristics of this period has been the unprecedented expansion of sports infrastructure throughout the country. According to official statistics, since 2002 the number of sports facilities has increased by approximately 500%, while the number of licensed athletes has grown by nearly 1000% (Sunay, 2024). These developments reflect a significant geographical democratization of access to sport and sporting opportunities. More importantly, the underlying philosophy of sport policy increasingly shifted toward viewing sport not merely as a recreational activity, but as a vital mechanism for social integration and public welfare. For instance, the programme of the 61st Government explicitly emphasized that sport should be regarded as an important instrument of socialization rather than solely as a leisure activity (Aykın & Bilir, 2013; Sunay, 2024).

Consequently, one of the central objectives of Turkish sport policy since 2002 has been the protection of youth from various social risks through greater integration into sporting and social life. At the municipal level, sport policy initiatives have particularly focused on the establishment of neighbourhood sports facilities and community-based programmes intended to steer young people away from harmful habits and social exclusion (İnci, 2011). In this regard, contemporary sport policy in Türkiye increasingly functions as a mechanism for promoting public health, regulating social behaviour, strengthening social cohesion, and facilitating the integration of youth into active and healthy lifestyles.

3. SPORT AS AN INVESTMENT INSTRUMENT: PUBLIC AND PRIVATE SECTOR DYNAMICS IN THE NEOLIBERAL ERA

From the public sector perspective, investments in sports infrastructure have increasingly evolved into strategic investment instruments, valued not only for their public-good dimension but also for their capacity to stimulate economic activity. Public investment in sports infrastructure can generate economic benefits through multiple channels, including employment creation, tourism development, urban regeneration, and broader regional economic revitalization. In this regard, the benefits of infrastructure development often extend beyond the sporting sector itself and "trickle down" to wider segments of society, particularly through employment opportunities generated for local communities during both the construction and operational phases (Jones, 2001).

Moreover, the construction of large-scale sports facilities, such as stadiums and training complexes, has the potential to attract external audiences, investors, and commercial activity into the host region, thereby generating additional inward investment and broader economic spillover effects (Gratton et al., 2005). However, given the highly costly nature of sports infrastructure projects, the optimization of planning, financing, and implementation processes remains critically important. In this context, public-private partnership (PPP) models have increasingly emerged as important mechanisms through which governments seek to combine the resources, expertise, and managerial capacities of both the public and private sectors (Gaafar et al., 2025), while simultaneously protecting the long-term interests of taxpayers (Kennedy & Rosentraub, 2000).

Particularly within Build-Operate-Transfer (BOT) models, which constitute a subcategory of broader PPP arrangements, the responsibility for financing and constructing facilities is transferred to private actors. This often enables states to obtain sports infrastructure projects more rapidly, cost-effectively, and with higher maintenance standards. A notable example can be observed in the case of the 2014

FIFA World Cup in Brazil. Reis and Cabral (2017) demonstrate that stadium projects implemented through PPP mechanisms generated more favourable outcomes in terms of cost-per-seat indicators when compared to projects financed exclusively through public resources. Furthermore, the same study highlights that in three out of five Brazilian PPP projects, major construction-related risks—including delays and cost overruns—were transferred almost entirely to private sector partners (Reis & Cabral, 2017).

Taken together, these examples illustrate how PPP mechanisms can enable governments to align sports infrastructure investments more effectively with principles of efficiency, fiscal sustainability, and risk optimization.

On the other hand, mega sporting events such as the FIFA World Cup, the Olympic Games, and the UEFA Champions League have increasingly been regarded since the 1980s as strategic investment instruments capable of generating both economic and geopolitical leverage for host states and cities. The growing importance of mega sporting events coincided with two broader historical developments: the acceleration of globalization and the 1984 Los Angeles Olympic Games.

The rise of globalization marked the intensification of global economic, political, and cultural interconnectedness, facilitating the transnational flow of capital, knowledge, ideas, and people across borders. This period also witnessed the increasing integration of emerging states into the international system, as countries sought new mechanisms through which they could enhance international visibility, competitiveness, and geopolitical influence (Grix & Lee, 2013). Within this broader context, mega sporting events increasingly became attractive strategic platforms for states aiming to project national prestige and strengthen their position within global politics.

The 1984 Los Angeles Olympic Games represented another major turning point in the organization and financing of mega sporting events. Unlike previous Olympic Games, the Los Angeles Olympics relied predominantly on private financing and consequently generated substantial economic returns while requiring comparatively limited levels of direct public expenditure on sports and transportation infrastructure (Preuss, 2004). This experience contributed significantly to the growing perception that mega sporting events could function not only as cultural spectacles but also as economically viable investment projects.

Nevertheless, it is important to emphasize that mega sporting events are neither inherently economically profitable nor inherently unprofitable. Their economic outcomes depend largely on the extent to which host governments and cities are able to manage infrastructure costs effectively and define realistic economic objectives capable of ensuring long-term financial sustainability (Baade & Matheson, 2006). Consequently, the academic literature concerning the economics of mega sporting events remains divided. While some studies emphasize the limited and often short-term nature of economic gains, others adopt a more positive perspective by highlighting long-term benefits such as urban regeneration, infrastructure modernization, tourism development, and enhanced international visibility.

However, reducing the success of mega sporting events solely to monetary outcomes would provide an incomplete assessment. As Gratton et al. (2006) argue, the significance of mega sporting events cannot be evaluated merely through calculations of economic profit and loss. More importantly, hosting such events increasingly functions as an instrument of soft power, enabling states and cities to shape global perceptions, strengthen international standing, and generate diplomatic advantages (Alshikhy et al., 2025).

The literature frequently emphasizes that mega sporting events produce a range of intangible benefits, including nation branding, image management, and broader "feel-good effects" among domestic populations (Baade & Matheson, 2006). In many cases, expectations regarding these intangible returns may even outweigh expectations of direct economic profitability. Despite the immense financial costs associated with hosting mega sporting events, states continue to compete intensely for hosting rights precisely because of the symbolic and geopolitical advantages such events may provide.

The experience of Barcelona following the 1992 Summer Olympics offers a notable example. Through the successful international marketing and urban transformation associated with the Games, Barcelona eventually became the fifth most visited city in Europe by 2010 (Baade & Matheson, 2006). Similarly, Germany experienced a significant improvement in its international image following the 2006 FIFA World Cup. According to nation-branding indices, Germany rose from seventh place in 2004 to first place in 2007, maintaining a leading position in subsequent years (Grix & Houlihan, 2014).

These examples demonstrate how mega sporting events can substantially enhance international perceptions, strengthen national branding strategies, and reinforce a country's soft power beyond immediate economic outcomes.

As a social policy tool, it is given that sport predominantly comes to the forefront with its said use-value. However, starting with the advance of globalization from the 1980s onward, sport has increasingly become a multidimensional realm of strategic investment for not only states but also private initiatives in the neoliberal era. There is a great variety of means through which sport is considered to be an investment tool for private initiative, two of which will be examined in this chapter: sports club acquisitions and sport sponsorships.

Historically, sports clubs around the world emerged primarily as voluntary, community-based member associations that operated without explicit profit-seeking motives. However, the processes of corporatization, stock exchange listings, and the internationalization of sports clubs developed over time not only as responses to financial pressures and sustainability concerns, but also as a consequence of the strategic opportunities identified by investors within the rapidly expanding sports economy. As sport increasingly evolved into a large-scale commercial sector, traditional organizational models became insufficient for managing growing financial and operational demands.

In this regard, the transition from conventional revenue sources such as ticket sales toward more diversified financial structures—including sponsorship agreements, broadcasting revenues, merchandising, and commercial partnerships—necessitated greater corporatization and professionalization within sports clubs (Yerlikaya, 2012; Aydın et al., 2007). Particularly in football, clubs increasingly came to be viewed by companies, business elites, and investment funds as strategic investment instruments due to the continuous growth of UEFA Champions League prize revenues, the expansion of global broadcasting rights markets, and the rising influence of sports marketing and brand visibility (Rohde & Breuer, 2017).

One of the principal economic rationales behind sports club ownership lies in player development and transfer markets. In many cases, investors seek to develop athletic talent and subsequently generate financial returns through player sales, thereby positioning talent production as a key component of the club's economic model (Metelski et al., 2026).

Nevertheless, the motivations driving sports club acquisitions cannot be reduced solely to direct financial returns. As Plumley et al. (2025) argue, investors acquire football clubs for a variety of economic, political, and strategic reasons, many of which extend beyond immediate profitability. In their study examining Japanese corporations that acquired foreign football clubs, Marin and Lee (2020) demonstrate that four out of five firms achieved little or no direct return on investment. Such findings suggest that, despite the substantial financial risks associated with sports club ownership, investors may continue to pursue acquisitions because of broader strategic advantages that are not strictly monetary in nature.

In this context, Bull and Whittam (2021) identify two major investor archetypes: first, owners primarily motivated by economic and political interests; and second, owners who utilize football clubs as vehicles for broader global and strategic objectives. Particularly within the latter category, sports club ownership can serve as a mechanism for enhancing domestic sporting systems, facilitating knowledge transfer, and strengthening international networks. For example, in the Chinese context, firms acquiring foreign football clubs have used these investments as platforms for transferring expertise, developing youth academies, and establishing coaching programmes within China itself (Lee & No, 2022). These examples illustrate that sports club ownership increasingly functions not merely as a commercial activity, but also as a strategic instrument connected to broader objectives of branding, internationalization, knowledge acquisition, and long-term sporting development.

Another important mechanism through which sport functions as an investment instrument for private actors is sports sponsorship. The primary objectives of sports sponsorships generally extend beyond direct short-term financial returns and instead focus on the creation of brand value, global visibility, corporate image, reputation, and market expansion opportunities (Amis et al., 1999; Reiser et al., 2012). Nevertheless, it is important to note that sports sponsorships may also generate indirect revenue streams and long-term commercial benefits. For instance, telecommunications and media companies frequently invest in sports content and sponsorship agreements in order to distribute sports-related media products across digital broadcasting platforms and expand consumer engagement (Santomier, 2008).

Moreover, facility naming rights—despite representing one of the most expensive forms of sports marketing investment—provide sponsoring firms with an exclusive and highly visible association with major sports venues and teams (Varea-Calderón et al., 2025; Reiser et al., 2012). Through these forms of sponsorship, companies invest in the construction of intangible assets such as brand recognition, prestige, consumer loyalty, and corporate reputation, all of which are increasingly regarded as crucial components of long-term competitive advantage.

Sports sponsorship possesses a unique strategic value because it enables brands to transcend national borders and expand their visibility within global markets. Professional sports organizations often possess international supporter bases, while major sporting competitions are broadcast to worldwide audiences. Consequently, sponsoring sports entities creates opportunities for firms to establish strong global brand awareness by associating themselves with sports institutions that carry significant prestige, emotional attachment, and symbolic value. Football club sponsorships, for example, are frequently described as powerful public relations mechanisms through which sponsoring firms seek to improve corporate image and increase public affinity toward their brands (Amis et al., 1999).

In this context, one of the most significant outcomes of sports sponsorship is what the literature conceptualizes as "meaning transfer." This refers to the process through which the positive emotions, loyalty, trust, and symbolic meanings associated with a sports team are transferred to the sponsoring company in the perceptions of supporters and consumers (Koronios et al., 2016; Henseler et al., 2011). Since sporting events are typically broadcast during peak viewing periods to highly engaged mass audiences, sports sponsorship also provides marketing exposure that is difficult to replicate through traditional advertising methods. Mega sporting events and professional sports competitions offer private actors valuable platforms through which marketing messages can be communicated to millions of viewers in a relatively seamless and emotionally engaging manner.

Furthermore, sports clubs and their supporter communities often possess exceptionally strong emotional bonds, which may become valuable assets for sponsoring firms seeking to benefit from the goodwill, loyalty, and sense of identity associated with those clubs. However, despite these advantages, sports sponsorship does not automatically translate into increased sales, stronger reputation, or improved financial performance. In this respect, sports sponsorship cannot be regarded as a guaranteed investment mechanism. As Farrelly et al. (1997) argue, the effectiveness of sponsorship largely depends on the existence of a strong strategic fit between the sponsoring brand and the sports entity being sponsored. Without such compatibility, the intended positive outcomes of sponsorship may remain limited or fail to materialize altogether.

REFERENCES

Akın, Y. (2005). Ana hatları ile Cumhuriyet döneminde beden terbiyesi ve spor politikaları. *Toplum ve Bilim, 103*, 53–92.

Alev, A., Alemdar, U., Alemdar, B., Yaman, S., & Sığırtmaç, Y. (2021). Türk spor yönetiminin dünden bugüne yapısal analizi: Yeni kamu yönetimi ve yönetişim yaklaşımları açısından bir değerlendirme. *Beden Eğitimi ve Spor Bilimleri Dergisi, 23*(2), 103–124.

Alshikhy, T., O'Sullivan, H., Polkinghorne, M., & Gennings, E. (2025). The role and impact of sporting mega-events in the context of soft power. *Encyclopedia, 5*(1), 31. DOI: 10.3390/encyclopedia5010031

Amis, J., Slack, T., & Berrett, T. (1999). Sport sponsorship as distinctive competence. *European Journal of Marketing, 33*(3/4), 250–272. DOI: 10.1108/03090569910253044

Antonie, A., Begović, M., & Petracovschi, S. (2024). Sport policy in Romania. *Sports Law. Policy and Diplomacy Journal, 2*(2), 17–35.

Aydın, A. D., Demir, H., & Yetim, A. (2007). Türk spor politikalarında öngörülen hedeflerin gerçekleşme düzeylerinin belirlenmesi üzerine bir araştırma: GSGM örneği. *Beden Eğitimi ve Spor Bilimleri Dergisi, 1*(2), 87–96.

Aydın, A. D., Turgut, M., & Bayırlı, R. (2007). Spor kulüplerinin halka açılmasının Türkiye'de uygulanan modeller açısından incelenmesi. *Gazi Üniversitesi Ticaret ve Turizm Eğitim Fakültesi Dergisi, 1*, 59–70.

Aykın, A. G., & Bilir, F. P. (2013). Hükümet programları ve spor politikaları. *Çukurova Üniversitesi Sosyal Bilimler Enstitüsü Dergisi, 22*(2), 239–254.

Ayvaz, Z. (2022). Erken Cumhuriyet Türkiyesinde uygulanan öjenik politikaların spora yansıması: Beden Terbiyesi Kanunu üzerine bir inceleme. *Journal of Sport Sciences Research, 7*(1), 174–196. DOI: 10.25307/jssr.1116251

Baade, R. A., & Matheson, V. A. (2006). Have public finance principles been shut out in financing new stadiums for the NFL? *Public Finance and Management, 6*(3), 284–320. DOI: 10.1177/152397210600600301

Begović, M. (2020). The development of sport policy in Montenegro. *International Journal of Sport Policy, 12*(2), 321–330. DOI: 10.1080/19406940.2020.1719186

Bull, M., & Whittam, G. (2021). Sustainable value creation? Entrepreneurial orientations in the football industry. *International Journal of Entrepreneurial Behaviour & Research, 27*(1), 27–44. DOI: 10.1108/IJEBR-07-2020-0498

Choi, Y. D., Jo, S. H., & Ok, G. (2019). Evolution of the sports for all policy in National Sports Promotion Plan in South Korea, 1962–2017. *The International Journal of the History of Sport*, *36*(9–10), 876–891. DOI: 10.1080/09523367.2019.1675643

Coalter, F. (2007). *A wider social role for sport: Who's keeping the score?* Routledge. DOI: 10.4324/9780203014615

Coalter, F. (2017). Sport and social inclusion: Evidence-based policy and practice. *Social Inclusion (Lisboa)*, *5*(2), 141–149. DOI: 10.17645/si.v5i2.852

Comeau, G. S. (2013). The evolution of Canadian sport policy. *International Journal of Sport Policy*, *5*(1), 73–93. DOI: 10.1080/19406940.2012.694368

Ekholm, D. (2016). *Sport as a means of responding to social problems: Rationales of government, welfare and social change* (Doctoral dissertation, Linköping University).

Farrelly, F. J., Quester, P. G., & Burton, R. (1997). Integrating sports sponsorship into the corporate marketing function: An international comparative study. *International Marketing Review*, *14*(3), 170–182. DOI: 10.1108/02651339710170249

Gaafar, A., Al-Yaaribi, A., Al Droushi, A. R., Al Kitani, M., Al Jadidi, K., & Al Maqbali, D. H.. (2025). Public-private partnerships in supporting talented athletes: Enhancing sports development in educational institutions. *International Journal of Human Movement and Sports Sciences*, *13*(4), 750–758. DOI: 10.13189/saj.2025.130410

Gratton, C., Shibli, S., & Coleman, R. (2005). Sport and economic regeneration in cities. *Urban Studies (Edinburgh, Scotland)*, *42*(5–6), 985–999. DOI: 10.1080/00420980500107045

Gratton, C., Shibli, S., & Coleman, R. (2006). The economic impact of major sports events: A review of ten events in the UK. *The Sociological Review*, *54*(2_suppl, s2), 41–58. DOI: 10.1111/j.1467-954X.2006.00652.x

Green, M. (2006). From "sport for all" to not about "sport" at all? Interrogating sport policy interventions in the United Kingdom. *European Sport Management Quarterly*, *6*(3), 217–238. DOI: 10.1080/16184740601094936

Grix, J., & Houlihan, B. (2014). Sports mega-events as part of a nation's soft power strategy: The cases of Germany (2006) and the UK (2012). *British Journal of Politics and International Relations*, *16*(4), 572–596. DOI: 10.1111/1467-856X.12017

Grix, J., & Lee, D. (2013). Soft power, sports mega-events and emerging states: The lure of the politics of attraction. *Global Society*, *27*(4), 521–536. DOI: 10.1080/13600826.2013.827632

Güler, E., & Yaman, M. (2023). Siyasal partiler ve spor politikaları. *New Era International Journal of Interdisciplinary Social Researches*, *8*(18), 19–34.

Hartmann-Tews, I. (2006). Social stratification in sport and sport policy in the European Union. *EJSS European Journal for Sport and Society*, *3*(2), 109–124. DOI: 10.1080/16138171.2006.11687784

Heggie, V. (2016). Bodies, sport and science in the nineteenth century. *Past & Present*, *231*(1), 169–200. DOI: 10.1093/pastj/gtw004

Henseler, J., Wilson, B., & Westberg, K. (2011). Managers' perceptions of the impact of sport sponsorship on brand equity: Which aspects of the sponsorship matter most? *Sport Marketing Quarterly*, *20*(1), 7–21. DOI: 10.1177/106169341102000104

Houlihan, B., Bloyce, D., & Smith, A. (2009). Developing the research agenda in sport policy. *International Journal of Sport Policy*, *1*(1), 1–12. DOI: 10.1080/19406940802681186

Houlihan, B., & Green, M. (Eds.). (2011). *Routledge handbook of sports development*. Routledge.

Houlihan, B., & White, A. (2003). *The politics of sports development: Development of sport or development through sport?* Routledge. DOI: 10.4324/9780203478547

İnci, H. (2011). *Avrupa Birliği ülkeleri ve Türkiye'de yerel yönetimlerin spora katkıları ve spor politikalarının karşılaştırılması* (Master's thesis, Sakarya University).

Jarvie, G. (2023). Sport policy in Scotland. In *Sport policy across the United Kingdom* (pp. 40–59). Routledge. DOI: 10.4324/9781003241232-3

Jones, C. (2001). A level playing field? Sports stadium infrastructure and urban development in the United Kingdom. *Environment & Planning A*, *33*(5), 845–861. DOI: 10.1068/a33158

Kang, T., & Kwon, S. Y. (2024). Development of sport policy in South Korea: Historical and institutional analysis. [Yayınevi/journal bilgisi eksik.]

Kasapoğlu, M. M., & Öçal, M. (2021). Türkiye'de spor yatırımlarının tabana yayılması politikasının sosyal adalet açısından önemi. *Yönetim ve Ekonomi Araştırmaları Dergisi*, *19*(3), 173–191. DOI: 10.11611/yead.991462

Kennedy, S. S., & Rosentraub, M. S. (2000). Public-private partnerships, professional sports teams and the protection of the public's interests. *American Review of Public Administration*, *30*(4), 436–459. DOI: 10.1177/02750740022064768

Koronios, K., Psiloutsikou, M., Kriemadis, A., Zervoulakos, P., & Leivaditi, E. (2016). Sport sponsorship: The impact of sponsor image on purchase intention of fans. *Journal of Promotion Management, 22*(2), 238–250. DOI: 10.1080/10496491.2016.1121739

Lee, S., & No, S. (2022). China's overseas financial direct investment (ODI) in European football clubs: Revisiting ODI in the context of sport industry. *Journal of Global Sport Management, 7*(3), 391–405. DOI: 10.1080/24704067.2020.1805163

Marin, B., & Lee, C. (2020). Exploring new trends of sport business: Japanese companies' investment in ownership of foreign football clubs. *Sport in Society, 23*(12), 2031–2054. DOI: 10.1080/17430437.2020.1817897

Meir, D., Brown, A., Macrae, E., & McGillivray, D. (2024). Country profile: Sport and physical activity policy in Scotland. *International Journal of Sport Policy, 16*(1), 181–197. DOI: 10.1080/19406940.2023.2271940

Metelski, A., Jarosz, O., & Kornakov, K. (2026). Multi-club ownership: A new business model in football. *Journal of Global Sport Management*, 1–19. https://doi .org/DOI: 10.1080/24704067.2025.2459921

Narin, M. (2025). Sekiz ülke politikasında sporun performanstan toplumsal refaha evriminde sosyolojik analiz. *Fenerbahçe Üniversitesi Spor Bilimleri Dergisi, 5*(2), 3–13.

Öçal, M., ve Kutlu, Ö. (2024). İstihdamın karanlık yüzü: Ter atölyelerine (sweatshop) insani bir bakış ve ter indeksi ile bir kıyaslama. Çalışma ve Toplum, 2024/4, 1391-1424. .DOI: 10.54752/ct.1569636

Öçal, M., & Kutlu, Ö. (2023). A study on welfare and living conditions of disadvantaged groups: The case of Burdur province. *Yönetim ve Ekonomi Araştırmaları Dergisi, 21*(3), 410–425. DOI: 10.11611/yead.1333231

Öçal, M., & Kutlu Dönmez, Ö. (2022). Ruhsal engeli olan bireylerin evsizlik sorununa insani bir bakış ve çözüm önerisi: "Önce konut yaklaşımı". *Mehmet Akif Ersoy Üniversitesi İktisadi ve İdari Bilimler Fakültesi Dergisi, 9*(3), 2006–2026. DOI: 10.30798/makuiibf.1097609

Öğüt, E. (2014). Türkiye'de spor yönetiminin neoliberal dönüşümü. *Amme İdaresi Dergisi, 47*(4), 1–26.

Plumley, D., Faulkner, T., & Ioannidis, G. (2025). Inside the deal: Analysing the investment strategy behind UK football club acquisitions—Sport finance and sports law in action. *International Sports Law Review*, 32–43.

Preuss, H. (2004). Calculating the regional economic impact of the Olympic Games. *European Sport Management Quarterly*, *4*(4), 234–253. DOI: 10.1080/16184740408737479

Reis, C. J. O. D., & Cabral, S. (2017). Public-private partnerships (PPP) in mega-sport events: A comparative study of the provision of sports arenas for the 2014 FIFA World Cup in Brazil. *Revista de Administração Pública*, *51*(4), 551–579. DOI: 10.1590/0034-7612158071

Reiser, M., Breuer, C., & Wicker, P. (2012). The sponsorship effect: Do sport sponsorship announcements impact the firm value of sponsoring firms? *International Journal of Sport Finance*, *7*(3), 232–248. DOI: 10.1177/155862351200700303

Rohde, M., & Breuer, C. (2017). The market for football club investors: A review of theory and empirical evidence from professional European football. *European Sport Management Quarterly*, *17*(3), 265–289. DOI: 10.1080/16184742.2017.1279203

Santomier, J. (2008). New media, branding and global sports sponsorship. *International Journal of Sports Marketing & Sponsorship*, *10*(1), 9–22. DOI: 10.1108/IJSMS-10-01-2008-B005

Saydam, Ç. (2024). Türkiye'de spor politikaları ve İstanbul planlarında spor. *Journal of Social. Humanities and Administrative Sciences*, *7*(46), 2352–2363. DOI: 10.31589/JOSHAS.858

Sivrikaya, K., & Demir, A. (2019). Türkiye'de 2001 yılı ve sonrasında uygulanan spor ekonomisi politikalarına yönelik bir değerlendirme. *Süleyman Demirel Üniversitesi Vizyoner Dergisi*, *10*(23), 126–136. DOI: 10.21076/vizyoner.451499

Spaaij, R., Magee, J., & Jeanes, R. (2014). *Sport and social exclusion in global society*. Routledge. DOI: 10.4324/9780203066584

Stewart, B., Nicholson, M., Smith, A., & Westerbeek, H. (2004). *Australian sport-better by design?: The evolution of Australian sport policy*. Routledge. DOI: 10.4324/9780203462928

Sunay, H. (2024). Spor ve politika ilişkisi perspektifinde Türk spor politikası. In *Yeni Türkiye: Beden Eğitimi ve Spor Özel Sayısı-I* (pp. 58–78). Yeni Türkiye Yayınları.

Thibault, L., & Harvey, J. (2013). The evolution of federal sport policy from 1960 to today. In *Sport policy in Canada* (pp. 11–35).

Tokatlıoğlu, A. E. (2021). Cumhuriyet modernleşmesinde devletin spor üzerinden bedene bakışı ve spor politikaları. *Journal of Applied and Theoretical Social Sciences*, *3*(2), 125–143. DOI: 10.37241/jatss.2021.29

Uçar, A. (2016). *Türkiye'de spor ve rekreasyon politikalarının oluşumu ve bu hizmetlerin sunumu.* [Tez/kitap bilgisi eksik.]

Varea-Calderón, A. D., Rejón-Guardia, F., Ramírez-Hurtado, J. M., & Berbel-Pineda, J. M. (2025). Impact and development of sport sponsorship: A three-decade bibliometric analysis (1993–2024). *Sport, Business and Management, 15*(2), 176–203. DOI: 10.1108/SBM-09-2024-0134

Yerlikaya, B. (2012). *Spor kavramında dönüşüm ve sporun bir sosyal politika aracı olarak kullanımı* (Master's thesis, Marmara University).

Chapter 4
Sport in the Fight Against Poverty:
A Social Policy Tool or a Symbolic Substitute for the Welfare State?

Ozal Cicek
http://orcid.org/0000-0002-2741-3003
Suleyman Demirel University, Turkey

ABSTRACT

This study critically examines how sports help combat poverty, particularly in the context of welfare-state changes and social policy. While sports often empower disadvantaged groups and promote well-being, this focus usually obscures deeper causes of poverty, like income inequality and unstable work. The impact of sports policies on poverty depends on welfare regime types. In social democratic regimes, sports complement universal rights. In conservative models, they build local solidarity. In liberal regimes, they are mainly a symbolic, low-cost tool stressing individual responsibility rather than addressing structural roots. The study argues that sports can foster a sense of belonging and provide short-term well-being. However, when used instead of comprehensive social mechanisms, sports make poverty manageable and less visible rather than reducing it. If sports do not align with core welfare responsibilities, they risk becoming a symbolic substitute rather than a structural solution.

INTRODUCTION

The historical evolution of social policy has witnessed structural changes in the state's protective measures since the Industrial Revolution. These measures were

DOI: 10.4018/979-8-2600-3174-2.ch004

designed to address market failures and social risks. Over time, the classical welfare state model emerged, reaching its golden age in the mid-20th century, and assumed a central role in providing citizens with universal rights, such as social security, healthcare, and education from cradle to grave. However, in the late 1970s, the global rise of neoliberalism brought about a radical shift in social policy. The state shifted from being the sole provider of welfare to a new structure known as "active welfare." In this model, social services were marketized, and civil society and local governments took on greater responsibility. Over the past two decades, sports have gained recognition as an innovative social policy tool. Sports have been used to increase participation of disadvantaged groups in social life, promote individual empowerment, and support overall well-being.

In current political discourse, sports are portrayed not merely as a realm of physical activity, but as a "magic wand" that enhances social capital, reduces crime rates, protects public health, and offers cost-effective solutions in the fight against poverty. International organizations and national governments, emphasizing the unifying power of sports, are funding sports-based programs to integrate young people at risk of poverty and marginalized groups into society. However, this optimistic rhetoric also carries deep structural tensions and academic skepticism. Poverty has its roots in macro-structural factors such as income inequality, precarious employment models, and inadequacies in social protection systems. Sports-based interventions, by their very nature, focus on an individual's physical capacity, psychological resilience, and personal motivation; in other words, they are micro-individual-focused. At this point, the fundamental issue is whether sports can address these deep-rooted structural causes of poverty—or merely render them invisible.

This study raises a central issue in discussing the role of sports in combating poverty: Is sports a tool that supports the core responsibilities of the welfare state, or a "symbolic substitute" that entirely replaces them? The theory of symbolic substitution suggests that, in an economic climate marked by cuts to public spending and the erosion of social rights, sports risks becoming a mechanism that renders poverty manageable and less socially visible, rather than serving as a transformative force capable of eliminating it. Under these conditions, sports—by replacing comprehensive social policy mechanisms and direct financial support—instill in impoverished communities a sense of short-term well-being, collective belonging, and social visibility; yet they may deprive them of the real economic tools needed to break free from the cycle of poverty.

To analyze this complex relationship on a sound basis, it is critical to interpret the impact of sports not as a universal and fixed phenomenon, but through the lens of the country's welfare regime typology. The impact of sports within social policy is strongly dependent on the political context. In social democratic welfare systems, sports have become institutionalized as an integral component of universal social rights and the state's responsibility for public welfare; in conservative models, however, they serve as a secondary tool that supports the family, the community, and local solidarity networks. In liberal welfare regimes, however, sport emerges as a relatively low-cost and symbolic policy domain that prioritizes individual responsibility over addressing the structural dimensions of poverty, within a context where public obligations have been scaled back. This distinction is the key factor in determining whether sports are viewed as a social right or a charitable activity.

Especially during economic crises and periods of austerity measures, the marketing of sports under the banner of "social inclusion" can become a rhetorical device that masks the retreat of the welfare state. The ability of sports to foster a sense of collective belonging is undeniable; however, it is debatable to what extent this sense of belonging masks pressing realities such as unemployment or housing shortages. If a sports program is designed merely to "get a poor young person off the streets" and "keep them occupied" rather than to improve their educational and employment opportunities, then we are not talking about the transformative power of sports, but rather about a public safety-focused approach to managing poverty. Consequently, this analysis examines sports policies from a comparative perspective, arguing that sports are neither a miraculous panacea nor a wholly ineffective practice, but rather can become a symbolic illusion when detached from the welfare state's fundamental obligations.

In the subsequent sections of this study, the analysis will be expanded under three main headings, built on this theoretical foundation. In the first main section, typologies of welfare regimes and the institutional role of sports within them will be examined comparatively. In the second main section, the tension between the short-term benefits of sports for groups experiencing poverty and the structural constraints of poverty will be examined in light of the empirical and theoretical literature. In the third main section, we will examine the current manifestations of the risk of symbolic substitution and the processes by which sports are being used as substitutes for social policy mechanisms. This roadmap aims to redefine the role of sports within social policy, navigating the fine line between a "transformative tool" and a "symbolic substitute," and to provide policymakers with a critical perspective.

Ultimately, this study positions sport not merely as a physical activity but as a political response to the crisis of the modern welfare state. The social transformative power of sports can only become a genuine social policy tool when integrated with macroeconomic social protection measures; otherwise, it will remain nothing more than an aesthetic facade that masks the structural causes of poverty and a symbolic substitute for the welfare state.

THEORETICAL FRAMEWORK: SPORT AND WELFARE REGIMES

Examining the history and function of modern social policies shows that welfare state regimes are more than economic redistribution mechanisms. They are also ideological frameworks that set the scope of citizens' rights and shape power dynamics among the state, the market, and the family. Gosta Esping-Andersen's 1990 work, "*The Three Worlds of Welfare Capitalism,*" is a key reference in understanding these structures. *In classifying welfare states, Esping-Andersen centers his analysis on two concepts: "decommodification" and "stratification".* Decommodification refers to the extent to which people rely on selling their labor in the market to maintain their standard of living. In other words, it reflects how much social rights offer individuals a "safety net" beyond the market. Stratification describes how the welfare state manages class distances and pursues social equality (Esping-Andersen, 1990, pp. 21–23).

Although sports are generally viewed as a "soft" area in traditional social policy analyses, interdisciplinary studies conducted in recent years have revealed that sports is a clear arena reflecting the fundamental ideological differences of welfare regimes. Sports policies serve as a silent witness to a country's conception of citizenship. The question of whether sports are framed as a "public right" or as a "market commodity" that individuals must purchase with their own resources is directly linked to the country's welfare regime architecture. The fact that the development of sports cannot be considered independent of political and social processes, and that the institutionalization of sports is shaped by regime priorities, is a fundamental debate in this field. For example, in systems where social rights are protected from commodification, sports are provided as a universal service alongside education and healthcare, whereas in regimes dominated by market logic, sports become either a luxury accessible only to those with sufficient socio-economic capacity or an instrumental intervention tool used to "discipline" the poor (Hylton & Bramham, 2008).

In this context, comparative analyses conducted by Bergsgard et al. (2007) reveal the extent to which changes and stability in sports policies depend on welfare regime typologies. The social role of sports changes with the state's regulatory power over the market and the family's position in social production. The social democratic model views sports as a collective space for rights and equality. As researchers such as Seippel (2006, p. 170) emphasize, voluntary sports organizations constitute the largest segment of civil society. However, the social significance of sports and the way it generates social capital vary depending on welfare systems. In the models described by Ferrera (1996, pp. 17–18), the "Southern Model"—where the income security system exhibits a fragmented and corporatist structure—and the conservative model, in which family and local solidarity occupy a central position, offer critical perspectives for understanding sports' place among social services. In contrast, the liberal model leaves sports to the market, viewing them as reflections of individual responsibility and competition.

Against this background, describing sports as a single social policy model can be academically misleading. Instead, analysis must explore how sports differ across welfare-state types. When critically evaluating sport's "broader social roles" (crime prevention, health, social inclusion), it is important to question the weak empirical basis for portrayals of sport as a "cost-effective solution" to complex issues such as poverty (Coalter, 2007). This framework will ground an analysis of sport's structural potential in poverty reduction and its susceptibility to "symbolic substitution."

Universal Rights and Sport in Social Democratic Regimes

The social democratic welfare state is regarded in the literature on social policy as the ideal type in which citizens' rights are maximally independent of market mechanisms—that is, where the level of decommodification is highest. This model, which has crystallized particularly in Scandinavian countries such as Sweden, Norway, Denmark, and Finland, is characterized by a structure in which the state is not merely a "safety net" but also the primary architect of social equality and collective welfare (Esping-Andersen, 1990, pp. 27–28). In this system, social rights are based not on an individual's ability to work or pay premiums, but directly on citizenship status. Sport is conceived not merely as a marginal "recreational" activity within this broad universe of rights, but as a universal public service supporting citizens' physical and social development. "Sport for All," the fundamental motto of the social democratic model's sports policies, is not merely a political slogan but a social policy objective to which the state is financially and institutionally committed. The success of this model relies on institutionalized cooperation between public authorities and the voluntary sector, as well as the collective financing of sport as a "public good" (Bergsgard et al., 2007).

The Scandinavian sports model is built on four pillars: a strong tradition of volunteerism, a uniform organizational structure across countries, close ties with public institutions, and a universal egalitarian philosophy (Tuastad, 2019). In this model, the institutionalization of sports is based on the principle of a "voluntary partnership" between the state's central regulatory role and the autonomy of local sports clubs. This tradition of voluntarism is recognized not merely as a geographically specific characteristic but as a structural component of the democratic welfare system (Krieger & Nordhagen, 2025). The shaping of sports' developmental form by regime priorities is one of the fundamental debates in this field; indeed, in social democratic regimes, sports are provided as a universal public service, akin to education and health, and access is guaranteed regardless of an individual's socio-economic status (Hylton & Bramham, 2008). Removing sports from the realm of a "market commodity" through public funding plays a vital role in combating poverty; in this way, sports become a space for social integration, where different classes come together on a shared public ground. In this context, this unique structure—where sports clubs both maintain their autonomy and serve public objectives—is defined as "democratic corporatism" (Ibsen & Seippel, 2010, pp. 594–595).

The most fundamental difference distinguishing the social democratic regime's approach to sports from other models is the recognition of sports' capacity for "social inclusion" as a structural component of the overall welfare system. The high levels of social trust and social cohesion at the core of the Nordic model are continuously reproduced through sports organizations (Koivunen et al., 2021). In this system, the participation of an individual at risk of poverty in a sports club is supported not merely as a leisure activity, but as a "social right" aimed at preserving social capital. The fact that voluntary sports organizations are the largest stakeholders in civil society demonstrates how deeply the way these structures produce social capital is integrated with welfare systems (Seippel, 2006, p. 170). In this context, sports serve as a "preventive social policy" tool against social exclusion triggered by poverty. Consequently, in Scandinavian societies, sports are not merely a realm of physical activity; they are designed as a strategic mechanism to prevent social exclusion for minorities and disadvantaged groups (Bergsgard et al., 2020).

However, this universalist framework is not entirely immune to the structural crises and neoliberal pressures facing the welfare state. The weakness of the evidence-based policies underpinning the presentation of sports as a "cost-effective antidote" to complex problems, such as poverty risks, is that this field will become a symbolic facade that replaces structural reforms (Coalter, 2007). In social democratic regimes, this risk is sought to be curbed through strong public oversight and universal access principles. In this context, sports are not a low-cost substitute for managing poverty; rather, they function as a physical and social extension of the broad protective umbrella provided by the welfare state. Indeed, despite the transformations undergone by Scandinavian welfare states, sports remain an integral part of "social citizenship" (Geyer, 2000).

Particularly in strategies to combat poverty, social democratic regimes' definition of sports as a "civil right" minimizes the individual's dependence on the market. When examining the impact of institutional differences in welfare models on the distribution of social services, the inclusive nature of universal models is decisive (Ferrera, 1996, p. 29). The widespread availability of neighborhood-level sports facilities and public subsidization of membership fees prevent sports from becoming a marker of social status. In this regard, the state's direct financial assistance to sports clubs eliminates the financial barriers to active participation for disadvantaged groups (Bergsgard et al., 2007). Such institutional support ensures that sports serve as an effective "social buffer," mitigating the disadvantages associated with poverty.

Social democratic welfare states reflect the ideal of "equality for all" in the realm of sports. The state's regulatory role and financial weight largely prevent market-based inequalities from seeping into this sphere, transforming sports' fight against poverty from a "symbolic act" into a structural welfare service. When compared to the limited approaches of conservative and liberal models, the "universal access" framework offered by social democratic regimes best represents the potential for sports to serve as a genuine tool of social policy. Indeed, the Scandinavian experience is recognized as one of the strongest global examples of how the democratization of sports can be intertwined with social justice policies (Da Costa & Miragaya, 2002).

Solidarity and Subsidiarity: Sport in Conservative Welfare Models

The conservative or corporatist welfare regime is a model, exemplified in Continental European countries such as Germany, France, and Austria, that bases social rights on employment status and the family unit. In this regime, the state's primary role is not to fully replace market mechanisms, but rather to preserve social status differences and provide security based on working life through social insurance systems. Esping-Andersen notes that in this model, the state intervenes only when the capacity of family and civil society networks (church, unions, local associations) has been exhausted; this situation is defined in the literature as the principle of "subsidiarity" (Esping-Andersen, 1990, p. 27). Within this framework, sports policies are shaped not as a direct state service but rather to strengthen local solidarity networks and preserve the status quo among social strata.

In conservative models, the institutionalization of sports is carried out through autonomous sports federations and local associations (Vereine in the German example) rather than through direct state management (Bergsgard et al., 2007). In this system, the role of sports is to preserve social bonds and strengthen local identity. While sports do not carry the same status as a "universal right" as in the social democratic model, nor are they a pure market commodity as in the liberal model, they are rather an area of social responsibility evaluated within the framework of the "common good" (Hylton & Bramham, 2008). Particularly in Southern European variants (the Southern Model), the fragmented structure of income security systems and corporatist privileges has placed the family and local solidarity networks at the center of the distribution of social services (Ferrera, 1996, pp. 17–18). In this context, sports clubs serve not only as venues for physical activity but also as a social "cement" that reinforces family values and community bonds.

In the fight against poverty, conservative models view sports not as a tool for structural transformation, but rather as a mechanism for strengthening social cohesion (Bergsgard et al., 2007). In these regimes, the fundamental strategy is not to produce direct solutions to the structural problems of poor groups, but to prevent these groups from becoming detached from the social fabric by facilitating their integration into traditional solidarity networks. In such models, it is acknowledged that sports serve as a social safety valve by reinforcing family values and a sense of local belonging (Heinemann, 2005, p. 185). The central role of sports clubs in the production of social capital demonstrates that individuals' potential for integration into social networks is directly linked to the characteristic structure of the welfare regime (Seippel, 2006, p. 170). However, in systems dominated by status-preserving tendencies, sports' ability to reach disadvantaged groups may be limited by various institutional barriers (Hylton & Bramham, 2008). Particularly within a welfare structure based on social insurance contributions, the "new poor" —those on the margins of the labor market—rely on the limited capacity of local aid organizations to access sports services (Bergsgard et al., 2007).

The rise of sports as an instrumental figure in social policy has found a place even in conservative regimes, as it has been framed as an area of intervention in disadvantaged neighborhoods through social inclusion projects (Bergsgard et al., 2007). The presentation of sports as a "cost-effective antidote" to complex problems such as poverty has been criticized for the weak evidence base of such interventions (Coalter, 2007). This risk emerging in conservative regimes manifests not through the replacement of core social protection mechanisms — i.e., "symbolic substitution" — but rather through the framing of sports as a supplementary element supporting them (Hylton & Bramham, 2008). While the alignment of sports' institutional structure with the state's vision of welfare is being questioned, it is noteworthy that this fragmented structure within the conservative model hinders the development of a comprehensive strategy to combat poverty (Krieger & Nordhagen, 2025).

The role of sports in conservative welfare regimes is seen as a concrete reflection of the delicate balance among family, civil society, and state institutions (Esping-Andersen, 1990, p. 27). In this structure, which is built on the principles of solidarity and mutual aid, sports, while not constituting a universal right of citizenship within the scope of the fight against poverty, seek to establish a protective space through local networks of belonging (Tuastad, 2019). However, this protective shield relies largely on civil society's existing capacity rather than on the welfare state's inclusive power. This limitation restricts sports' ability to fundamentally eliminate structural poverty and positions it as a "symbolic instrument of stability" aimed at establishing social peace (Koivunen et al., 2021).

Individual Responsibility and Market Logic: Sport in Liberal Welfare Regimes

In Gøsta Esping-Andersen's (1990) classic typology, the liberal welfare regime is defined by the absolute dominance of market mechanisms over social protection. In this regime, state intervention takes on a "residual" character, intervening only when the market fails, and social rights are structured around individual merit and means-testing rather than as a universal right of citizenship. Such a regime effectively limits the scope of social rights, leads to a relative equalization of poverty among those receiving social assistance, produces social assistance at varying levels within a market-based framework, and creates a stratification order on the class level. Typical examples of this model include the United States, Canada, and Australia (Esping-Andersen, 1990, pp. 26–27). The sports sector is not independent of this ideological framework; in liberal regimes, sports are conceived not as a public right but as an individual choice, a market service, and an instrumental mechanism for addressing social issues.

In liberal models, the state's role in sports is "selective" and "instrumental" in nature. In countries like the United Kingdom, it is emphasized that sports are used solely as a "tool" to achieve specific social goals (such as combating crime and fighting obesity). Accordingly, the state provides limited funding not for sports themselves, but for the secondary benefits they generate (Houlihan & Green, 2009, p. 685). The current situation has led to sports being transformed into a low-cost tool for managing poverty under the guise of "social inclusion." Along with defining this process as the "fetishization of sports," it is argued that sports serve as a veil covering structural problems (Coalter, 2007). Particularly over the past decade, the "austerity" policies implemented in these regimes have further eroded sports' status as a social right and pushed it entirely into market dynamics (Parnell et al., 2018).

In liberal models, the financing and organization of sports are largely left to market logic. In these systems, the process of "commodification" is quite pronounced in the sports sector, and individuals can access sports services only to the extent of their purchasing power. The current situation presents a picture that is the exact opposite of the Scandinavian sports model, in which sports are conceived as a democratic right. It is emphasized that while the Scandinavian model presents sports as a collective good through its strong tradition of volunteerism and state support (Krieger & Nordhagen, 2025), the liberal model, lacking this structure, reduces sports to an arena of individual performance. While it is noted that the "sports for all" ideal in the Scandinavian model may at times be shrouded in myths (Tuastad, 2019), it is acknowledged that market pressures in liberal systems render the risk of social exclusion far more concrete and institutionalized.

In this market-oriented structure, sports infrastructure is shaped by economic efficiency rather than social needs. When examining the impact of sports infrastructure on participation, it has been demonstrated that the availability of facilities is directly linked to individual demand for sports (Hallmann et al., 2012, p. 526). However, in liberal regimes, the adoption of the "user-pays" principle in the operation of sports facilities creates a structural barrier that hinders the participation of low-income groups in sports. It is argued that the tendency of neoliberal policies to privatize sports has led to the transfer of the operation of sports facilities to profit-driven third-party providers, which in turn has resulted in the exclusion of the "new poor" from sports services (Parnell et al., 2018).

In the liberal model, sports risk becoming nothing more than a "symbolic substitute" in the fight against poverty. In a liberal context where public spending is cut, efforts are made to manage discontent among impoverished populations by funding soccer tournaments or short-term youth projects rather than pursuing massive social reforms (Green, 2006). It is noted that in these regimes, sports serve as a tool to instill "discipline" and "personal responsibility" in the poor. If an individual is poor, they are expected to "strengthen their character" through sports and become competitive in the market (Nichols, 2007). Thus, the function of sports in this regime is not to reduce inequalities, but to manage their consequences in an aesthetically pleasing manner (King, 2009).

In liberal regimes, sports clubs have begun to be managed more like commercial enterprises than as part of civil society. Although it is noted that sports clubs, as "voluntary organizations," occupy an autonomous position between the state and the market, it is noteworthy that, in liberal regimes, this autonomy generally implies a lack of public support (Heinemann, 2005, pp. 181–182). The current structure also directly affects sports' capacity to produce "social capital." It is argued that while sports have the potential to strengthen bonding among individuals and bridge between different groups, this production of social capital may weaken in liberal and market-oriented systems because sports serve commercial purposes (Seippel, 2006, p. 171). It is stated that the volunteer-based sports structure in Scandinavia encourages democratic participation (Ibsen & Seippel, 2010, p. 594), whereas in liberal models, participation is framed through a "consumer" identity.

In summary, it appears that in liberal welfare regimes, sports strive to strike a balance between market logic, individual responsibility, and limited public resources. In the context of the challenges faced by modern welfare states, attention is drawn to the fact that the "individualized" sports experience offered by the liberal model weakens social belonging (Koivunen et al., 2021). It is noteworthy that, alongside the state's withdrawal and the weakening of the social protection shield, sports have increasingly become a consumption object tied to socio-economic status (Hallmann et al., 2011). In the liberal model, it is understood that sports' capacity for social integration is constrained by the individual's position in the market and the limited resources of civil society.

SPORT AS A TOOL FOR FIGHTING POVERTY: POTENTIALS AND LIMITS

The structural transformation of modern welfare states and the decisive influence of the neoliberal paradigm on public policies have turned sports from a mere recreational activity into a strategic and instrumental component of social policy. Today, when poverty is defined not merely as a lack of income but as social exclusion, alienation, and limited access to public resources, sports are being promoted as a "cost-effective" and "rapid" intervention against this complex web of problems. On one hand, sports are promoted as a tool to foster social cohesion, prevent crime, instill individual discipline, and generate social capital. On the other hand, there is a persistent tension between the promises of sports and the structural realities they confront. Where welfare regimes differ—such as the "residualist" approach of liberal regimes versus the "universalist" vision of the Scandinavian model—sports' ability to address poverty also diverges. This section thus highlights a fundamental contrast: the "potentials" of sports, like empowerment and collective belonging, stand in sharp opposition to "structural constraints" such as income inequality and precarious employment. The central question then becomes whether sport acts as a real solution to poverty or primarily as a symbolic gesture that makes poverty appear more manageable. By examining the gap between theoretical promises and actual socio-economic realities, we can better clarify the true role of sport in social policy.

Potentials: Collective Belonging and Psychosocial Well-Being

The potential of sports in the fight against poverty is generally defined not so much by macroeconomic indicators as by the micro-transformations it brings about in the individual's social and psychological world. In this context, sports—particularly for disadvantaged groups—go beyond being merely a venue for physical activity; they are also presented as a "soft" social policy tool that fosters social capital, a sense of collective belonging, and psychosocial well-being. Conceptualized in the literature as *"sport for good,"* this approach focuses on sport's capacity to repair social bonds fractured by poverty and reintegrate the individual into the social fabric (Coalter, 2007).

One of the most fundamental potentials offered by sports is the generation of social capital, as examined *from a Putnamian perspective*[1]. Poverty does not merely deprive individuals of material resources; it also pushes them outside of social networks, trapping them in a state of "social isolation" and "alienation." Sports clubs and organizations provide the *"bonding"* and *"bridging"* social capital necessary to break this isolation. Bonding social capital weaves a network of internal solidarity and trust among individuals with similar socio-economic backgrounds; bridging social capital enables impoverished individuals to engage with different social classes and resources (Putnam, 2000; Seippel, 2006, p. 171).

The principle of voluntarism, which lies at the heart of the Scandinavian sports model, fosters a sense of *"collective belonging"* by bringing individuals together around shared goals (Ibsen & Seippel, 2010, p. 594). In this model, sports clubs serve as a "democratic laboratory" where individuals perceive themselves as valuable, functional, and equal members of society (Krieger & Nordhagen, 2025). For individuals living below the poverty line in particular, joining a sports club means breaking free from a sense of social exclusion and integrating into a collective identity. Poverty often brings with it social stigma; those living in disadvantaged areas are labeled by the rest of society solely as "needy" or "at-risk." At this point, sports have the potential to alleviate—even if only temporarily—the stigma associated with poverty by offering individuals positive, respected roles such as "athlete," "teammate," or "volunteer" (Tuastad, 2019). As part of a team, the individual breaks free from the cycle of failure and transforms into an active agent striving toward a common goal. This process strengthens the individual's connection to social norms while replacing the sense of "deprivation" caused by poverty with a sense of social "existence" and "belonging" (Bergsgard et al., 2020).

For disadvantaged groups, sports provide *"social visibility"* by offering opportunities to establish a positive identity in the public sphere. A young person from a poor neighborhood who succeeds in a tournament can shed the label of "someone from a poor neighborhood" and be recognized as a "talented individual" (Hylton & Bramham, 2008). This visibility not only strengthens the individual's self-esteem but also transforms society's perspective on them. The success-oriented nature of sports gives individuals a sense of control over their lives, serving as a significant antidote to the helplessness stemming from poverty.

The release of endorphins through physical activity provided by sports creates a tangible "breathing space" for coping with the chronic stress and anxiety caused by poverty (Coalter, 2007). Since poverty is a constant struggle for survival, it depletes an individual's mental resources. The "flow" experience and *short-term psychosocial well-being* offered by sports provide the individual with a temporary escape from this heavy burden. This situation enhances the individual's psychological resilience, thereby sustaining their motivation to participate in social life (Parnell et al., 2018).

Sports possess a powerful "micro-potential" to combat poverty by generating social capital, fostering a sense of collective belonging, and promoting psychosocial well-being. However, while this potential makes a vital impact at the individual level, it is constrained by structural barriers to social participation and economic constraints (access to facilities, equipment costs, etc.) (Hallmann et al., 2012, p. 530). While the well-being promised by sports may successfully alleviate the symptoms of poverty, its capacity to create lasting social change at the macro level without structural support remains debatable.

Structural Limits: Social Insecurity and Welfare State Constraints

The potential of sports to combat poverty faces a serious risk of becoming ineffective when it confronts the macro-structural barriers created by today's neo-liberal order. Income inequality, precarious employment, and inadequacies in social protection systems limit sports' capacity to create "structural transformation" as a tool of social policy. From the perspective of welfare regimes institutionalized by Esping-Andersen (1990), for a state to fundamentally resolve poverty, it must focus on "de-commodification." In other words, an individual's basic living standards must be freed from dependence on the sale of labor power in the market (Esping-Andersen, 1990, pp. 21–22). However, under liberal and conservative regimes, sports largely remain a "commodified" service left to market dynamics; this turns access to this field into a systemic barrier for disadvantaged groups.

For low-income individuals, the decision to participate in sports is more shaped by financial constraints and infrastructure availability than by individual motivation. Multilevel analyses have demonstrated that the availability of facilities is a critical prerequisite for participation (Hallmann et al., 2012, p. 541). However, the primary structural barrier here is not the existence of facilities but their accessibility. The "user pays" logic, which has become widespread in liberal regimes, leads to the exclusion of low-income groups from public sports venues. For a poor individual, sports represent not merely a physical activity but a *"series of economic barriers"* —such as transportation costs, equipment expenses, and membership fees—that must be overcome (Hallmann et al., 2011; Hallmann et al., 2012, p. 530). For a household living in material deprivation, sports expenditures are a luxury item that takes a backseat to primary needs like food and shelter, and can be easily sacrificed.

The *austerity policies* implemented in the aftermath of the 2008 global economic crisis led to dramatic cuts in local government budgets and social assistance programs. It is emphasized that the most severe impact of these cuts was felt in public services in disadvantaged areas. As the scope of social policy narrows, sports are expected to fill this void and function as a kind of social "savior." However, in an environment where public resources and state support are being withdrawn, sports' capacity to bring about structural change at the macro level is being crippled. This "era of austerity," in which the state's protective umbrella has weakened, carries the risk of stripping sports of its role as a strategic tool in the fight against poverty and reducing it to mere rhetoric that masks budget cuts (Houlihan & Green, 2009, p. 678; Parnell et al., 2018).

Sports programs often promise to prepare disadvantaged youth for the labor market by instilling skills such as "character building," "discipline," and "leadership." However, this approach systematically overlooks the macro-structural causes of unemployment and precarious employment. It is argued that the values instilled by sports—such as discipline and self-control—do not alter the mechanisms of exploitation in the labor market or the harsh reality of low-wage, *precarious jobs* (Kelly, 2011, pp. 140–142). No matter how disciplined and self-confident an individual may be, without a strong social safety net and employment security, they cannot escape the "working poor" cycle. Consequently, the micro-improvements offered by sports are constantly undermined by the market's structural inequalities and gaps in the social security system (Hylton & Bramham, 2008; Kelly, 2011, p. 145).

While sports' capacity to generate social capital and foster a sense of collective belonging offers a vital "micro-level impact," the sustainability of this success depends on macro-level welfare policies. Shortcomings in social protection and insufficient state intervention to address income inequality limit the impact of sports to a "temporary respite." For structural transformation, it is imperative that sports be provided as a public service free from the commodifying effects of the market, and that this process be supported by robust redistributive policies. Otherwise, sports are doomed to remain a marginal activity that fails to address the structural roots of poverty and offers solace only through individual success stories.

Managing Poverty: The Symbolic Substitution of Sports

Although sports are often presented in modern social policy discourse as a central element in the fight against poverty and as a social "savior," a thorough analysis reveals that these interventions serve to make poverty *"manageable"* and *"less visible"* rather than eliminating it (Coalter, 2007). Poverty is not merely a material deprivation; it is a multi-layered phenomenon that must be addressed in terms of its symbolic, cultural, and political dimensions. In this context, the process of *"managing poverty"* reduces a structural injustice issue to a technical and behavioral problem, while transforming sports into a symbolic substitution mechanism that dampens social unrest and integrates disadvantaged groups into the existing system (Hartmann & Kwauk, 2011; Jarvie, 2011).

The first step in the strategy for managing poverty is to conceal or sanitize *poverty through aesthetic management* (Nichols, 2007; King, 2009) from the public sphere. Sports projects render the most visible manifestations of poverty (homelessness, petty crime) invisible by taking young people from poor neighborhoods off the streets and into "safe" and "controlled" spaces. During the era of austerity policies, sports served as a tool to mask the social devastation caused by budget cuts with an aesthetic veil (Parnell et al., 2018). Especially in the Global South, mega-events and sports infrastructure projects costing billions of dollars are designed as tools for gaining national prestige by managing the legitimacy crisis caused by poverty and authoritarian regimes (Gunter, 2014, p. 41; Liu & Qi, 2024). Here, sports aim not to solve poverty but to manage the negative image it creates and to mask structural inequalities through the "rhetoric of promise" (Rein & Shields, 2007, p. 80; Levermore, 2011, pp. 886–887).

Sports-based interventions create an *"individual responsibility trap"* by shifting the causes of poverty from structural inequalities to individual shortcomings. These programs label poor youth as *"at-risk individuals"*; concepts such as "discipline," "self-confidence," and "leadership" instilled in them construct a logic that holds the individual solely responsible for their own failure (Kelly, 2011, p. 126; Hartmann & Kwauk, 2011). This approach, which frames poverty not as a lack of material resources but as a *"moral and behavioral deviation"* (MUD) *(moral underclass discourse)* (Levitas, 2005, p. 7), disregards structural barriers and transforms young people into neoliberal subjects. Thus, poverty is presented not as a human rights violation that the state must resolve, but as a personal test that the individual must overcome by developing their character through sports (Green, 2006; Darnell, 2012).

In the management of poverty, sports *weaken class consciousness* and *alienate* individuals from their own realities. While promising "imagined mobility" to poor individuals, sports sever them from a shared class struggle and confine them to a world of individual competition (Coalter, 2007; Boehl & Ignácio, 2023). By instilling a sense of "competitiveness," sports facilitate the acceptance of exploitation mechanisms rather than challenging them (Green, 2006; Kelly, 2011, p. 132). This leads individuals to become alienated from the social causes of poverty and to internalize this situation as a result of their own "inadequacy." While the commodification of social rights subjects the individual to market forces, sports aestheticizes this subjugation through a process of voluntary discipline and conformity.

In a system where redistributive policies that could fundamentally resolve poverty have been abandoned, sports step in as a symbolic substitute (Green, 2006; Coalter, 2007). While real constraints such as difficulties in accessing facilities and economic barriers persist, the micro-improvements offered by sports fall short of resolving macro-level problems (Hallmann et al., 2011; Hallmann et al., 2012, p. 530). Given the reality that "social exclusion is not something children do to themselves, but something society does to them," it is impossible for sports coaches to change society (Kelly, 2011, p. 142). Sports-based interventions push structural inequalities into the background while highlighting individual failings, thereby legitimizing the symbolic management of poverty rather than resolving it (Green, 2006; Kelly, 2011, p. 126).

Consequently, focusing on individual success stories (myths of redemption through sports) rather than collective political action to address structural issues erodes the political nature of poverty. While managing poverty in this way ensures the system's continuity by distracting impoverished individuals through symbolic consumption and identity construction (Unsal Yılmaz & Şahin, 2023), it falls far short of enabling the masses to genuinely break free from the structural trap (Andrews et al., 2014).

In order to transform the symbolic potential of sports into a genuine tool for transformation, it is imperative that sports policies be redesigned within the framework of an "interventionist approach" that addresses the structural causes of poverty and challenges colonial legacies and power imbalances (Hartmann & Kwauk, 2011; Adamson et al., 2022).

CRITICAL DISCUSSION: A SOCIAL POLICY TOOL OR A SYMBOLIC SUBSTITUTE?

The social function of sports and its role on the policy agendas of modern states present a profound paradox in the context of strategies to combat poverty and promote social integration (Hartmann & Kwauk, 2011). On the one hand, there is an unshakable, even romantic belief in the positive effects of sports on individual empowerment, social integration, peacebuilding, and national identity—one that views sports as a "low-cost, high-impact tool" (Lindsey et al., 2017). On the other hand, serious academic critiques are emerging regarding whether this practice of instrumentalization serves as a symbolic substitute that masks structural inequalities, reinforces existing power relations, and merely renders deep-seated social problems "manageable" (Coalter, 2007; Darnell, 2012). This debate is not merely a matter of theoretical curiosity but an issue with profound practical implications for policy design, resource allocation, and social justice (Hartmann & Kwauk, 2011).

The Decline of the Welfare State and the Role of Sports in the Neoliberal Order

The transition from the golden age of the welfare state to the neoliberal "austerity" regime has fundamentally transformed the nature of social policy instruments and the state's role in this area (Parnell et al., 2018). While the traditional welfare state model aimed to protect the individual from market risks through collective safety nets, today's "post-welfare" order centers on a discourse of "active citizenship" and "individual responsibility" that individualizes risk management (O'Malley, 1992, pp. 260–261). In this process of transformation, sports have become a tool for social engineering and poverty management through a complex linkage between civil society and the state apparatus (Kaal, 2021, p. 376).

While austerity policies have led to dramatic cuts, particularly in local government budgets and direct public services, the state has shifted its primary responsibilities in the fight against poverty to civil society and volunteer networks. In this social vacuum, sport functions as a temporary "social band-aid" that absorbs the social damage caused by poverty rather than resolving structural issues (Parnell et al., 2018). The modernization of institutions such as Sport England and UK Sport in the UK has established sports as a central issue serving policy objectives such as health, social integration, and economic development (Houlihan & Green, 2009, p. 685). However, in this process, sport faces the risk of being severed from its civil society roots and of masking the state's primary responsibility in the fight against poverty (Green, 2006). In particular, the strong tradition of volunteerism in the Nordic model can sometimes provide a basis of legitimacy that masks the state's withdrawal from professional services (Ibsen & Seippel, 2010, p. 602).

Symbolic Substitution: The Risk of Using Sports as a Substitute for Comprehensive Social Reforms

The most critical risk for sports within social policy is that it becomes a symbolic facade that replaces genuine, lasting structural reforms (Coalter, 2007). At this point, poverty is stripped of its status as an issue of economic distribution and reduced to a technical public order problem suppressed through "visibility management" and aesthetic governance (Wacquant, 2009; Parnell et al., 2018).

The symbolic substitution function of sports becomes evident in the aesthetic concealment of poverty's traces in the public sphere and in the masking of authoritarian practices. Mega-sports events and urban renewal projects are instrumentalized to "clean up" the "undesirable" sights in poor neighborhoods and sterilize the city for global capital (Gunter, 2014, pp. 42–43). In the Athletes' Village project in Johannesburg, the rhetoric of fighting poverty was superimposed on the need for urban growth, yet in reality, no structural improvement was achieved in the lives of the poor (Gunter, 2014, p. 49). This dynamic aligns with the concept of *sportswashing*[2], which describes efforts to conceal human rights violations in international relations behind the glamour of sports (Brannagan et al., 2026).

Sports serve as a powerful symbolic foundation for promoting nationalism and patriotism in the construction of national identity. In countries like China, athletes are turned into symbols of nationalism, and the sports infrastructure is designed to serve this purpose (Liu & Qi, 2024). In postmodern consumer culture, sports alienate individuals from their own reality by weakening class consciousness. Masses unable to access real economic capital acquire a false sense of status by forming symbolic identifications with famous athletes, and this symbolic economy transforms the collective struggle against the structural causes of poverty into an individual competition for success (Coalter, 2007; Boehl & Ignácio, 2023).

Policy Implications: Integrating Sports Policies with Social Rights

For sports to move beyond being a symbolic substitute and become a genuine tool of social policy, they must be deeply integrated with universal social rights and comprehensive protection mechanisms (Adamson et al., 2022). Current evidence indicates that sports alone have a limited capacity to address macro-level issues and that there is a "symbolic implementation" gap between policy commitments and practical application (Green, 2006; Ali et al., 2024).

Policy makers must acknowledge that sports' potential to reduce poverty is meaningful only when supported by basic livelihood security, quality education, and the right to employment (Green, 2006; Coalter, 2007). Micro-programs focused solely on "character building" may perpetuate hierarchies while constituting acts of "symbolic violence" against individuals. Therefore, an "interventionist approach" that views marginalized communities not merely as passive recipients but as informed agents must be adopted (Hartmann & Kwauk, 2011). Inequities in the distribution of sports facilities (facility quality, economic barriers) should be viewed as a human rights violation in and of themselves, and spatial inequalities must be addressed (Hallmann et al., 2012, p. 530).

While the commodification of social rights subjects the individual to market forces, sports policies should not aestheticize this subjugation; rather, they should be designed as an integral part of the law of citizenship. As seen in the example of sports towns in China, the use of sports as a tool to combat poverty is only possible with the full participation of the local population in employment and decision-making processes (Liu & Qi, 2024). Otherwise, sports will continue to serve as a symbolic veil that "manages" poverty (Tak et al., 2018).

Sports hold genuine potential as a tool of social policy; however, realizing this potential depends on a policy design that directly addresses structural inequalities, challenges power relations, and goes beyond symbolic discourse (Hartmann & Kwauk, 2011; Adamson et al., 2022). Current practices indicate that sports often serve as symbolic substitutes that mask structural problems (Connell, 2018). Practitioners must design appropriate programs that transform rather than reproduce the existing social order. A social justice-focused approach to sports should aim to amplify the voices of the silenced and position sports as a radical complement to comprehensive social protection systems (Hartmann & Kwauk, 2011; Adamson et al., 2022).

CONCLUSION AND RECOMMENDATIONS

The effectiveness of sports in addressing social issues is not a universal constant but rather depends on the welfare regime and ideological architecture of the state in question. While the positioning of sports as a universal right of citizenship in Scandinavian models relatively shields it from market pressures, in liberal regimes, it is framed as a tool focused on individual responsibility and public order. These regime-based differences constitute the fundamental distinction that determines whether sports function as a subject of rights or as a low-cost control mechanism in the fight against poverty. However, there is always the risk that sports will serve as a symbolic veil, making the negative symptoms of poverty manageable and less visible, rather than producing a structural solution that eliminates poverty. Especially during periods of austerity, the state uses sports like a band-aid to fill the void left by its withdrawal from core responsibilities; it transforms poverty from an issue of economic distribution into a matter of aesthetic image management and individual behavior.

To mitigate these risks, *sports-based social inclusion projects* should be designed not as an alternative to fundamental rights—such as employment, income security, and quality education, which are core obligations of the welfare state—but as a complementary element that reinforces the effectiveness of these rights. For policymakers, the primary goal should be to address access to sports infrastructure in low-income neighborhoods not merely as the construction of physical facilities, but as a *matter of spatial justice*. The quality of facilities and the availability of free access should be defined not as a charitable favor granted to disadvantaged groups, but as a standard required by citizenship law. This integrated approach will transform sports' role within social policy from a symbolic substitute into a genuine social force.

In addition, interventions must be resolutely free of moralistic discourses that label poor individuals as undisciplined or morally deficient. Social inclusion strategies should aim to *remove the structural barriers facing individuals* and *broaden the distribution of social capital*, rather than focusing on changing individual behavior. At the same time, *transparent oversight mechanisms* must be established to measure the actual social impacts of projects, preventing national and international sports investments from being used as a mask of legitimacy to cover up authoritarian practices or societal failures. Such a structural transformation will ensure that sports serve social justice by *preventing them from becoming a tool for "sportswashing."*

It is critically important for future academic research to move beyond one-sided narratives centered on the magical healing power of sports and instead examine its impact on participants' long-term life prospects using *longitudinal and critical datasets. The tensions between countries' sports policies and their different welfare models must be analyzed*, and the transferability of successful practices from specific regions to different social contexts must be questioned. Research should focus on the subjective sports experiences of individuals living below the poverty line, migrants, and marginalized groups—rather than the rhetoric of administrators or bureaucrats—to develop a perspective that *centers the voices of the excluded.* This approach will contribute to the development of a deep social justice literature that goes beyond statistical data when measuring the social impact of sports.

Sports can only realize their potential as a genuine tool of social policy when they are combined with a commitment to establishing social justice and integrated with the fundamental responsibilities of the welfare state. A conception of sports detached from comprehensive social protection systems will remain nothing more than a symbolic substitute that reproduces the status quo by aestheticizing poverty rather than eliminating it. Ultimately, the transformative power of sports will only gain meaning to the extent that it can amplify the voices of the voiceless and challenge the systems that perpetuate inequalities rather than rendering them invisible.

REFERENCES

Adamson, B., Adamson, M., Clarke, C., Richardson, E. V., & Sydnor, S. (2022). Social justice through sport and exercise studies: A manifesto. *Journal of Sport and Social Issues*, *46*(5), 407–444. DOI: 10.1177/01937235221099150

Ali, A. E., Millington, R., Darnell, S. C., & Smith, T. (2024). Policy vs. practice in sport and climate change: The perspectives of key actors in global sport and international development. *Frontiers in Sports and Active Living*, *6*, 1297739. Advance online publication. DOI: 10.3389/fspor.2024.1297739

Amnesty International. (2023, February 14). *Saudi Arabia: FIFA's award of the World Cup to Saudi Arabia is blatant sportswashing*. https://www.amnesty.org/en/latest/news/2023/02/saudi-arabia-fifas-award-of-the-world-cup-to-saudi-arabia-is-blatant-sports-washing/

Andrews, D. L., Batts, C., & Silk, M. (2014). Sport, glocalization and the new Indian middle class. *International Journal of Cultural Studies*, *17*(3), 259–276. DOI: 10.1177/1367877913487531

Bergsgard, N. A., Bratland-Sanda, S., Giulianotti, R., & Tangen, J. O. (Eds.). (2020). *Sport, outdoor life and the Nordic world*. Routledge. DOI: 10.4324/9781003009047

Bergsgard, N. I., Houlihan, B., Mangset, P., Nødland, S. I., & Rommetvedt, H. (2007). *Sport policy: A comparative analysis of stability and change* (1st ed.). Routledge., DOI: 10.4324/9780080498218

Boehl, W. R., & Ignácio, M. C. (2023). Talent in top-flight football: Concept, recruitment and predictive models for identification. In Wojda, T. (Ed.), *Technology in sports - Recent advances, new perspectives and application.*, DOI: 10.5772/intechopen.1002431

Boykoff, J. (2022). Toward a theory of sportswashing: Mega-events, soft power, and political conflict. *Sociology of Sport Journal*, *39*(4), 342–351. DOI: 10.1123/ssj.2022-0095

Brannagan, P. M., Grix, J., & Norrito, A. (2026). Demystifying sportswashing: An assemblage theory perspective on authoritarian states' investment in global sport. *British Journal of Politics and International Relations*, *28*(1), 144–164. DOI: 10.1177/13691481251352321

Canniford, R., & Hill, T. (2022, January 17). *Sportswashing: How mining and energy companies sponsor your favourite sports to help clean up their image*. The Conversation. https://theconversation.com/sportswashing-how-mining-and-energy-companies-sponsor-your-favourite-sports-to-help-clean-uptheir-image-173589

Coalter, F. (2007). *A wider social role for sport: Who's keeping the score?* Routledge. DOI: 10.4324/9780203014615

Connell, J. (2018). Fiji, rugby and the geopolitics of soft power. Shaping national and international identity. *New Zealand Geographer*, *74*(2), 92–100. DOI: 10.1111/nzg.12184

Da Costa, L. P., & Miragaya, A. (2002). *Worldwide experiences and trends in sport for all*. Meyer & Meyer Sport.

Darnell, S. C. (2012). *Sport for development and peace: A critical sociology*. Bloomsbury Academic., DOI: 10.5040/9781849665896

Esping-Andersen, G. (1990). *The three worlds of welfare capitalism*. Princeton University Press.

Ferrera, M. (1996). The 'southern model' of welfare in social europe. *Journal of European Social Policy*, *6*(1), 17–37. DOI: 10.1177/095892879600600102

Fruh, K., Archer, A., & Wojtowicz, J. (2023). Sportswashing: Complicity and corruption. *Sport, Ethics and Philosophy*, *17*(1), 101–118. DOI: 10.1080/17511321.2022.2107697

Geyer, R. R. (2000). *Exploring European social policy*. Polity Press.

Green, M. (2006). From 'sport for all' to not about 'sport' at all?: Interrogating sport policy interventions in the United Kingdom. *European Sport Management Quarterly*, *6*(3), 217–238. DOI: 10.1080/16184740601094936

Grix, J., & Brannagan, P. M. (2024). *Sports mega-events as foreign policy: Sport diplomacy, "soft power," and "sportswashing". American Behavioral Scientist*. Online First., DOI: 10.1177/00027642241262042

Gunter, A. (2014). Mega events as a pretext for infrastructural development: the case of the All African Games Athletes Village, Alexandra, Johannesburg. In Szymańska, D., & Biegańska, J. (Eds.), *Bulletin of geography: Socio-economic series* (Vol. 23, pp. 39–52)., DOI: 10.2478/bog-2014-0003

Hallmann, K., Wicker, P., Breuer, C., & Schönherr, L. (2012). Understanding the importance of sport infrastructure for participation in different sports – findings from multi-level modeling. *European Sport Management Quarterly, 12*(5), 525–544. DOI: 10.1080/16184742.2012.687756

Hallmann, K., Wicker, P., Breuer, C., & Schüttoff, U. (2011). Interdependency of sport supply and sport demand in German metropolitan and medium-sized municipalities – findings from multi-level analyses. *EJSS European Journal for Sport and Society, 8*(1–2), 65–84. DOI: 10.1080/16138171.2011.11687870

Hartmann, D., & Kwauk, C. (2011). Sport and development: An overview, critique, and reconstruction. *Journal of Sport and Social Issues, 35*(3), 284–305. DOI: 10.1177/0193723511416986

Heinemann, K. (2005). Sport and the welfare state in Europe. *European Journal of Sport Science, 5*(4), 181–188. DOI: 10.1080/17461390500344347

Houlihan, B., & Green, M. (2009). Modernization and sport: The reform of sport England and UK sport. *Public Administration, 87*(3), 678–698. DOI: 10.1111/j.1467-9299.2008.01733.x

Human Rights Watch. (2024, January 17). *Saudi government uses European football to sportswash its reputation.* https://www.hrw.org/news/2024/01/17/saudi-government-uses-european-football-sportswash-its-reputation

Hylton, K., & Bramham, P. (2008). *Sports development: Policy, process and practice* (2nd ed.). Routledge.

Ibsen, B., & Seippel, Ø. (2010). Voluntary organized sport in Denmark and Norway. *Sport in Society, 13*(4), 593–608. DOI: 10.1080/17430431003616266

Jarvie, G. (2011). Sport, social division and social inequality. *Sport Science Review, 20*(1-2), 95–109. DOI: 10.2478/v10237-011-0049-0

Kaal, H. (2021). Boundary disputes: New approaches to the interaction between sport and politics in the postwar years. *Journal of Modern European History, 19*(3), 362–379. DOI: 10.1177/16118944211014418

Kearns, C., Sinclair, G., Black, J., Doidge, M., Fletcher, T., Kilvington, D., Liston, K., Lynn, T., & Santos, G. L. (2024). 'Best run club in the world': Manchester City fans and the legitimation of sportswashing? *International Review for the Sociology of Sport, 59*(4), 479–501. DOI: 10.1177/10126902231210784

Kelly, L. (2011). 'Social inclusion' through sports-based interventions? *Critical Social Policy, 31*(1), 126–150. DOI: 10.1177/0261018310385442

King, N. (2009). *Sport Policy and Governance: Local Perspectives* (1st ed.). Routledge., DOI: 10.4324/9780080942476

Koivunen, A., Ojala, J., & Holmén, J. (Eds.). (2021). *The Nordic economic, social and political model: Challenges in the 21st century*. Routledge. DOI: 10.4324/9780429026690

Krieger, J., & Nordhagen, S. E. (2025). The Scandinavian sport model. In García, B., & Smokvina, V. (Eds.), *The European model of sport: Myth or reality?* (1st ed.). Routledge., DOI: 10.4324/9781032665153-10

Levermore, R. (2011). Sport-for-development and the 2010 football world cup. *Geography Compass*, *5*(12), 886–897. DOI: 10.1111/j.1749-8198.2011.00460.x

Levitas, R. (2005). *The inclusive society? Social exclusion and new labor*. Palgrave Macmillan., DOI: 10.1057/9780230511552

Lindsey, I., Kay, T., Jeanes, R., & Banda, D. (2017). Sport for development in policy, practice and research. In Lindsey, I., Kay, T., Jeanes, R., & Banda, D. (Eds.), *Localizing global sport for development* (pp. 17–51). Manchester University Press., DOI: 10.7765/9781526104991.00008

Liu, S., & Qi, W. (2024). Sports poverty alleviation: Concept and model innovation for the development of Chinese sports towns in the new era. *Frontiers in Sports and Active Living*, *6*, 1423767. Advance online publication. DOI: 10.3389/fspor.2024.1423767

Nichols, G. (2007). *Sport and Crime Reduction: The Role of Sports in Tackling Youth Crime* (1st ed.). Routledge., DOI: 10.4324/9780203089156

O'Malley, P. (1992). Risk, power and crime prevention. *Economy and Society*, *21*(3), 252–275. DOI: 10.1080/03085149200000013

Parnell, D., Millward, P., Widdop, P., King, N., & May, A. (2018). Sport policy and politics in an era of austerity. *International Journal of Sport Policy*, *10*(1), 1–5. DOI: 10.1080/19406940.2018.1432672

Putnam, R. (2000). *Bowling Alone: The Collapse and Revival of American Community*. Simon & Schuster.

Putnam, R. D. (1993). *Making Democracy Work: Civic Tradition and Modern Italy*. Princeton University Press.

Rein, I., & Shields, B. (2007). Place branding sports: Strategies for differentiating emerging, transitional, negatively viewed and newly industrialised nations. *Place Branding and Public Diplomacy*, *3*(1), 73–85. DOI: 10.1057/palgrave.pb.6000049

Seippel, Ø. (2006). Sport and social capital. *Acta Sociologica*, *49*(2), 169–183. DOI: 10.1177/0001699306064771

Skey, M. (2023). Sportswashing: Media headline or analytic concept? *International Review for the Sociology of Sport*, *58*(5), 749–764. DOI: 10.1177/10126902221136086

Tak, M., Sam, M. P., & Jackson, S. J. (2018). The politics of countermeasures against match-fixing in sport: A political sociology approach to policy instruments. *International Review for the Sociology of Sport*, *53*(1), 30–48. DOI: 10.1177/1012690216639748

The Guardian. (2023, October 8) *The Guardian view on World Cup sportwashing: Money talks- and what it says is troubling*. https://www.theguardian.com/commentisfree/2023/oct/08/the-guardian-view-on-world-cup-sportwashing-money-talks-and-what-it-says-is-troubling

The Independent. (2019, August 9). *What are Man City? Premier League champions, the greatest team ever and a 'sportswashing instrument' of a foreign state*. https://www.independent.co.uk/sport/football/premier-league/manchester-city-premier-league-season-preview-champions-greatest-team-eversportswashing-abu-dhabi-a9046866.html

Tuastad, S. (2019). The Scandinavian sport model: Myths and realities. Norwegian football as a case study. *Soccer and Society*, *20*(2), 341–359. DOI: 10.1080/14660970.2017.1323738

Unsal Yılmaz, B., & Şahin, M. (2023). Overview of sports metaphors through visual rhetoric classification in the context of the postmodern consumer culture. *Spormetre Journal of Physical Education and Sport Sciences*, *21*(3), 89–106. DOI: 10.33689/spormetre.1251664

Wacquant, L. (2009). *Punishing the poor: The neoliberal government of social insecurity*. Duke University Press.,

ENDNOTES

1 One of the most significant contributions to the discourse on social capital and voluntary organizations comes from Robert Putnam (1993, 2000). In his seminal study of regional government performance in Italy, Putnam identified a strong positive correlation between the intensity of civic participation and the effectiveness of established political institutions and democratic attitudes. He later applied this approach to the United States, arguing that social ties had

weakened and that there had been a steady decline in many forms of social capital; he opened up a discussion on the causes of this decline and the risks it posed to democratic life. Although Putnam's works touch on the "dark side" of social capital—which includes its exclusionary elements—they have helped spread an optimistic perspective that generally focuses on the positive impact of civil society on democratization. In this vein, a widely accepted "common sense of social capital" has emerged that establishes a direct link between a vibrant association life and the success of democratic processes (Seippel, 2006, p. 172).

2 The growing popularity of the term "sportswashing" serves as a reaction to the rise of new non-Western sports powers. Although there is no universally agreed-upon definition yet, this concept generally focuses on the phenomenon described as "the fundamental dynamic at play." This dynamic involves using investments in sports as a *"valuable strategic tool"* to divert attention from a known moral violation on the one hand, and to diffuse interest in that violation on the other. Drawing from the literature on *"greenwashing"* (companies exaggerating or fabricating their environmental virtues or the environmental qualities of their products to capitalize on consumers' eco-friendly sentiments) and *"whitewashing"* (presenting something or someone in a positive light despite the presence of questionable traits, while covering up negative traces against it), the term "sportswashing" (Fruh et al., 2023, pp. 102–103) reflects the strategic efforts of state leaders to associate themselves and their countries with the positive, clean, and healthy values of elite sports. The primary aim of these initiatives is to *eliminate negative associations stemming from environmental degradation and human rights violations* (Canniford & Hill, 2022). Today, these strategic initiatives are criticized by three main groups, each with concrete examples. *International civil society organizations* view Saudi Arabia's investment in the Saudi Pro League by signing stars like Cristiano Ronaldo (Human Rights Watch, 2024) and its hosting of the 2023 FIFA Club World Cup as an attempt to divert attention from the country's human rights record (Amnesty International, 2023); *global media* views Manchester City FC, owned by the Abu Dhabi United Group, as a "sportswashing tool" for a foreign state (The Independent, 2019), and has characterized the 2022 World Cup hosted by Qatar as a "sportswashing summit" aimed at covering up a poor human rights record (The Guardian, 2023). Meanwhile, *academics* and *some sports critics* interested in the subject have focused on developing the scientific framework of the concept by scrutinizing sportswashing practices from both theoretical and practical perspectives (Boykoff, 2022; Skey, 2023; Grix & Brannagan, 2024; Kearns et al., 2024).

Chapter 5
Social Welfare and Sports Policies:
An Evaluation of Türkiye and Welfare Societies

Mehmet Ulaş
http://orcid.org/0000-0002-5633-542X
Burdur Mehmet Akif Ersoy University, Turkey

ABSTRACT

This chapter examines the relationship between social welfare levels and sports policies within a socio-economic and structural framework. Sport is considered not merely as a field promoting physical activity, but also as a significant public policy instrument contributing to social integration, equality, public health, and the development of social capital. In this context, the chapter analyzes how sports policies are shaped in high-welfare societies and evaluates their effects on social participation through a comparative perspective with Türkiye.

1. INTRODUCTION

Social welfare is a multidimensional concept that is not limited to economic magnitudes alone; it encompasses individuals' quality of life, health status, education level, and opportunities for social participation. In the modern welfare state concept, supporting individuals' physical, psychological, and social well-being, not just increasing their income levels, is among the fundamental goals (Gøsta Esping-Andersen, 1990; Organisation for Economic Co-operation and Development, 2011). In this context, sport and physical activity have become one of the areas that

DOI: 10.4018/979-8-2600-3174-2.ch005

improve individuals' quality of life and are considered an important component of social welfare.

When the social functions of sport are examined, it is seen that its effects are not limited only to physical health; it also has a broad scope of impact, including social integration, social belonging, reduction of crime rates, and support for the psychological well-being of individuals (Sherry & Coalter, 2009; World Health Organization, 2018). In particular, maintaining regular physical activity plays a critical role in preventing chronic diseases, protecting mental health, and extending lifespan (Warburton & Bredin, 2017). In this respect, sport is considered today not only an individual choice but also a social policy tool that should be supported through public policies.

With the development of welfare states, sports policies have also undergone a transformation. Policies traditionally focused on elite sporting achievement have given way to a "sport for all" approach encompassing all segments of society (Houlihan & White, 2002). This approach envisions sports not only as a means of performance and competition, but also as a strategic tool for increasing social welfare, reducing inequalities, and ensuring social inclusion. In this context, sports policies are evaluated within an integrated framework with health, education, and social services policies.

From the perspective of welfare regimes, the ways in which different countries shape their sports policies also vary. In social democratic welfare regimes, the state's role in sports is more prominent and inclusive, while in liberal regimes, sports are organized more through market mechanisms and the private sector (Gøsta Esping-Andersen, 1990). In conservative welfare models, it is noteworthy that sports are conducted through club-based structures and local organizations. These differences directly affect the capacity and accessibility of sports to generate social welfare.

When evaluated specifically in Turkey, it is observed that sports policies have historically focused more on elite sporting achievement, but in recent years, policies aimed at promoting physical activity and improving public health have gained importance. However, various studies show that the capacity of sports to generate social welfare in Turkey is still limited and that structural improvements are needed in this area (Sunay, 2024; Devecioğlu, Çoban, Karakaya, & Karataş, 2012). The effective use of sports as a social policy tool requires the integration not only of the sports system but also of health, education, and local government policies.

The aim of this chapter is to examine the relationship between social welfare and sports policies from a theoretical and comparative perspective; to analyze sports policies implemented in societies with high levels of welfare and to evaluate the current situation in Turkey. Accordingly, the effects of sports on social welfare will be discussed, the sports policies of different welfare regimes will be examined, and Turkey's position within this framework will be debated.

1.2. Literature Review

The relationship between social welfare and sports policies has become one of the important focus areas of interdisciplinary studies in recent years. The approach that welfare cannot be explained solely by economic indicators, but is a multidimensional structure encompassing the physical, psychological, and social well-being of individuals, has made the role of sport within this structure more visible. Indeed, the well-being framework developed by the Organisation for Economic Co-operation and Development shows elements such as health, life satisfaction, and social connections among the basic components of welfare; and considers physical activity as a factor directly related to these components (OECD, 2011).

In the welfare state literature, the welfare regimes approach put forward by Gøsta Esping-Andersen (1990) provides a basic framework for understanding the social policies of countries. This approach reveals that social democratic, liberal, and conservative welfare regimes have different policy tools and priorities. Sports policies also differ within this framework; Social democratic regimes tend to implement more inclusive and egalitarian sports policies by the state, while liberal regimes see sports organized more through market mechanisms (Bergsgard et al., 2007). This difference directly affects sports' capacity to generate social welfare.

When examining the effects of sport on social well-being, the health aspect stands out. The protective effect of regular physical activity against cardiovascular diseases, obesity, diabetes, and some types of cancer has been strongly demonstrated scientifically (Warburton & Bredin, 2017). In this context, the World Health Organization (2018) defines physical activity as one of the fundamental elements of global public health policies and encourages countries to develop national strategies in this area. Increasing physical activity levels is considered a critical policy tool for reducing healthcare costs and improving quality of life.

However, the effects of sport are not limited solely to health. Sport is also an important tool for developing social capital, ensuring social integration, and increasing the participation of disadvantaged groups in social life. Sherry & Coalter (2009), examining the effects of sport on social inclusion, state that it plays a significant role in reducing crime rates, developing social skills, and strengthening the sense of social belonging, especially among young people. Similarly, Putnam (2000), within the framework of social capital theory, emphasizes that participation in sport and physical activity strengthens interpersonal trust and social bonds.

International literature shows that sports policies in countries with high levels of welfare tend to be more inclusive and sustainable. In Scandinavian countries, in particular, sport is considered a right and is widely supported by the state. Policies developed in these countries in line with the "sport for all" approach are notable for their high participation rates and strong infrastructure systems (Bergsgard et al.,

2007). In contrast, in liberal welfare regimes, the financing and organization of sport are largely carried out through the private sector and civil society organizations, which can lead to inequalities in access to sports services (Houlihan & White, 2002).

Another important dimension examining the relationship between sports policies and welfare is the economic impact of sports. The sports sector contributes to job creation, increased tourism revenue, and the revitalization of local economies (Gratton & Taylor, 2000). However, the impact of elite sports investments on social welfare is a controversial topic in the literature. Some studies argue that the economic returns of large sports organizations and elite sports investments are limited and that public resources should be directed more towards grassroots sports policies (Coates & Humphreys, 2008).

When studies conducted in the Turkish context are examined, it is seen that sports policies have historically focused more on elite sports success. Devecioğlu (2012) states that the sports management system in Turkey has a centralized structure and that policies aimed at popularizing sports are not sufficiently developed. Similarly, Sunay (2024) states that in order for sports to be used effectively as a social policy tool, institutional structures should be strengthened, local governments should be more actively involved in the process, and a sports culture should be spread throughout society.

Although there have been various policy initiatives in Turkey in recent years aimed at increasing physical activity, there are limitations regarding the sustainability and effectiveness of these policies. In particular, the inadequacy of school-based sports programs, inequalities in access to facilities, and the limited integration of sports into the education system are among the main factors that limit the capacity of sports to generate social welfare (Öztürk and Koca, 2018).

In conclusion, the literature reveals that sports are an important component of social welfare and that effective sports policies play a critical role in improving the quality of life of individuals. However, the level of this effect is directly related to the welfare regimes, policy priorities, and institutional structures of countries. This situation necessitates a reassessment of Turkey's sports policies from a welfare-oriented perspective and the utilization of international best practices.

2. CONCEPTUAL FRAMEWORK

2.1. What is Social Welfare?

Social welfare is a multidimensional concept that expresses the level of well-being of individuals not only economically but also in physical, psychological, and social dimensions. While traditional approaches mostly evaluate welfare through per capita income and economic growth indicators, the modern understanding of welfare has expanded to include individuals' quality of life, health status, educational opportunities, and levels of social participation (Stiglitz, Sen & Fitoussi, 2009). In this context, welfare is associated not only with "how much one possesses" but also with "how one lives."

2.2. The Concept of the Welfare State

The welfare state refers to a state structure that aims to meet the basic life needs of individuals and protect them against social risks. In this model, the state aims to reduce social inequalities by taking an active role in areas such as health, education, social security, and employment. The concept of the welfare state developed especially after World War II and, with the institutionalization of social policies, has become an important component of modern state structures.

Gøsta Esping-Andersen (1990), a prominent figure in the welfare state literature, classified welfare states under three main regimes: social democratic, liberal, and conservative. This classification is based on criteria such as the level of state intervention in social policies, the role of market mechanisms, and the impact of family structure on social welfare. In the social democratic model, the role of the state is strong and inclusive, while in the liberal model, market mechanisms are prominent. In the conservative model, social policies are shaped more through family and occupation-based structures. These different welfare regimes directly affect individuals' welfare levels and their access to public services.

2.3. Well-Being Indicators

Measuring social well-being is a complex process due to its multi-dimensional nature. Although gross domestic product (GDP) has traditionally been used as the primary indicator of well-being, this measure provides limited information about individuals' quality of life. Therefore, more comprehensive indicators are used in measuring well-being today.

Well-being indicators can generally be grouped under the following headings:

- **Income and economic security:** Per capita income, income distribution, poverty rate
- **Health:** Life expectancy, disease rates, access to health services
- **Education:** Schooling rates, education level, lifelong learning opportunities
- **Quality of life:** Housing conditions, environmental factors, security
- **Social participation:** Community ties, volunteer activities, social security

These indicators allow for the assessment of individuals' social and psychological well-being, not just their economic well-being. Approaches focused on quality of life, in particular, tend to measure the subjective dimensions of well-being (such as life satisfaction).

2.4. OECD and United Nations Well-being Measures

One of the most comprehensive frameworks for measuring societal well-being today is the "Better Life Index" and "How's Life?" reports developed by the Organisation for Economic Co-operation and Development (OECD). The OECD (2011) focuses not only on economic indicators but also on factors that directly affect the quality of life of individuals when measuring well-being. In this context, the OECD's well-being measures include dimensions such as income, employment, housing, health, education, environment, civic participation, life satisfaction, and work-life balance. This approach reveals the multidimensional nature of well-being, offering policymakers a more comprehensive assessment opportunity. Similarly, the Human Development Index (HDI), developed by the United Nations, is another important indicator widely used in measuring well-being. Developed by the United Nations Development Programme (UNDP), this index is based on three fundamental dimensions: life expectancy, education level, and per capita income (UNDP, 2020). HDI assesses countries' development levels not only through economic growth but also from a human-centered perspective.

These criteria, developed by the OECD and the United Nations, reveal the multifaceted nature of well-being, contributing to the adoption of more comprehensive and holistic approaches in policy-making processes. Within this framework, sport and physical activity are considered one of the important determinants of societal well-being, particularly due to their direct relationship with health, quality of life, and social inclusion.

2.5. The Relationship Between Sports Policies and Social Policy

When we talk about sports policy, we think of "the approach to sports, its principles and goals, the ways and methods of achieving these goals, infrastructure, facilities, equipment and training understanding, the perspective on sports at the national and international levels, and the philosophy of organization and implementation of sports" (Ekici, 2002). Sports policies refer to the entirety of public policies developed to encourage individuals' participation in physical activity, increase elite sports success, and support the social functions of sports. While traditionally sports policies were mostly addressed within a performance and competition-oriented framework, this approach has changed significantly today, and the use of sports as a social policy tool has come to the forefront. This transformation has progressed in parallel with the development of the welfare state concept.

Social policy encompasses policy areas aimed at improving individuals' living conditions, reducing social inequalities, and ensuring social justice. In this context, sport is considered an important component of social policy due to its direct relationship with areas such as health, education, and social services (Houlihan & White, 2002). The use of sport as a social policy tool is of great importance, especially in terms of the integration of disadvantaged groups into society, the social development of young people, and the improvement of public health. The relationship between sport and social policy can be examined in three main dimensions: health, social integration, and education. Firstly, in the health dimension, it has been scientifically shown that regular physical activity increases the physical and mental health levels of individuals, reduces the risk of chronic diseases, and improves quality of life. Accordingly, the World Health Organization (2018) defines physical activity as one of the fundamental components of global health policies and encourages countries to develop policies in this area.

Secondly, sport is an important tool for social integration. Sports activities increase social interaction among individuals, strengthen the sense of belonging to society, and contribute to the formation of social capital. Especially for young people and disadvantaged groups, sport stands out as a mechanism that reduces social exclusion and increases participation in society (Sherry & Coalter, 2009). In this respect, sport is not only an activity that provides individual benefit, but also a social policy tool that strengthens the social structure.

Thirdly, the relationship between sport and education is noteworthy. School-based sports programs enable individuals to acquire physical activity habits at an early age, while also contributing to the development of social skills such as discipline, teamwork, and responsibility. Therefore, implementing sports policies in an integrated manner with education policies is critically important for long-term social welfare.

In international literature, the integration of sports policies with social policy is addressed within the framework of the "sport for development" and "sport for all" approaches. The "sport for all" approach aims to ensure equal access to sports for all segments of society, while the "development through sport" approach refers to the use of sport as a tool contributing to social, economic, and cultural development (Coalter, 2013). These approaches reveal that sport is not only a competitive activity but also a strategic tool that increases social welfare. In this context, the effectiveness of sports policies should be evaluated not only through athlete success but also through outcomes such as increasing the level of physical activity in society as a whole, improving health indicators, and reducing social inequalities. Indeed, the Organisation for Economic Co-operation and Development (2011) lists the quality of life and social participation levels of individuals as key criteria when measuring the success of welfare policies. This situation makes the role of sports policies in welfare production even more important. In conclusion, sports policies should be considered an integral part of the social policy field. The multifaceted impacts of sport on health, education, and social integration make it a crucial component of welfare state policies. Therefore, sport policies should not only focus on performance but also adopt an inclusive perspective aimed at enhancing societal well-being.

2.6. The Welfare Regimes Approach

One of the most effective theoretical frameworks developed to understand how social welfare is produced and distributed is the welfare regimes approach. This approach makes it possible to analyze the social policies of countries not only through economic indicators but also within the framework of the relationships between the state, the market, and the family. The welfare regimes approach has gained widespread acceptance in the literature, particularly with the classification put forward by Gøsta Esping-Andersen (1990).

Esping-Andersen (1990) examines welfare states under three basic regimes: social democratic, liberal, and conservative (corporatist) welfare regimes. This classification is based on criteria such as the scope of social rights, the role of the state in social policies, and the effectiveness of market mechanisms. In this context, welfare regimes are considered as fundamental structures that determine the level of access of individuals to social services and how social inequalities are managed.

2.6.1. Social Democratic Welfare Regime

The social democratic welfare regime stands out as the model where the state's role in social policies is strongest. In this regime, welfare is considered a universal right and is provided equally to all citizens by the state. The Scandinavian countries (Sweden, Norway, Denmark) are among the most typical examples of this model. In this model, sports policies are also addressed with an inclusive understanding. Sport is not only considered a field for elite achievement, but also a public service that increases the general welfare of society. The "sport for all" approach is one of the fundamental characteristics of this regime. State-supported sports infrastructure, high participation rates, and strong local organizations increase the capacity of sport to generate social welfare (Bergsgard et al., 2007). In this context, in social democratic regimes, sport is implemented in an integrated manner with health policies and education systems.

2.6.2. Liberal Welfare Regime

In a liberal welfare regime, the state's role in social policies is limited, and market mechanisms are paramount. In this model, the well-being of individuals largely depends on their individual efforts and market conditions. The US and the UK are the best-known examples of this regime. In this regime, sports policies are also largely shaped by the private sector and civil society organizations. In the US, in particular, the university sports system and professional leagues play a central role in the organization of sports. While this structure is quite effective in increasing elite sports success, it can lead to unequal levels of sports participation across society (Houlihan & White, 2002). Therefore, in liberal regimes, the capacity of sports to generate welfare varies depending more on economic access and individual resources.

2. 6. 3. Conservative (Corporatist) Welfare Regime

The conservative welfare regime is based on a more balanced relationship between the state, the market, and the family. In this model, social policies are generally implemented through occupation-based structures and social insurance systems. Germany, France, and Italy are among the leading examples of this regime. In this regime, sports policies are largely organized through club-based structures. The "Verein" system in Germany, in particular, stands out as an important mechanism for the widespread adoption of sports at the societal level. This system supports individuals in developing regular sports habits while also contributing to the strengthening of social ties. In this respect, sports are considered an important tool for the production of social capital in conservative regimes (Putnam, 2000).

2.7. The Relationship Between Welfare Regimes and Sport Policies

The welfare regimes approach offers an important analytical framework for understanding why sport policies differ from country to country. In social democratic regimes, the popularization and increased accessibility of sport are prioritized, while in liberal regimes, performance and the production of economic value are more decisive. In conservative regimes, sport stands out as an activity that strengthens the social structure and is sustained through local organizations. These differences directly affect the capacity of sport to generate social welfare. In social democratic countries with high participation rates, the effects of sport on health and quality of life are more pronounced; while in liberal regimes, despite high elite sporting success, inequalities at the societal level are noticeable. In conservative regimes, the effects of sport on social integration are stronger.

When evaluating Turkey's current structure, it can be said that there is a hybrid model exhibiting characteristics of different welfare regimes in certain aspects. However, the fact that sports policies are predominantly conducted through a centralized structure and focused on elite sporting success stands out as a significant factor limiting sports' capacity to generate social welfare. This situation indicates that Turkey needs to restructure its sports policies with a more inclusive and welfare-oriented perspective.

Table 1. Welfare Regimes and Sports Policies

Country	Welfare Regime	Sports Policy Model	Public Expenditure (Sport)	Sport Participation Rate	Olympic Success	Key Feature
Sweden	Social Democratic	State-supported "Sport for All"	High	Very high (70%+)	Medium-High	Equal access, widespread sport culture
Norway	Social Democratic	Club + state-supported model	High	Very high (70%+)	High (especially winter sports)	Child and youth-oriented system
Germany	Conservative	Club-based (Verein system)	Medium-High	High (60%+)	High	Strong local club structure
France	Conservative	State + federation-oriented	Medium	Medium-High (50%+)	High	Central planning + elite sport
United Kingdom	Liberal	Market + state hybrid model	Medium	Medium (40–50)	Very high (especially recent years)	Strong elite sport investment
USA	Liberal	Private sector + university system	Low (public) / high (private)	Medium (40–50)	Very high	NCAA and professional sport system
Türkiye	Conservative Hybrid / Developing	Centralized + state-oriented	Medium	Low (20–30)	Low-Medium	Elite sport-focused, limited participation

This comparative analysis reveals that sports policies in countries with high levels of welfare tend to be more inclusive and sustainable. Particularly noteworthy are countries with social democratic welfare regimes (e.g., Sweden and Norway), where sport is considered a right and widely supported by the state. High participation rates in sports in these countries increase sport's capacity to generate social welfare.

In conservative welfare regimes, however, sport is more often organized through a club-based structure. In the case of Germany, the "Verein" system stands out as a significant institutional structure ensuring the regular participation of individuals in sports activities. This model supports sport's function of generating social capital by creating strong social ties at the local level.

In liberal welfare regimes (USA and UK), the sports system is largely shaped by market mechanisms and the private sector. While this may increase elite sporting success, it can lead to inequalities in access to sports services.

In the United States, the collegiate sports system (NCAA) serves as an effective model for developing elite athletes, while overall physical activity participation in society remains limited. In Turkey, sports policies are largely centralized and focused on elite sporting success. Low sports participation rates are a significant factor limiting the capacity of sports to generate social welfare. This situation indicates the need for sports policies to be transformed into a more inclusive and grassroots structure. The findings of this study reveal that the relationship between sports policies and social welfare is strong but contextually variable. Particularly in countries with high levels of welfare, sports are positioned not only as a field that promotes physical activity but also as a tool of social policy. This is consistent with the multifaceted impacts of sports on health, social integration, and quality of life (Sherry & Coalter, 2009; World Health Organization, 2018).

From the perspective of welfare regimes, the classification put forward by Gøsta Esping-Andersen (1990) appears to be decisive in shaping sports policies. In social democratic welfare regimes, the treatment of sport as a public service is directly related to high participation rates. In these countries, the active role of the state ensures that sport is accessible to all segments of society, thus increasing its capacity to generate welfare. This finding aligns with the work of Bergsgard et al. (2007), who emphasize that sports policies are closely related to institutional structure. In contrast, in liberal welfare regimes, the organization of sport primarily through market mechanisms, while increasing elite sporting success, can deepen inequalities at the societal level. Particularly in the US, the university-based sports system, while highly successful in producing elite athletes, shows that participation in physical activity remains limited in society as a whole. This situation demonstrates that the welfare-generating function of sport cannot be achieved solely through performance-oriented policies (Houlihan & White, 2002).

In conservative welfare regimes, club-based sports structures are prominent and play a significant role in the production of social capital. The "Verein" system in Germany supports individuals in developing regular sports habits while simultaneously strengthening social ties at the local level. This finding reveals that sport is an important tool not only for individual health but also for social integration (Putnam, 2000).

The findings obtained specifically for Turkey show that sports policies have not yet sufficiently developed from a welfare-oriented perspective. The largely centralized structure of the sports system and its focus on elite sporting success limit the spread of sport to the grassroots level. This situation parallels the structural problems frequently highlighted in the literature for Turkey (Devecioğlu, 2012; Sunay, 2024). In particular, the low sports participation rates reveal that the potential effects of sport on public health and social welfare are not being fully realized.

One of the fundamental problems facing sports policies in Turkey is the lack of policy continuity and inter-institutional coordination. The failure to integrate sports with education, health, and local government policies limits the effective use of sports as a social policy tool. However, as emphasized by the Organisation for Economic Co-operation and Development (2011), holistic policy approaches are critically important in increasing welfare. Nevertheless, various initiatives aimed at increasing physical activity have been observed in Turkey in recent years. However, for these initiatives to be sustainable and to create widespread impacts throughout society, more systematic and data-driven policies need to be developed. Repositioning sports to contribute not only to elite achievement but also to public health and social development would be an important step towards increasing welfare levels. In this context, it can be said that the most suitable approach for Turkey is a hybrid sports policy model that combines the strengths of different welfare regimes. By combining the inclusiveness of the social democratic model, the club-based structure of the conservative model, and the resource diversity of the liberal model, a sustainable sports policy specific to Turkey can be developed. This approach will make it possible to both popularize the sport and improve performance levels.

In conclusion, the impact of sports policies on social welfare is directly related not only to the existence of sport but also to how it is structured. Reconsidering Turkey's current sports policies from a welfare-oriented perspective will yield significant gains at both individual and societal levels. At this point, leveraging international best practices and restructuring sports policies in light of scientific data is a critical necessity.

3. CONCLUSION AND POLICY RECOMMENDATIONS

This study examines the relationship between social welfare and sports policies from a theoretical and comparative perspective, demonstrating that sport is not only a field of physical activity but also a powerful tool for social policy. The findings show that sports policies in countries with high levels of welfare are more inclusive, sustainable, and holistic. In particular, in social democratic welfare regimes, the treatment of sport as a right and its widespread state support are directly related to high participation rates and positive health outcomes. In contrast, in liberal welfare regimes, the market-based structure of sport, while increasing elite sporting success, can deepen inequalities at the societal level. In conservative welfare regimes, club-based structures are seen to play a significant role in popularizing sport and generating social capital. These findings reveal that the welfare-generating capacity of sports policies is directly related not only to economic resources but also to institutional structure and policy approach.

Assessments specific to Turkey show that sports policies exhibit a significantly centralized structure and are primarily focused on elite sporting achievement. This situation limits the widespread adoption of sports throughout society and leads to low rates of physical activity participation. However, frameworks established by the World Health Organization (2018) and the Organisation for Economic Co-operation and Development (2011) clearly demonstrate that increasing physical activity is a critical indicator of well-being in terms of both health and quality of life.

In this context, sports policies in Turkey need to be restructured and addressed from a welfare-oriented perspective. The following policy recommendations stand out in this transformation process:

3.1. Policy Recommendations

1. Adopting a “Sport for All” Approach

Sport policies should be transformed from an elite, achievement-oriented structure into a model that includes all segments of society. Accessible sports programs should be developed, especially for children, youth, women, and disadvantaged groups.

2. Strengthening the Role of Local Governments

Local governments play a critical role in the dissemination of sports. Increasing sports facilities at the local level, developing neighborhood-based sports programs, and encouraging community participation are necessary.

3. Integration with the Education System

School-based sports programs should be strengthened to ensure that individuals acquire physical activity habits at an early age. Sports should be made an integral part of the education system.

4. Data-Driven Sports Policies

Sports participation rates, physical activity levels, and health indicators should be regularly monitored, and policy development processes should be based on scientific data.

5. Developing a Club-Based Structure

The institutional capacities of local sports clubs should be increased and sustainable structures should be created, particularly in a manner similar to club models in Europe.

6. Ensuring Inter-Institutional Integration

Sports policies should be addressed in an integrated manner with health, education, and social services policies. In this regard, a multi-stakeholder management model should be developed.

A Model Proposal for Turkey (Original Contribution)

The approach proposed for Turkey within the scope of this study can be defined as a "Hybrid Sport Welfare Model" that combines the strengths of different welfare regimes. This model:

- The inclusiveness of the social democratic approach
- The club-based structure of the conservative model
- The resource diversity of the liberal model

offers a sustainable sports policy framework by bringing these elements together. The main goal of this model is to use sport not only to produce performance but also to improve public health, strengthen social integration, and enhance quality of life.

4. GENERAL ASSESSMENT

In conclusion, the impact of sports policies on social welfare is directly related not only to the existence of sports activities, but also to how these activities are planned, managed, and which segments of society they reach. Reconsidering Turkey's current sports policies from a welfare-oriented perspective will yield significant gains at both individual and societal levels. In this regard, utilizing international best practices and restructuring sports policies in light of scientific data will be a strategic step in increasing Turkey's welfare level.

REFERENCES

Bergsgard, N. A., Houlihan, B., Mangset, P., Nødland, S. I., & Rommetvedt, H. (2007). *Sport policy: A comparative analysis of stability and change*. Butterworth-Heinemann.

Coalter, F. (2013). *Sport for development: What game are we playing?* Routledge. DOI: 10.4324/9780203861257

Coates, D., & Humphreys, B. R. (2008). Do economists reach a conclusion on subsidies for sports franchises, stadiums, and mega-events? *Econ Journal Watch, 5*(3), 294.

Devecioğlu, S., Çoban, B., Karakaya, Y. E., & Karataş, Ö. (2012). Türkiye'de spor kulüplerinin şirketleşmeye yönelimlerinin değerlendirilmesi. *SPORMETRE Beden Eğitimi ve Spor Bilimleri Dergisi, 10*(2), 35–42. DOI: 10.1501/Sporm_0000000218

Ekici, S. (2002). *Türkiye'de spor federasyonlarını oluşturan fahri(gönüllü) çalışanların spor politikalarının oluşumu ve uygulamalarına yaklaşımları, Yayınlanmamış doktora tezi*. Gazi Üniversitesi Sağlık Bilimleri Enstitüsü.

Gøsta Esping-Andersen, G. (1990). *The Three Worlds of Welfare Capitalism*. Princeton University Press.

Gratton, C., & Taylor, P. (2000). *Economics of sport and recreation*. Spon Press.

Houlihan, B., & White, A. (2002). *The politics of sports development: Development of sport or development through sport?* Routledge.

Organisation for Economic Co-operation and Development. (2011). *How's Life? Measuring Well-being*. OECD Publishing., DOI: 10.1787/9789264121164-

Öztürk, P., & Koca, C. (2018). Uluslararası politika belgeleri kapsamında spor ve toplumsal cinsiyet politikaları. *Spor Bilimleri Dergisi, 29*(3), 114–130. DOI: 10.17644/sbd.364514

Putnam, R. D. (2000). Bowling alone: America's declining social capital. In *Culture and politics: A reader* (pp. 223–234). Palgrave Macmillan US.

Sherry, E., & Coalter, F. (2009). A Wider Social Role for Sport: Who's Keeping the Score? *Sport Management Review, 12*(4), 273–274. DOI: 10.1016/j.smr.2009.05.002

Stiglitz, J. E., Sen, A., & Fitoussi, J. P. (2009). Report by the Commission on the Measurement of Economic Performance and Social Progress.

Sunay, H. (2024). *Spor ve Politika İlişkisi Perspektifinde Türk Spor Politikası. Yeni Türkiye (Beden Eğitimi ve Spor Özel Sayısı-I).* Yeni Türkiye Yayınları.

United Nations Development Programme (UNDP). (2020). Human Development Report.

Warburton, D., & Bredin, S. S. D. (2017). Health benefits of physical activity: A systematic review. *Current Opinion in Cardiology*, *32*(5), 541–556. DOI: 10.1097/HCO.0000000000000437 PMID: 28708630

World Health Organization. (2018). Global action plan on physical activity 2018–2030.

Chapter 6
Tax Incentives for Sport in Türkiye:
Economic Outlook and Policy Assessment

Hülya Kabakçı Karadeniz
http://orcid.org/0000-0003-3321-4905
Pamukkale University, Turkey

ABSTRACT

This study evaluates the distribution and public-interest orientation of sports-related tax incentives in Türkiye, using TÜİK's 2024 Industry and Services Statistics and Revenue Administration tax-expenditure data. In 2024, 13,022 sports enterprises employed 45,097 people. Although sports clubs represented a small share of enterprises, they generated 43.6% of sectoral value added; value added per paid employee was about 9.4 times the annual gross minimum wage. Fitness and bodybuilding centres comprised nearly half of enterprises, yet their corresponding ratio was only 0.84. Türkiye supports national sport through wage exemptions, sponsorship deductions, reduced withholding rates, and income, corporate and value-added tax exemptions. However, insufficient beneficiary-level data prevent reliable evaluation of effectiveness and distributional fairness. The study recommends redirecting support toward community programmes, amateur clubs, young people and persons with disabilities; providing conditional incentives to small fitness centres and sports entrepreneurs; and regularly assessing the cost-effectiveness and distributional impact of all sports-related tax expenditures.

DOI: 10.4018/979-8-2600-3174-2.ch006

INTRODUCTION

In today's modern economies, sport is not merely an individual recreational activity. Sport has also become a significant and ever-growing industry, characterised by club budgets, massive transfer fees, sponsorship networks and global advertising revenue (Gürek, 2018, p. 1). The increasing global significance of sport over time has also brought its role in the sports economy to the fore. The sports industry, with its global structure, ranks among the rapidly growing economic sectors (Değer, 2022:68). The significant growth of the sports industry has brought with it a need for funding. Governments have begun to adopt hybrid models based on tax incentives and private-sector partnerships, rather than direct subsidies, to support sport. Tax incentives for sport are among the key public policies implemented by governments to promote the widespread participation in sport, strengthen infrastructure and foster the growth of the sports industry. These incentives are implemented through various mechanisms, such as tax reductions, exemptions, the deduction of sponsorship expenditure from tax, or the channelling of donations made via income and corporation tax to sports clubs. Policies aimed at building a productive and socially developed society should place greater emphasis on high-quality investments in children and young people, including education, healthy lifestyles and participation in sport (Tugal et al., 2025: 38).

In Türkiye, the promotion of sport is among the state's duties under Article 59 of the Constitution. This provision of the Constitution mandates that the state take measures to improve the physical and mental health of citizens of all ages and encourage the widespread participation in sport, whilst also providing protection for successful athletes (Çeribaş, 2020, p. 577). In Türkiye, the tax advantages provided to amateur sports clubs in particular, and the tax deductibility of sponsorship expenditure, are notable features. It is expected that financial incentives for sport will contribute to an increase in the number of young athletes, growth in infrastructure investment and the wider dissemination of sport. However, if financial incentives for sport are distributed unevenly or if the expected economic returns are not achieved, these objectives may not be realised. Research on the scale of tax expenditure on sports incentives in Türkiye, the public benefit they provide, the types of sporting activities and clubs supported by these incentives, and Türkiye's sports and health policy objectives is quite limited. This study aims to contribute to filling this gap.

1. Purpose and Methodology of the Study

The primary objective of this study is to examine tax incentives for sport in Türkiye; to determine the economic scale of these incentives using data from the Turkish Statistical Institute (TÜİK) on Industry and Services Statistics and the

Revenue Administration (GİB) on tax expenditure and to assess the current tax incentives structure from public-interest and policy alignment perspective. The study examines differences in the number of enterprises, employment and value added across the sub-sectors of the sports sector (sports clubs, sports facilities, fitness centres). In doing so, it analyses which types of clubs and activities are supported by the current tax incentive structure. Furthermore, the study assesses the alignment of tax incentives with the development of amateur sport, under-supported areas such as sport for people with disabilities, and the health objectives of the Twelfth Development Plan (obesity, diabetes, tobacco use). The study aims to identify areas for improvement in the current system regarding the wider dissemination of sport and to develop recommendations for a tax policy that promotes the widespread participation in sporting activities.

2. The Economic Outlook of the Sports Activities Sector in Türkiye

The most important database that can be used to assess the economic outlook of the sports industry is the Turkish Statistical Institute's (TÜİK) Industry and Services Statistics database (TÜİK, 2024; Ağazade, 2025). When examining the sub-sectors related to sports activities, fitness centres and bodybuilding centres constitute the most widespread sub-sector in terms of the number of businesses. There are 6,546 businesses in this sub-sector, accounting for approximately 50.2 per cent of the total number of businesses. The same sub-sector accounts for 41.8 per cent of total employment, with 18,861 employees. By contrast, its share of value added stands at 11.9 per cent. This indicates that whilst fitness and bodybuilding centres have a widespread business and employment structure, they lag behind sports clubs and sports facilities in terms of value-added production.

According to 2024 data, there are a total of 13,022 businesses, 45,097 employees and 34,344 paid employees within the 93.1 Sports Activities sector in Türkiye. The sector's value added at factor cost stands at 22.4 billion TL.

The activities of sports clubs, however, account for only 133 enterprises, representing approximately 1 per cent of the total. Despite this, they generate 9.8 billion TL in value added, accounting for 43.6 per cent of the sector's total value added. This concentration of value added may partly reflect the economic scale of a limited number of professional sports clubs. The sub-sector of sports facility management, meanwhile, accounts for more than one-third of salaried employees and approximately 40 per cent of value added. Ağazade's (2025) findings for the 2003–2022 period reveal that the sports activities sector has demonstrated growth in terms of production, turnover and value added that exceeds the general growth performance of the Turkish economy. The study indicates that, during the 2003–2022 period, the sports activities sector grew by an average of 9.1 per cent annually in real production value, 9.3 per cent in turnover and 8.9 per cent in value added; these rates exceeded Türkiye's GDP growth rate for the same period.

Table 1. Key Economic Indicators for the Sports Activities Sector in Türkiye, 2024

Sector	Number of Enterprises	Number of Employees	Number of paid employees	Value added, TL	Value added per employee, TL	Value added per paid employee, TL
93.1 Total for sports activities	**13,022**	**45,097**	**34,344**	**22,447,380,271**	**497,758**	**653,604**
Operation of sports facilities	2,588	14,401	12,553	8,787,138,608	610,176	700,003
Activities of sports clubs	133	4,375	4,350	9,797,626,725	2,239,458	2,252,328
Fitness centres and bodybuilding gyms	6,546	18,861	13,278	2,667,838,778	141,447	200,922
Other sporting activities	3,755	7,460	4,163	1,194,776,160	160,158	286,999

Source: Calculated from the TÜİK Industry and Services Statistics Database

At this point, the value added per paid employee in professional sports clubs is almost three times that of sports facility operations. Whilst the value added per paid employee in sports clubs is approximately 9.4 times the annual minimum wage, the corresponding ratio for the operation of sports facilities is 2.92 (Table 2). Fitness centres, however, represent a sector where the value added per employee and per paid employee remains below the minimum wage. The fact that the value added per employee in fitness and bodybuilding centres falls below the annual gross minimum wage may indicate issues in this sub-sector regarding low productivity, the prevalence of small-scale businesses, cost pressures and the sustainability of formal employment.

Table 2. Ratio of Value Added per Employee and per Wage-Earning Employee to the Annual Gross Wage in the Sports Activities Sector, 2024

	Value added per worker / annual gross minimum wage	**Value added per salaried employee / annual gross minimum wage**
Total Sports Activities	2.07	2.72
Operation of sports facilities	2.54	2.92
Activities of Sports Clubs	9.33	9.38
Gyms and Bodybuilding Centres	0.59	0.84
Other Sports Activities	0.67	1.2

Source: Calculated using data from the TÜİK (Turkish Statistical Institute) Industry and Services Statistics Database, taking into account the Minimum Wage Data from the Ministry of Labour and Social Security (ÇSGB, n.d.).

The targets set out in the Twelfth Development Plan (SBB, n.d.), for sports policy in Türkiye include the widespread promotion of sport and the support of performance-based professional sport. During the plan period, the aim is to increase the number of licensed athletes from 14.8 million to 20 million, the number of athletes with disabilities from approximately 49,000 to 100,000, and the number of sports clubs serving people with disabilities from 2,278 to 3,500 (SBB, n.d.). These targets are significant in that they demonstrate the need to consider not only economic scale but also public interest criteria—such as social inclusion, access to sport for people with disabilities, engaging young people in sport, and strengthening local sports clubs—when allocating public funding for sport. In this regard, tax expenditure on sport must also be consistent with these targets.

The health objectives of the 12th Development Plan reinforce the public health dimension of sports policies. The Plan aims to reduce the obesity rate from 31.5 per cent in 2022 to 27 per cent, the diabetes rate to 11 per cent, and the prevalence of tobacco use from 32.2 per cent to 27 per cent by 2028 (SBB, n.d.). These targets demonstrate that sports-related tax incentives, in particular, should be assessed not only in terms of club funding or sporting performance success, but also within the context of preventive health policy. Given the role of regular physical activity in reducing the risk of obesity and diabetes, it is in the public interest to link sports incentives to school sports, local sports facilities, sports for people with disabilities and community-based physical activity programmes. In this regard, there is a particular need to support gyms aimed at fitness maintenance.

3. Tax Incentives for Sport in Türkiye

Nowadays, tax expenditure is utilised in many countries to achieve targeted economic and social objectives. Tax expenditure essentially refers to tax revenue that is foregone or reduced. In practice, these can be categorised as tax exemptions and exceptions, deductions, offsets, reduced tax rates, tax incentives and tax deferrals (Eriçok, 2019:321). Within the Turkish tax system, sport is supported through various mechanisms of exemptions, reliefs and deductions via income tax, corporation tax and specific statutory provisions. The Income Tax Act provides for exemptions for amateur sportspeople (Article 23/15), competition prizes (Article 29/3) and referees' fees (Article 29/4), as well as a reduced withholding tax rate on professional athletes' earnings (Transitional Article 72) and a deduction for sponsorship expenditure (Article 89/8). The Corporation Tax Act, on the other hand, contains provisions granting exemption to the commercial operations of sports clubs (Article 4(1)(j)) and a sponsorship expenditure deduction (Article 10(1)(b)). Furthermore, Law No. 5894 grants the Turkish Football Federation exemption from corporation tax. These provisions will be examined below under separate headings.

Income Tax Incentives

Article 23 of the Income Tax Act No. 193, titled 'Miscellaneous Exemptions' (ITA Art. 23), lists the remuneration exempt from income tax. Paragraph 15 of the relevant article stipulates that remuneration paid to amateur sportsmen (provided it does not exceed twice the minimum wage) is exempt from income tax, subject to proof of their participation in national competitions each year. This exemption applies to one amateur sportsman in workplaces employing 100 or fewer workers, and to two amateur sportsmen in workplaces employing more than 100 workers (Income Tax Code, Article 23(15)). Furthermore, certain bonuses and rewards paid for incentive purposes are exempt from income tax (Income Tax Code, Article 29). These include prizes and bonuses paid to amateur athletes participating in sports competitions, and fees paid to referees officiating in amateur sports competitions (excluding those officiating in the top leagues of basketball and volleyball) (Income Tax Code, Article 29/3-4).

Incentives are not limited solely to tax exemptions on the fees of athletes and referees. Furthermore, expenditure on sports facilities, aimed at supporting and promoting sport, may also be deducted from the income tax base. The relevant legislation states that, when determining the income tax base, certain deductions may be made from the income declared in the income tax return (Income Tax Code, Article 89). All expenditure incurred on the construction of youth centres and youth and scouting camps belonging to the Ministry of Youth and Sport, carried out under the authorisation and supervision of local administrative authorities, is deductible from the income tax base. Furthermore, all donations and contributions of any kind made to these organisations for the construction of such facilities are deductible from the income tax base. All forms of monetary and in-kind donations and contributions made to enable these sports facilities to continue their activities are fully deductible from the income tax base (Income Tax Code, Article 89/5). Sponsorship expenditure incurred under the Law on the Establishment and Duties of the Turkish Football Federation is fully deductible from the income tax base for amateur sports, and 50 per cent of such expenditure is deductible for professional sports (Income Tax Code, Article 89/8).

Pursuant to the provision added by the transitional article (Income Tax Code, Article 72), income tax withholding shall be applied at the following rates on remuneration paid to athletes until 31 December 2028. In sports governed by a league system: a 20 per cent withholding tax applies to those in the top league, 10 per cent to those in the six leagues below the top, and 5 per cent to those in other leagues; a 5 per cent withholding tax applies to payments made to athletes in sports not governed by a league system, as well as to national athletes in return for their participation in international competitions.

For many years, Türkiye has applied a flat-rate withholding tax system for the taxation of athletes' earnings that has been well below European standards (Çeribaş, 2020, p. 576). Prior to the amendments introduced in 2020, the comparatively low withholding rate applied to top-league athletes led Türkiye to be characterised in the literature as offering tax-haven-like advantages to high-income professional athletes (Öz & Akçay, 2013, p. 45; Ergür & Köstekçi, 2021, pp. 2947–2948).Following the fundamental changes introduced by Law No. 7194, athletes whose annual salary income exceeds a certain threshold (500,000 TL for 2020) were made obliged to submit an annual tax return, and the withholding tax rate for the top leagues was raised to 20 per cent (Çeribaş, 2020, p. 568). Under this system, whilst taxes deducted by clubs are paid to the tax office on behalf of the athletes, in accordance with Additional Article 12 of Law No. 3289, a portion of these taxes is refunded to the clubs via a special account for the purpose of supporting amateur sports (Çeribaş, 2020, p. 567).

Corporation Tax Incentives

The entities listed in the article entitled 'Exemptions' in the Corporate Tax Law No. 5520 (CTL, Art. 4) are exempt from corporation tax. This article (CTA, Art. 4/j) covers the economic enterprises of sports clubs registered with the General Directorate of Youth and Sport and autonomous sports federations that are engaged in training and sporting activities, as well as public limited companies engaged solely in training and sporting activities. Under the section of the same Act entitled 'Other Deductions' (CTA, Art. 10), expenses deductible from corporate profit are listed for the purposes of determining the corporate tax base, provided that they are specifically indicated on the corporate tax return. Under the Law on the Establishment and Duties of the Turkish Football Federation, sponsorship expenditure is fully deductible from corporate profit for amateur sports, and 50 per cent of such expenditure is deductible for professional sports (Corporate Tax Law, Article 10/b). Donations made to public administrations with general and special budgets, provincial special administrations, local authorities and villages, foundations granted tax exemption by the President, and associations operating in the public interest, as well as institutions and organisations engaged in scientific research and development activities, The full amount of aid and donations made towards the construction costs of youth centres and youth and scouting camps belonging to the Ministry of Youth and Sport may be deducted from the corporate tax base. Furthermore, all cash and in-kind donations and contributions made to enable existing facilities to continue their operations may also be deducted in full from the corporate tax base (Corporate Tax Law, Article 10/ç).

In Türkiye, sports clubs may operate legally either as associations or as public limited companies (Karataş Durmuş, 2016, p. 245). With the aim of supporting the development of sport , the legislator has, under Article 4/1-j of the Corporation Tax Act, exempted the economic enterprises belonging to sports clubs and joint-stock companies engaged solely in training and sporting activities from corporation tax (Karataş Durmuş, 2016, p. 245). However, the exemption is limited solely to sporting activities; non-sporting commercial enterprises operated by clubs, such as restaurants, car parks, petrol stations or hotels, are subject to corporation tax (Gürek, 2018, p. 70).

Sponsorship is one of the most critical elements in the financing of sport in Türkiye and is incentivised through the Income Tax and Corporation Tax Acts (İmamoğlu, 2009, p. 72). Under the applicable legislation, sponsorship expenditure is deductible in full for amateur sports and at 50 per cent for professional sports (İmamoğlu, 2009, p. 85; Çınarlı & Ersöz, 2010, p. 150).

Value Added Tax Incentives

Article 13(k) of the Value Added Tax Law No. 3065, which exempts certain supplies and services from tax, also includes sports-related supplies and services (VAT Law, Art. 13(k)). Under the relevant provision, supplies and services provided to those making donations for the construction of youth centres and youth and scouting camps belonging to the Ministry of Youth and Sport—provided such donations are made to public administrations with general or special budgets, provincial special administrations, municipalities and villages—are exempt from VAT. Furthermore, in the article of the Value Added Tax Act listing other exemptions (VAT Act, Art. 17), there is an exemption applicable to sports facilities. General and special budgeted departments, provincial special administrations, local authorities, villages, universities, revolving fund organisations, public institutions and organisations, professional organisations with the status of public institutions, associations serving the public interest, and foundations granted tax exemption; the supplies and services they provide in connection with cultural and educational activities carried out through the operation or management of sports facilities are exempt from VAT. (VAT Law, Art. 17/1-b) From the perspective of Value Added Tax (VAT), whilst events in which professional sportspeople participate are subject to tax, services provided free of charge in amateur sports and certain activities of clubs with the status of associations operating in the public interest are exempt (Karataş Durmuş, 2016, p. 272).

It is observed that total tax expenditure on sport in Türkiye is projected to reach 1.5 billion TL by 2025. On the other hand, the exemptions granted to the commercial enterprises and public limited companies of sports clubs involved in training and sporting activities could not be calculated as the relevant data was unavailable. Yet sports clubs constitute the group that generates the highest added value within the sports industry.

Table 3. Tax Expenditures on Sports Activities in Türkiye

Tax type and legal provision	Explanation of incentive/exemption	Amount for 2024, TL	Amount for 2025, TL
Income Tax — Income Tax Code, Article 23/15	Exemption relating to remuneration paid by employers of amateur sportspeople to such sportspeople	122,498,000	159,259,000
Income Tax — Income Tax Code, Article 29/3	Exemption relating to prizes and bonuses awarded to amateur sportsmen and women participating in sporting competitions	31,147,000	40,494,000
Income Tax — Income Tax Code, Article 29(4)	Exemption relating to fees paid to referees officiating at amateur sports competitions	69,335,000	90,142,000
Income Tax — Income Tax Code, Article 89/8	Deduction for sponsorship expenditure incurred by income tax payers for amateur and professional sports	184,491,000	257,281,000
Income Tax — Transitional Article 72 of the Income Tax Code	Withholding tax at reduced rates on remuneration and payments treated as remuneration made to sportspeople	233,556,000	303,646,000
Corporation Tax — Article 4(1)(j) of the Corporation Tax Code	Exemption granted to the commercial enterprises and public limited companies of sports clubs engaged in training and sporting activities	Data not available	Data not available

continued on following page

Table 3. Continued

Tax type and legal provision	Explanation of incentive/exemption	Amount for 2024, TL	Amount for 2025, TL
Corporation Tax — Corporation Tax Law, Article 10(1)(b)	Deduction for sponsorship expenditure incurred by corporation tax payers	523,366,000	609,770,000
Other Legislation — Law No. 5894 on the Turkish Football Federation	Corporation tax exemption for the Turkish Football Federation	No tax expenditure has arisen	No tax expenditure has arisen

Source: Compiled using data from the Turkish Revenue Administration (GİB, 2025).

4. Policy Assessment of Tax Incentives for Sport in Türkiye

Although sports clubs account for a limited share of the number of enterprises within the 93.1 Sports Activities sector, they carry significant weight in terms of value added. However, the lack of detailed data on which types of clubs, which sports disciplines and which regions benefit from tax expenditure makes it difficult to assess the distributional fairness of the incentives. However, it should not be overlooked that tax incentive schemes cover major sports clubs. There is a need to restructure sports incentives so that they move away from being purely performance-oriented and instead take into account healthy living and social inclusion.

Disabled sports disciplines face significant difficulties in securing sponsors due to their limited reach and low advertising potential (Çınarlı and Ersöz, 2010, p. 153). The 100 per cent tax relief provided for amateur disciplines under current legislation does not generate sufficient motivation for these disciplines. Çınarlı and Ersöz (2010, p. 154) recommend offering more radical incentives to companies sponsoring para-sports, such as direct offsetting against tax liabilities or additional tax credits. Ultimately, one way to achieve the target set out in the 12th Development Plan of increasing the number of disabled athletes to 100,000 by 2028 (SBB, n.d.) is to increase tax incentives for this sector.

Under the previous investment incentive framework, sports tourism facility investments were assessed within the category of strategic investments (Günay & Enes, 2014, p. 6). Under the current legislation, sports facility investments with a minimum fixed investment amount of TL 15 million may qualify for VAT exemption and customs duty exemption (Cumhurbaşkanı Kararı No. 9903). These incentives may contribute to the development of sports facility infrastructure, sports tourism and tourism revenues.

Comparative data reported for 2017 indicate that tax rates applied to professional athletes in countries such as France, England and Italy were substantially higher than Türkiye's pre-2020 withholding rate. However, the amendments introduced by

Law No. 7194, including the obligation to submit an annual tax return above a specified income threshold and the increase in the top-league withholding rate, reduced this tax advantage to some extent (Çeribaş, 2020, pp. 575–576). The absence of a comparable improvement in sporting success despite favourable tax treatment also suggests that tax advantages alone are insufficient to address the structural problems of professional sport in Türkiye (Ergür & Köstekçi, 2021, p. 2949).

It has been argued that Türkiye's relatively low tax burden on professional athletes has encouraged clubs to recruit expensive foreign players nearing the end of their careers, without producing a comparable improvement in sporting success (Bay & İnneci, 2017, p. 211). This tax treatment has also been criticised on the grounds that it weakens tax equity and results in a loss of public revenue (Ergür & Köstekçi, 2021, p. 2947). From a long-term policy perspective, directing a greater share of tax support towards young domestic athletes and grassroots development could contribute more effectively to the sustainable development of sport.

A practical limitation of sponsorship deductions is that they operate through the tax base. Consequently, they provide little or no tax benefit to firms that do not generate sufficient taxable profits. Research on amateur sports clubs in Türkiye also indicates that difficulties in obtaining sponsorship constitute an important component of their financial problems and that sponsorship tends to be concentrated in more popular sports disciplines (Erturan-Öğüt & Şahin, 2017, pp. 105–106).For this reason, the contribution of tax incentives to the development of sport should be examined, and support should be provided to amateur sports clubs and companies that promote grassroots sport. As a policy option, targeted tax or social insurance contribution incentives could be considered for fitness centres that provide accessible, affordable and regularly monitored physical-activity services. Any such support should be conditional on measurable public-health and participation criteria rather than being granted as a general sector-wide exemption. Such a policy could be piloted in regions with low levels of physical activity or limited access to community sports facilities, and its effects should be evaluated before wider implementation.

CONCLUSION

The current tax treatment of professional athletes has been criticised on the grounds that it creates tax equity concerns and may lead to a loss of public revenue (Ergür & Köstekçi, 2021, p. 2949). In this study, it is argued that a greater share of sports-related tax support should be directed towards grassroots participation, amateur clubs and inclusive sporting activities. For sporting success to become sustainable, incentives must be linked *not* only to *'expenditure'-based* criteria but also to *'performance and* infrastructure'-focused criteria (Çeribaş, 2020, p. 578).

Tax incentives granted for sponsorship expenditure increase the private sector's interest in sport and also support amateur athletes. However, restructuring tax incentives for sponsorship expenditure to provide greater support to amateur sports clubs could contribute to the grassroots development of sport. Furthermore, structuring the low tax burden on athletes in a way that supports domestic athletes could help to discover new talent in sport. Furthermore, there is a need for greater incentives to support sports for people with disabilities. However, it should not be overlooked that tax advantages for sport may not always achieve their intended purpose, and that incentives need to be supported by public expenditure directed specifically towards the development of sport, in addition to tax advantages. In the absence of regular impact assessments, it is not possible to determine whether the economic and social benefits generated by sport-related tax incentives are proportionate to their fiscal cost. For this reason, sport-related tax expenditures should be subject to periodic cost-effectiveness and distributional-impact assessments.

Sport is also a fundamental tool for a healthy lifestyle. From a preventive-health perspective, policies that increase regular participation in physical activity may help reduce the incidence of health conditions associated with physical inactivity. In this regard, tax incentives for sport could be provided not only to professional sports clubs that support competitive success, but also to fitness centres that help people stay in shape. Turkish Statistical Institute (TÜİK) data on the sports industry indicates that, particularly in fitness and bodybuilding centres, the value added per employee remains below the annual minimum wage. Policymakers could consider a targeted support mechanism for small-scale fitness and physical-activity centres operating in neighbourhoods where access to public sports facilities is limited. Eligibility for such support could be linked to affordable membership fees, services for young people, older persons and people with disabilities, qualified staffing, and evidence of regular participation.. A complementary entrepreneurship programme could also be considered for graduates of sport sciences faculties who wish to establish small-scale physical-activity or fitness enterprises. Such support could include business-development training, access to start-up finance and temporary social security contribution relief, subject to professional qualification, service-quality and formal-employment requirements.

REFERENCES

Ağazade, S. (2025). An analysis of the Turkish sports industry based on data from the sports activities sector. In Günay, N. (Ed.), *Proceedings of the Turkish Sports Congress: From the Founding of the Republic to the Turkish Century* (25–27 April 2024). Turkish Historical Society Publications. https://ttk.gov.tr/wp-content/uploads/2025/10/46-Seymur-Agazde.pdf DOI: 10.37879/978-975-17-6294-8.2025.1015

Bay, H., & İnneci, A. (2017). The taxation of wage income in Türkiye from the perspective of tax justice. *International Journal of Public Finance*, *2*(2), 196–219. DOI: 10.30927/ijpf.327776

Çeribaş, D. (2020). The taxation of athletes' wages in Türkiye. *Hacettepe Law Faculty Journal*, *10*(2), 555–583. https://doi.org/10.32957/hacettepehdf.761172

Çınarlı, S., & Ersöz, G. (2010). Recommendations regarding sponsorship and tax regulations in terms of the development of sports services for people with disabilities. Journal of the Institute of Social Sciences. *Süleyman Demirel University*, (12), 141–156. https://izlik.org/JA38NX95DD

ÇSGB. (n.d.). https://www.csgb.gov.tr/poco-pages/asgari-ucret/ (Accessed Date:02/05/2026)

Değer, R. (2022). The Development of the Sports Economy in Turkey and State Support. *Scientific Journal of Finance and Financial Law Studies, 2*(1), 61-70. https://izlik.org/JA76NH54DY (Accessed Date:02/03/2026)

Ergür, O. K., & Köstekçi, A. (2021). Tax justice in the taxation of wage income in Türkiye: The case of athletes. *Journal of Human and Social Sciences Research, 10*(3), 2936–2951. https://doi.org/10.15869/itobiad.907247

Eriçok, R. E. (2019). The Evolution of Tax Expenditures in Turkey: 2015-2021. *Istanbul Journal of Economics, 69*(2), 321-355. https://doi.org/10.26650/ISTJECON2019-0012

Erturan-Öğüt, E., & Şahin, M. Y. (2017). Problems of amateur sports clubs: An exploratory study. *Journal of Sports Sciences*, *28*(2), 101–120. https://doi.org/10.17644/sbd.356710

GİB (Revenue Administration). (2025) *Tax Expenditure Report*. https://cdn.gib.gov.tr/api/gibportal-file/file/getFileResources?objectKey=arsiv/kurumsal/Vergi_Harcamalari_Raporu_2025.pdf (Accessed: 24/05/2026)

Günay, F., & Enes, K. (2014). *An analysis of incentives and support provided for sports tourism. 3rd Eastern Mediterranean Tourism Congress*. Congress Date 21-04-2014 / 23-04-2014, Mersin, 92-103. https://www.researchgate.net/publication/357484948_SPOR_TURIZMINE_SAGLANAN_TESVIK_VE_DESTEKLER_UZERINE_BIR_INCELEME (Accessed Date:01/05/2026)

Gürek, A. (2018). *Taxation of footballers and football clubs in Türkiye* [Master's thesis]. Istanbul Okan University. https://tez.yok.gov.tr/UlusalTezMerkezi/tezDetay.jsp?id=mWVegi4Y8dm1L-kP2wOFtA&no=x6LgKBRezeWFAQwolhPZ1w (Accessed Date:02/04/2026)

İmamoğlu, S. H. (2009). An evaluation of the legal framework regarding sports sponsorship. *Ankara University Faculty of Law Journal, 58*(1), 63–94. https://doi.org/10.1501/Hukfak_0000001564

Karataş Durmuş, N. (2016). Taxation of Sports Clubs. *Journal of the Turkish Academy of Justice, 27*, 245-278. https://izlik.org/JA86CW76RB

Öz, E., Akçay, F. (2013) Taxation of Athletes, with a Focus on Footballers. *Journal of Tax Issues, 300*, September, 35-54

SBB (n.d.). *Presidency of Strategy and Budget, Twelfth Development Plan.* On-Ikinci-Kalkinma-Plani_2024-2028_11122023.pdf (Accessed Date:24/05/2026)

Tugal, A., Özden, S., Türkay, H., & Şahin, O. (2025). Sport as an Investment Vehicle. *International Journal of Current Educational Research, 11*(1), 29-41. https://izlik.org/JA48PH88GR

TÜİK. (2024) *Industry and Services Statistics*. https://biruni.tuik.gov.tr/medas/?kn=129&locale=tr (Accessed: 24/05/2026)

Chapter 7
Targeting Sports Subsidies for Social Welfare:
Principles, Paradoxes, and Policy Implications

Komal Komal
http://orcid.org/0009-0007-1415-6857
Lakshmibai National Institute of Physical Education, India

Mahendra Kumar Singh
http://orcid.org/0000-0001-9989-9420
Lakshmibai National Institute of Physical Education, India

Sohom Saha
http://orcid.org/0009-0006-9438-1554
Lakshmibai National Institute of Physical Education, India

Sumit Kumar Singh
http://orcid.org/0009-0000-1728-8213
Lakshmibai National Institute of Physical Education, India

ABSTRACT

This chapter examines whether government spending on sport truly improves social welfare. While sport is often promoted as a way to enhance health, social inclusion, and community development, evidence shows that its benefits are uneven and sometimes overstated. Public funding frequently supports elite and commercially successful sports rather than community-based activities that benefit wider populations. A key concept discussed is the "subsidy paradox," where funding intended

DOI: 10.4018/979-8-2600-3174-2.ch007

to help disadvantaged groups often benefits already advantaged individuals due to barriers such as cost, access, and social support. The chapter applies theories from economics and social justice to evaluate when sport subsidies are justified. It proposes a capability-based framework that focuses on improving real opportunities for participation, especially for disadvantaged groups. Overall, the chapter calls for fairer distribution, better evaluation, and policy reforms to ensure sport funding genuinely contributes to social welfare.

1. INTRODUCTION: SPORT, STATE, AND THE WELFARE QUESTION

There few areas of public investment that enjoy as wide political support as sport. Whether in social democratic welfare states or liberal market economies, governments invest public funds in sport infrastructure, elite performance and participatory sport for all, and do so in the name of sport's unique social value: its ability to promote health, community, identity and inclusion. Yet empirical evidence of these effects is far more contestable than the rhetoric of political justification, and the distributional outcomes of state investment in sport are often at odds with the presumed welfare benefits that are invoked to justify such investment (Madsen, 2009). The disjuncture between rhetorical justification and welfare reality is the central concern of this chapter, and a gap that has become more politically significant as austerity policies in many developed countries have heightened the focus on the value of public investment in sport for individual citizens, communities and the welfare of nations.

When, if ever, and for whom state intervention in sport delivers social welfare benefits is not just an empirical question. It is indeed a normative question about the appropriate ends of public spending and the appropriate metrics by which public investment should be assessed. But sport policy research has lagged behind other fields of social policy in its rigorous engagement with the theoretical traditions (welfare economics, political philosophy, public goods theory) that are used widely in other areas of social policy to examine the links between public intervention and social welfare (Sam, 2009). In other areas of policy, including education policy, housing policy and health policy, well-developed theoretical traditions link public investment to welfare outcomes through robust normative argumentation. By contrast, sport policy has often invoked rather than theorised, and its assertion of the social benefits of sport has not been grounded in the evaluative frameworks that are required to determine whether particular patterns of public investment function to advance the welfare goals that are claimed in its name. This chapter seeks to redress that deficiency and in so doing provides theoretical context for the volume in which it appears.

To grasp the full implications of this theoretical shortfall, we need to understand the magnitude of public investment in sport sustained by governments in a range of national settings. For example, in the United Kingdom, billions of pounds are spent on sport and physical activity each year by the state in the form of facility investment, support for national governing bodies, elite performance support and mass participation programs (De Castro et al., 2025; Schausteck De Almeida et al., 2018). In Australia, Canada, Germany, the Netherlands and in the Nordic countries, similar levels of public investment in sport are premised by a political consensus that public investment in sport is justified by commensurate public value. Yet the lack of robust theoretical and evaluative frameworks for gauging that value means that the consensus is grounded in very tenuous intellectual foundations - foundations that are seldom tested because the social desirability of sport is so widely taken for granted that, for many policy practitioners, it seems superfluous, if not counterintuitive, to subject it to welfare-theoretic inquiry. This taken-for-grantedness is the principal claim of this chapter; it is a political achievement of those who stand to benefit from the status quo in sport investment, and it is incumbent on good and transparent sport policy to undo it.

This chapter puts forward three related arguments. First, it contends that sport is a complex and contested public/private good and that the principled application of public goods theory yields both principled grounds for sport subsidy and principled grounds against it, which are conveniently ignored in policy debates. Second, it theorises the subsidy paradox: the systematic tendency for public investment in sport to benefit the already advantaged, reversing the redistributive justification for public sport investment. Third, building on the work of Sen (2009), the chapter offers a normative framework - the welfare-alignment criteria - for assessing when sport subsidies can and cannot be justified as public policy, and when they cannot. Combined, these arguments represent a call for a theoretical reorientation in the field of sport policy and a tool for assessing sport investment for its social welfare effects.

The chapter proceeds as follows. Section 2 explores public goods analysis of sport and develops a typology of sport provision and welfare outcomes. Section 3 looks at social cohesion claims, separating theoretical from empirical dimensions. Section 4 explores the political economy of the sport subsidy and elite capture of public investment. Section 5 theorises the subsidy paradox in sport. Section 6 proposes the capability-based approach to welfare-aligned sport subsidy. Section 7 offers the welfare-alignment criteria as a normative scorecard. Section 8 concludes with an analysis of the changed ideology that welfare-aligned policy demands of sport.

2. PUBLIC GOODS THEORY APPLIED TO SPORT: A TYPOLOGICAL ANALYSIS

The traditional framework for analysing state provision of goods and services draws on Samuelson's (1954) seminal theory of public expenditure, which identified two characteristics of public goods: non-rivalry in consumption (use of the good by one person does not limit the availability of the good to others) and non-excludability in access (it is impossible to exclude non-paying users from enjoying the good) (Samuelson, 1954). Samuelson's analysis laid the groundwork for the modern discipline of public finance, and offered the central economic argument for state provision of goods that the market tends to under-provide. The argument is simple: if goods are non-rival and non-excludable, it is in the self-interest of individuals to avoid the costs of providing goods and to free-ride on the provision of others, resulting in systematic undersupply of socially valuable goods unless the state intervenes to provide the goods and fund provision through compulsory taxation (Musgrave, 1987). Built on this framework by introducing the notion of merit goods: goods whose social value is greater than the value as determined by private consumption, therefore justifying state subsidy on paternal or distributional grounds, despite their potential provision by the market.

This analysis immediately runs into problems when applied to sport. The term sport covers a myriad of activities, institutional arrangements, and provision arrangements; each of these fall at different points along the spectrum of public/private goods. Elite spectator sport (professional football, Olympic athletics, international cricket) displays considerable degrees of rivalry and excludability: major events are capacity constrained and access is often made exclusive through ticketing, broadcasting and high prices. The economics of professional sport has thoroughly examined the private good aspects of elite spectator sport events and the economic merits of public subsidies to privately owned stadiums and sport franchises (Hassan & Lewis, 2007). The sport economics consensus is strong: that the direct economic benefit of public stadium subsidy is routinely overestimated by promoters and that the methodological flaws inherent to commissioned economic impact studies (lack of attention to substitution, time switching effects and leakage) result in inflated multiplier estimates that do not pass muster (Crompton, 2006). This reliance on such studies as the justification for major, publicly subsidised sport infrastructure is less a matter of welfare-economic analysis than political theatre, a display of economic rigour that obscures the degree to which subsidy is based on the preferences of organised sporting and commercial elites rather than the welfare needs of the citizenry whose taxes are used to fund the investment.

But this critique of elite sport subsidy is not the whole story on public goods in sport. Public goods characteristics of community-scale sport infrastructure (public parks, municipal swimming pools, community sports halls, public access to recreational facilities) are more pronounced, especially where investment is structured to avoid exclusion (through price) from its benefits. Further, the benefits of all levels of sport have what are called positive externalities: benefits to non-participants and the broader public that are not priced in the market and therefore under-supplied. The externalities of physical activity health benefits are well documented (Clays et al., 2014): reductions in health-care expenditure relating to chronic diseases linked with physical inactivity represent a non-excludable benefit of public investments in sport participation which the market fails to supply. The social externalities of sport - community integration, identification, youth participation, reduction in delinquency - are less empirically clear but are potential candidates for non-excludable social benefits from public sport provision (Sherry & Coalter, 2009). The welfare-economic argument for public sport provision is therefore not black-and-white but nuanced: strongest when the public health externalities are well known, the provision of sport is non-excludable and the benefits flow to those with the greatest unmet welfare need.

This analysis leads to an analytical typology of sport provision with policy implications. At one extreme, elite professional sport provision by private profit-making entities fails both tests of public goods status and creates no welfare-economic case for unconditional public subsidy: its externalities, if they exist at all, are limited and the benefits are enjoyed by an elite few. At the other pole, community sport facilities available to all, with known health and social externalities, provide a compelling case for public provision on welfare-economic grounds. In between lie modes of provision (elite national sport, semi-professional leagues, national governing body pathways) whose public goods status is open to question and whose social value is to be empirically determined, case by case, rather than claimed a priori. A proper public goods approach to sport policy would require that each mode of public investment be assessed in terms of the market failure it claims to address, with the standard of evidence commensurate with the size of the public investment.

Even if sport fails the technical tests for public goods, the state is justified in subsidy if it can be shown that individuals systematically underestimate the health, social and other benefits of physical activity compared to its welfare consequences. Behavioural welfare economics has supported this argument: present-bias, information asymmetries and social norm effects generate systematic biases in individual sport participation choices relative to socially optimal levels of participation that merit good reasoning can justify remediation through public subsidy (Watson, 2011). The work of Kahneman and others in behavioural economics has shown that humans are generally poor at valuing future social and health benefits against the present costs of participation, a well-known cognitive bias that results in participation levels that are lower than they would be if individuals were fully informed and able to act on their long-term welfare expectations. The merit good justification is, however, explicitly paternalistic and its application to sport must be separated from an egalitarian welfare justification: a merit good justification for sport subsidy is compatible with subsidising the participation of anyone, while a welfare-egalitarian justification is solely concerned with overcoming barriers to participation by the structurally disadvantaged. The normative implications of these alternative justificatory paths are quite different, as later sections of this chapter reveal.

3. SOCIAL COHESION REVISITED: BONDING, BRIDGING, AND THE LIMITS OF SPORT CAPITAL

Social cohesion is one of the most politically resilient rationales for public investment in sport: that there is something about common participation in sport culture that produces the social connections across ethnic, class and generational divisions that are essential to democratic politics. This claim has enjoyed remarkable political longevity across ideological and national boundaries, furnishing sport with a mode of expression that is widely palatable to public and political opinion. Its empirical and theoretical underpinnings are somewhat less resilient (Sherry & Coalter, 2009);(Putnam, 2000a). The social cohesion claim's political resilience is no guarantee of its truth. It is a reflection of the political attractiveness of the claim to a broad constituency of political actors: for the political right, sport's capacity for social cohesion associates itself with themes of community self-organization and voluntary action; for the political left, it associates itself with themes of inclusion and social solidarity. The multi-faceted political utility of the social cohesion claim should be a cue for critical reflection rather than unreflective acceptance.

The most theoretically advanced approach to the analysis of the cohesive potential of sport is offered by the distinction between bonding and bridging social capital (Putnam, 2000a). Bonding social capital refers to the high-trust relationships that exist within relatively closed, similar groups (for example, people of similar social class, ethnic background or personal identity), and is associated with strong within-group solidarity and mobilisation. Bridging social capital is the lighter, more diverse network of intergroup relationships that promote civic participation, tolerance and integration. For Putnam, a democratic society needs both, but policymaking tends to overlook the more challenging task of investing in bridging capital, opting instead for the more naturally "self-organising" bonding capital. In terms of sport, Putnam's thesis is a sobering one. The evidence for sport's ability to generate bonding capital among relatively homogenous sporting communities is quite good: repeated participation in shared sporting activities generates trust, reciprocity, and shared identity among the co-participants (Nicholson & Hoye, 2008). The evidence for sport's capacity to generate bridging capital across social divisions is much more limited and contingent.

Kay & Bradbury (2009) systematic review of the evidence reveals that sport delivers social cohesion benefits primarily when it is explicitly designed to facilitate cross-cultural interaction, when facilitators of sport programs are given training in relationship-building, and when participants in sport activities possess approximately equal status. The absence of these conditions, which is often the case in competitive sport in which success and failure is ranked hierarchically, may result in social divisions being reinforced by sport. Competition creates winners and losers, and the ranking of athletic performance is an easy fit with pre-existing social hierarchies in ways that can support and validate them, rather than subvert them. The talented young working-class athlete who succeeds in a meritocratic sport structure may be celebrated as an example of sport's emancipatory potential; the failure of that structure to attract, retain, or nurture working class athletes who lack the cultural, social and financial capital of their middle-class counterparts is untold and undocumented.

Grusky & Szelényi (2006) theory of fields offers a more structurally oriented critique of sport and social reproduction. Bourdieu's view is that sport fields are not neutral, meritocratic settings of competition but sites where existing distributions of economic, social and cultural capital are reproduced and legitimated through competitive activity. The different sporting tastes and practices of the social classes, from working-class identification with collective team sports to upper-middle-class participation in individual sports requiring costly equipment and training, are emblematic of the distribution of economic, social and cultural capital across social class. The symbolic power of sport resides precisely in its ability to mask what are structural realities-differential participation in sporting culture-as the expression of individual taste, ability and effort: the "meritocratic myth." The brilliance of this cultural formation is that it conceals itself precisely by rendering invisible the structural impediments to participation in sport that those who have never experienced them do not see: hence, the sporting success of the advantaged can be explained by natural ability and effort, rather than by the advantages of class position.

Critical sport studies scholars have applied Bourdieu's insights to sport's role in the reproduction of race and gender inequalities (Hylton, 2009a), application of critical race theory to sport illustrates how seemingly race-neutral sports policies reproduce racial inequalities by privileging sports cultures and organisational structures that reproduce the norms of the white majority. The discourse of 'talent identification' in sport, for example, is always culturally weighted by racial assumptions such that the "natural talent" that sport gatekeepers recognise and reward is not neutral but shaped by assumptions about what kinds of bodies, athletic movement patterns, and sporting dispositions represent true athletic potential (Hylton, 2009b). Andrews & Silk (2012) explore how neoliberal approaches to sport policy, which frame individual participation in sport as an exercise of free will and individual responsibility, obscure the structural realities - poverty, segregation, lack of local sporting infrastructure - that limit access to the freedom of the field for large segments of the population.

The meritocratic mythology of sport has, in their view, not just an incidental but rather a constitutive role in sport policy: the political appeal of sport as a social policy vehicle is partly derived from its capacity to present structural welfare issues as subject to voluntary individual solutions that do not involve redistribution of income and power. If sport can promote social cohesion, health, and civic agency, then the social conditions that generate social division, ill-health, and powerlessness can be tackled via sport policy rather than more politically challenging avenues such as income redistribution, restructuring of housing and education policy, or ensuring economic and political power is devolved to marginalised communities. The social cohesion argument for sport, on this analysis, has the ideological purpose of displacing a politically unpalatable "structural" solution with an attractive "cultural" one. This critique does not mean that sport has no social cohesion potential. Rather, that the conditions for sport to generate genuine bridging capital and social integration (rather than the semblance of these outcomes) are specific, challenging and often absent in mainstream sport policy programmes (Sherry & Coalter, 2009).

This conditional proposition is supported by (Coakley, 2011) research on youth sport development. In his research on positive youth development in sport he found that the outcomes often claimed for sport participation - leadership, resilience, social responsibility - occur predictably only when the following conditions are met: when the goals of the sport program are developmental as well as competitive; when the adults who work with the young people prioritise their agency and voice; when participation is voluntary and free from coercive pressures; and when the structure of the program environment promotes, rather than reinforces, hierarchy. When these conditions are in place, sport can positively develop young people across a wide range of social backgrounds. When they do not, as is the case in most youth sport programmes that are organised to compete, the developmental claims attributed to sport are aspirational.

4. THE POLITICAL ECONOMY OF SPORT SUBSIDY: ELITE BIAS AND MARKET FAILURE

To understand why sport subsidies often fail to achieve their espoused welfare goals, it is necessary to consider not only the technical conditions for the supply of public goods but the political economy of sport governance: the constellation of institutional power, ideological belief and distributional struggle that informs public sport investment outcomes. While a welfare-economic analysis of market failure is a necessary condition for understanding the outcomes of sport subsidies, a political economy analysis is needed to explain why market failures that justify community sport subsidies are not addressed as generously as market failures (often much weaker) that justify elite sport subsidies.

The political economy of sport subsidy is determined in part by a number of structural aspects of sport governance that skew public investment in favour of elite and commercially organised sport at the expense of community and recreational sport. First, organised sports (national governing bodies, international federations, professional sport leagues) represent powerful, organised interests with direct access to policy processes and established lines of communication with government sport ministries, and the resources to lobby for preferred public investment priorities. In contrast, community sport provision is often represented by unstructured, less organised interests without such institutional access to policy-making (Houlihan & Green, 2011). This organisational bias in political representation favours the resource demands of powerful, elite sport interests over other forms of sport. The asymmetry is not coincidental, but is a consequence of patterns of past public investment: public support for organised sport has, over time, produced powerful institutions that are vested in extending and entrenching patterns of public resource allocation.

The path dependency of sport governance - that is, the ways in which past institutional arrangements shape future resource allocation - is a key but little understood aspect of sport policy systems. Second, the politics of elite sport success and national sporting glory creates enthusiasm in public and political circles that is not matched in community sport. Olympic medals, World Cup success and international sporting success trigger symbolic politics (national identity, pride, international standing) that mobilise political support for elite sport investment despite weak evidence of the welfare benefits of such investment (Houlihan & Green, 2011). The idea of 'trickle down' participation - that elite success stimulates mass participation - offers a politically convenient, but empirically questionable rationale for investing public resources in elite sport that primarily serves preselected talented athletes from upper-class backgrounds (Weed et al., 2015a). In their systematic review, Weed and colleagues found no evidence that major sport event hosting or elite success led to long-term increases in mass sport participation, but the trickle-down assumption remains a policy driver in several national settings, confirming its political utility despite the absence of evidence. Third, the infrastructure politics of major sport events (arena construction, urban development, transport infrastructure) create coalitions between sport governing bodies, urban developers, construction capital and municipal governments that can be mobilised to support large-scale public investment in sport (Crompton, 2006).

These coalitions are typically better organised and better funded than the coalitions that might emerge to advocate for community sport infrastructure investment, resulting in a systematic skew in sport capital expenditure towards large and profitable facilities in urban centres and away from accessible community facilities in areas where welfare needs are greatest. The winners from major event infrastructure investment (property developers, construction firms, hospitality and tourism providers) have clear financial interests in public investment in elite sport infrastructure and the organisational capacity to bring these interests to bear politically. The communities most in need of accessible local sport facilities tend not to have either.

There is a great deal of empirical evidence for this elite bias in sport subsidy. Evidence from a number of national settings (the United Kingdom, Australia, Canada, Germany and the Netherlands) has shown that the allocation of public sport investment is consistently biased in favour of performance sport development pathways, major event hosting and high-profile facility construction as opposed to community access infrastructure (Sam, 2009) (Houlihan & Green, 2011). In the United Kingdom, the Active People surveys by Sport England from 2005 to 2016 consistently found that sport participation was positively associated with income, education and social class, meaning that years of public investment in sport had not improved participation rates across the class divide. Similarly, the Australian government's post-Montreal Olympic Games (1976) audit of national sport investment revealed that most public funds had been spent on elite development pathways serving a pre-selected group of talented young athletes from middle-class families (Houlihan & Green, 2011).

This analysis does not mean that elite sport investment lacks any valid social functions or that there are no market failures in elite sport provision. It does imply that the welfare-theoretic justification of elite sport subsidy is much more precarious than its political salience would imply, that the welfare effects of elite sport investment are distributed in ways that are systematically inconsistent with the social welfare functions that justify public expenditure and that a rigorous, welfare-theoretic approach to sport policy requires a significant refocusing of sport subsidy priorities onto the forms of provision that actually generate allocatively efficient, equitably distributed welfare gains. The political economy analysis outlined in this section is not despondent about the prospects for reform but realistic about the institutional challenges confronting welfare-congruent reform. Knowing those obstacles is a precondition for overcoming them.

5. THE SUBSIDY PARADOX: STRUCTURAL TENSIONS IN SPORT WELFARE POLICY

The disconnect between the redistributive politics of sport policy and its distributive effects is not merely a consequence of implementation failure, sub-optimal program design or weak monitoring. It is an expression of what this chapter calls the subsidy paradox: a systemic characteristic of sport subsidy regimes that sees the political economy of sport governance work to distribute public resources in favour of already advantaged groups, even - and perhaps particularly - in circumstances where the policy goal is to improve the welfare of disadvantaged groups. The subsidy paradox is not an aberration to be eliminated by piecemeal reform but a structural element of sport governance that calls for structural, rather than technical, solutions. Its recognition and analysis are the main analytical contribution of this chapter.

The subsidy paradox manifests in a number of ways. First is what might be called the complementarity of sporting capital: the ability to participate in organised, subsidised sport is dependent on complementary resources - time, money, transport, equipment, social networks, physical literacy, confidence - which are highly correlated with social advantage (Bourdieu, 1984; Roberts, 2008). Price subsidies provided by governments (in the form of subsidised sporting facilities, reduced fees or free sport programs) serve those who already have the complementary resources required to turn price reductions into participation. Those most disadvantaged in terms of access to participation (low-income populations, single parents, the disabled, rural residents) tend not to have the complementary resources necessary to benefit from price subsidies, and therefore benefit least from the most common forms of sport subsidy (Kay & Bradbury, 2009b). The implication is counterintuitive but important: price subsidies in the absence of complementary support interventions (transport support, childcare, equipment provision, coaching, outreach) will underserve the populations most in need of welfare gain, even when ostensibly targeted at these populations.

The second mechanism is spatial targeting of sport infrastructure investment. Public sport facilities are unevenly distributed across regions with different levels of existing sport culture (typically well-urbanised areas, rich suburbs and university towns) due to both historical capital investment patterns and the political economy of facility location (in which organised sport cultures are better able to lobby for investment than unorganised, resource-poor communities). This results in a spatial pattern of subsidised access to sport that reproduces rather than offsets patterns of socioeconomic inequality. The geography of sport infrastructure does not simply reflect historical coincidence but also reproduces existing patterns of advantage: areas better endowed with political and economic resources are able to attract and retain more sport infrastructure, generating a snowball effect that reinforces existing inequalities. Sport infrastructure under-supply in impoverished communities is thus both a welfare problem (the communities that most need the welfare benefits of sport) and a public investment problem (the communities that least benefit from the geography of public sport investment).

The third is the governance capture of subsidy allocation. The institutions that receive public sport investment - national governing bodies, regional sport councils, sport facility operators - are typically governed by representatives of existing sport communities: participants, club members, volunteer board members. These institutions are seldom representative of the non-participating population, and their investment priorities reflect the interests of existing sport participants - not those most marginalised from sport culture. Roberts (2008) traces this governance capture in several contexts of national sport policy development, showing that there was systematic evidence of how publicly funded sport development initiatives were driven by the institutional interests of governing bodies rather than the social welfare of target populations. The democratic deficit in sport governance is not a secondary feature of the subsidy paradox but fundamental to it: when government institutions that manage public sport investment are captured by advantaged communities, the welfare logic of investment is undermined.

The fourth pathway is the measurement and evaluation bias toward participation numbers as the key indicator of sport policy success. If participation is the primary measure of programme success, policies that boost participation among already-inclined populations (those closest to participation, with lowest barriers) will have a higher return on investment than policies that target the most excluded populations, which demand more intensive and costly policy interventions to boost participation. This creates incentive-biased measurement to invest in lower marginal cost of participation gain (the already advantaged) than marginal need (the most excluded), creating a welfare-adverse targeting bias in sport policy (Weed et al., 2015b). This measurement distortion is compounded by the short funding cycles of most sport programmes, which generate pressure to deliver participation gains in the short-term rather than invest in the long-term, intensive and relational engagement with communities for whom barriers to participation are highest.

The normative implications of the subsidy paradox go beyond its empirical description that sport subsidies are socially inequitable. The paradox is political in the sense that welfare rhetoric that legitimates sport subsidy is actually used to justify patterns of investment that reproduce welfare inequality. When governments cite the social cohesion, public health, and community development potential of sport to justify public investment that overwhelmingly privileges middle- and upper-income communities, they are not simply making a mistake, they are mobilising an ideological rhetoric to the advantage of already-privileged sporting communities at the expense of the populations whose welfare needs legitimise their expenditure (Andrews & Silk, 2012; Coalter, 2007). Uncovering this paradox is not a theoretical point but a precondition of transparent sport policy. A sport policy framework that is unable to acknowledge the subsidy paradox cannot explain it, and a sport policy scholarship that cannot theorise it cannot fulfil its mandate to supply the information needed for democratic accountability of public institutions.

6. A CAPABILITY-BASED FRAMEWORK FOR WELFARE-ALIGNED SPORT INVESTMENT

Recognising the subsidy paradox poses a normative challenge: if current patterns of sport subsidy are structurally weighted against promoting welfare, what normative framework can guide an alternative approach to sport policy? This section provides such a framework, drawing on capability approach as the primary framework and supplementing it with the theories of distributive justice developed by Rawls (2020) and the list of capabilities developed by Nussbaum (2011). The capability approach is taken as the primary framework for three reasons: its focus on substantive freedom rather than formal access aligns with the structural analysis of participation barriers outlined in previous sections; its methodological priority of evaluating welfare outcomes by reference to individuals' lives (rather than aggregate data) represents an alternative to the aggregate participation counting of the subsidy paradox; and its compatibility with pluralist political philosophy means that it can be applied across different national and cultural contexts without imposing a substantive vision of the good life.

The capability approach recasts the normative question of welfare economics from 'what do individuals have?' to 'what can individuals do and be?'. Well-being, then, is not determined by income or resources, or the satisfaction of preferences, but by the substantive freedoms - capabilities - that individuals are able to exercise. An individual who has the formal right to play sport but cannot afford it (or does not have the time, transport, physical or cultural capital to do so) is not substantively free to play: formal access is not the same as substantive capability. This has significant implications for sport policy. Policies that increase formal access (via subsidised facilities or lower entry fees) but do not address complementary policies that make it harder for the most disadvantaged to participate may increase the number of participants, but not the substantive capability of the neediest. The capability approach requires a switch from the formal to the substantive in policy evaluation, away from the counting of participation toward its ability to create opportunities for people to be and do what they value as good.

To apply the capability approach to sport welfare, it's necessary to identify the capabilities supported by satisfying sport participation. Robeyns (2017) has shown that the extension of Sen's approach to policy analysis requires the identification of a policy-relevant capability set that can be used as the normative foundation for policy evaluation. Drawing on Sen's methodological flexibility and Nussbaum

(2011) more specific capabilities list, a set of sport-relevant capabilities might include: bodily health-the capability to be physically healthy, which sport contributes to through physical activity; bodily integrity-the capability to move freely and to have opportunities for physical recreation; affiliation-the capability to live with and toward others, to recognise and show concern for other human beings, and to engage in various forms of social interaction that sport can facilitate; and play-Nussbaum's specific inclusion of the capability to laugh, to play, to enjoy recreational activities as a central component of human flourishing (Nussbaum, 2011). All of these capabilities are curtailed for populations facing poverty, disability, geographical disadvantage, or social disadvantage, and it is in the expansion of these particular capabilities for these populations that sport investment can most plausibly claim welfare significance.

These are not just preferences to be satisfied but integral aspects of a fully human life whose loss or severe curtailment is a welfare loss with independent moral weight. This has profound implications for the evaluation of sport policy. A sport subsidy program that mainly serves already-healthy, socially-included people who already exercise broad sporting capabilities delivers low welfare gains in terms of capabilities. A programme which helps people who are poor, or disabled, or socially excluded, or geographically disadvantaged, to develop sporting capabilities that they otherwise would not have, generates significant welfare gains - precisely because it expands previously unavailable capabilities. The welfare gains from sport subsidy are greatest, then, where capability deficits are greatest. This turns the subsidy paradox on its head, which generates the smallest welfare gains where welfare need is greatest.

Sen's approach also calls for consideration of what he calls "conversion factors": the personal, social, and environmental conditions that affect the conversion of resources into capabilities (A. Sen, 2009). An individual with a physical disability may need much more sport-specific resources (specialised facilities, coaching, transport, social support) to achieve the same sporting capability as an able-bodied person. A woman living in a community where women do not participate in sport faces social conversion factors that cannot be addressed by resource provision. An isolated rural individual faces environmental conversion factor constraints that urban sport facility subsidies cannot overcome. Consequently, capability-sensitive sport policy must consider not just resource provision but also the personal, social and environmental all factors that determine whether resources can translate into effective capability for marginalised groups. This requires a more resource-intensive, context-sensitive and relationally attuned approach to sport policy program design than the generic, facility-focused models that currently predominate.

The theory of distributive justice proposed by Rawls (2020) offers a further principle for policy translation of the capability framework. The difference principle, that social and economic inequalities are just only if they maximally benefit the least-advantaged members of society, translates into a sport policy maximin criterion: public sport investment is only as distributively just as the structure of investment maximally enhances the sporting capabilities of the least-advantaged members of society (Rawls, 2020). This criterion does not rule out investment in elite sport or in already-active populations but requires that such investment can be justified by its benefits for the least-advantaged (for example, its trickle-down effects on participation or its public health benefits) rather than by its benefits to those who directly benefit themselves. If taken seriously, the Rawlsian criterion would require a significant shift in current priorities in sport investment: investment in elite development programs and major sporting events would need to be justified by their welfare effects on the least-advantaged before public money is spent, a test that most existing elite sport investment would not pass.

A sport policy framework that cannot justify the allocation of its subsidies to those who are excluded from the benefits of its investments (because the allocation of subsidies is determined by the preferences of existing sport communities and not the welfare needs of excluded groups) fails the impartiality criterion and therefore fails as a public policy framework. The impartiality criterion places a procedural condition on the distributive justice criterion: not only must sport investment lead to outcomes that benefit the least-advantaged, but the process of sport investment decision-making itself must be open to scrutiny by all parties, including those most excluded from the status quo of sporting culture. The welfare-alignment criteria developed in the next section operationalise this procedural criterion and the substantive welfare criteria developed above from the capability approach and Rawlsian justice.

7. WELFARE-ALIGNMENT CRITERIA: A NORMATIVE SCORECARD FOR SPORT POLICY

The theoretical framework developed so far furnishes a normative framework for real-world practice: a set of criteria for the "alignment" of sport subsidy policy with social welfare. These criteria are meant to be theoretically coherent (drawing on the welfare-economic, capability and distributional justice frameworks outlined above) and practically useful for assessing the contribution of actual sport policy programs in different national settings. These criteria are not a bureaucratic tool but a normative framework for public deliberation: they offer citizens, academics and policy-makers a common language through which to question whether public sport investment is being used to achieve the welfare ends claimed for it.

Table 1.Welfare-Alignment Criteria for Sport Subsidy Evaluation

Criterion	Assessment Question	Welfare-Alignment Indicator
Market Failure Correction	Does the subsidy address a demonstrable failure in private provision?	Evidence of positive externality or public good characteristic
Distributional Equity	Do participation gains accrue disproportionately to disadvantaged groups?	Disaggregated participation data by income, ethnicity, disability status
Capability Expansion	Does the intervention expand substantive freedoms, not merely formal access?	Capability assessment measures beyond participation counting
Spillover Measurability	Are claimed social benefits empirically measurable and independently verified?	Pre-registered evaluations; independent audit of social value claims
Governance Accountability	Are allocation decisions transparent and insulated from elite capture?	Published funding criteria; community representation in governance
Maximin Orientation	Is priority given to improving the welfare of the least-advantaged?	Resource allocation weighted toward underserved communities and groups

The first criterion, correction of market failure, relates to the welfare-economic basis of the subsidy case. A subsidy to sport is welfare-aligned to the extent it corrects a failure in private provision: a situation in which the market undersupplies a form of sport with positive externalities, or in which information asymmetries and/or behavioural constraints prevent individuals from participating in sport in their long-run welfare interests. This criterion explicitly rules out subsidies to profitable, privately profitable, sport enterprises - professional sport leagues, elite teams and franchises, major sporting events with high private sponsorship value - unless there is some specific market failure that the subsidy is intended to address. The level of proof required to meet this criterion is necessarily tougher than the level of rhetoric commonly invoked to justify sport subsidies: it is not enough to claim that sport is 'good for communities', it is necessary to demonstrate that it generates externalities and that undersupply exists. This standard demands pre-programme research to establish the presence and scale of a market failure that a subsidy is designed to correct, and post-programme evaluation to determine whether it has been corrected.

The second criterion, distributional equity, operationalises the Rawlsian maxim that investment decisions should be assessed on their impact on the 'worst off'. This criterion requires that sport subsidies generate disproportionate participation gains for disadvantaged groups, as indicated by disaggregated participation data that provides more detailed information about participation beyond headline participation figures; including by income, race/ethnicity, disability, gender, age and geographical area. Programmes that raise overall participation while leaving participation gaps between advantaged and disadvantaged unchanged do not satisfy this criterion, even if they boost headline participation. Meeting the distributional equity criterion requires not just that subsidised provision is accessible to disadvantaged groups but that the design, marketing, pricing and support systems of subsidy programmes address the barriers to participation faced by disadvantaged groups. That is, it requires a program model that is not geared to the convenience of the existing sporting population but to the barriers faced by the most disadvantaged.

The third criterion, capability expansion, requires that the evaluation of sport investment be not only based on whether people participate, the most common metric used to evaluate sport policy, but also on whether participation increases their substantive freedoms: their health, their social interactions, their self-esteem, their capacity to participate in a community of practice. This criterion demands evaluation frameworks that do more than count participation to measure increases in participant well-being, capability and life chances that result from participation. The operationalisation of this criterion is challenging but not impossible: the measurement frameworks used to evaluate well-being underpinning the OECD's Better Life Initiative and the Human Development Index offer methodological models for capability-sensitive policy evaluation that sport policy could borrow from. Robeyns (2017) research on operationalising the capability approach in particular policy contexts offers a methodological framework for developing capability measures specific to sport that go beyond counting participation without abandoning the empirical rigour of sound policy evaluation.

The fourth criterion, spillover measurability, relates to the empirical evidence for sport's social benefits. Subsidies for sport are often justified by reference to benefits (crime prevention, community harmony, mental health, health care cost savings) that are claimed rather than measured, and whose connection with particular sport interventions is often poorly evaluated. This criterion requires that social spillovers be measured, verified and audited, through pre-registered evaluation, longitudinal measurement of outcomes, and independent audit of social value claims. Coalter (2007) comprehensive survey of the evidence base for the social value of sport found the gap between policy claim and empirical data to be wide: sport policy routinely claimed benefits for which no evaluation evidence was available, and when such evidence was available it was often produced for the providers of the sport programs, who had incentives to produce positive findings. Independent evaluation capacity, similar to that of health policy - for instance, the UK's National Institute for Health and Care Excellence - is a prerequisite of welfare-aligned sport policy.

The fifth criterion, governance accountability, relates to the political economy of allocation. Welfare-aligned sport investment demands transparent and explicable allocation decisions based on explicit welfare criteria, free of the elite capture mechanisms outlined in Section 4. This criterion requires that funding criteria be published detailing the welfare objectives that guide allocation; governances' structures that provide representation for communities that might be excluded from allocation decisions that affect them; and independent oversight of allocation that ensures regulatory capture by the established sport elite does not occur. The institutional architecture of welfare-aligned sport governance builds on principles of participatory governance and deliberative democracy that demand the participation of affected communities in policy design (Fung, 2006). Fung's model of empowered participatory governance, in which affected communities are given decision-making power rather than merely consultative status in governance, is a model for overcoming the democratic deficit in sport governance discussed in Section 5.

The sixth criterion, maximin orientation, operationalises the Rawlsian difference principle, in that public investment in sport should be allocated in a way that prioritises the improvement of the sporting capabilities of those who at present have the least, and that subsidy allocation should be weighted in favour of communities, groups and areas where participation opportunities are the lowest. This is clearly a lexical criterion: it requires prioritisation of the most disadvantaged, and allocation of further investment to those already participating, rather than the spread of investment across all populations, or simply the most cost-effective allocation of participation gains. The maximin criterion is the most stringent of the six, and its application would require a substantial reallocation of current priorities in sport subsidy; it is hence also the most effective tool for welfare improvement. Its application would require not just the rhetorical prioritisation of inclusion but institutional mechanisms (funding formulas, allocation rules, governance criteria) that institutionalise the priority of the least-advantaged in the allocation of public sport resources.

The six criteria form an interrelated normative set. A sport subsidy package might meet the market failure correction criterion without meeting the distributional equity criterion (correcting an actual market failure while benefiting the advantaged). It might satisfy the participation measurability criterion without satisfying the capability expansion criterion - generating measurable increases in participation while generating no increase in the well-being or freedom of participants. The welfare-alignment criteria are intended to be applied as a whole, in a holistic evaluation of the extent to which a sport subsidy system is in fact aligned with social welfare objectives, as opposed to being rhetorically linked with such objectives in order to justify investments that are pursued for other reasons. In this respect, the criteria represent a welfare constitution for sport policy: a normative framework that circumscribes the boundaries of political discretion over sport investments that is democratically justified.

8. CONCLUSION: REPOSITIONING SPORT AS A WELFARE INSTRUMENT

This chapter has established a theoretical basis for the assessment of public sport subsidies as instruments of social welfare, suggesting that the stock-in-trade political justifications for investments in sport (the social cohesion potential of sport, the public good nature of sport, the health and community development benefits of sport) are both theoretically sound and practically contested in a way that calls for them to be subject to rigorous welfare-theoretic scrutiny rather than rhetorical approval. The theoretical journey that has been taken in this chapter - from Samuelson's (1954) public goods theory to Putnam (2000b) social capital theory, Bourdieu (1984) field theory, the political economy of sport governance, and Sen's (2009) capability approach to Rawlsian distributive justice - has yielded a complex picture of the promise and challenges of sport as a welfare instrument. Each theoretical approach casts a different light on the various aspects of the "sport-subsidy-welfare" relationship: the market failure aspect, the social capital aspect, the structural reproduction aspect, the political economy aspect, and the substantive freedom aspect. Theoretically, they represent a full suite of justifications for welfare-aligned sport policy.

The key analytic contribution of the chapter is the conceptualisation and theorisation of the subsidy paradox, the structural bias for public sport investment to favour the already-advantaged, thereby reversing the redistributive paradigm upon which it was justified. This paradox is not a curable problem of program implementation but a systemic pattern of the political economy of sport governance that reproduces elite capture of public investment into sport. It cannot be overcome by better programme design but by re-alignment of the governance, evaluation and normative structures that form the basis for the design and assessment of sport subsidy. The subsidy paradox will not be defeated by persuasion but by structural change: of funding formulae, of the composition of the governing boards, of the evaluation frameworks and of the ideological criteria through which the social value of sport is defined and claimed. Without such reform, progressive reform in programme design will be continually offset by the political economic factors that sustain elite capture of public sport investments.

The welfare-alignment criteria outlined in Section 7 offer a practical guide to this reorientation, based on the welfare-economic analysis of public goods and market failure, the sociological analysis of social cohesion and its limits, the capability approach's call for substantive rather than formal freedom, and Rawlsian distributive justice's demand that public investment be justified from the standpoint of the worst-off. We offer these criteria as an analytical framework for the empirical and comparative chapters of this book: as a common vocabulary and normative framework with which to evaluate the welfare claims of some of the many different sport policy programmes and systems in place. They are valuable not only as a means of assessing existing policy programs but also as a means of designing new ones: the criteria specify the conditions that must be met if welfare-aligned sport investment is to be made and they thereby provide guidance to policymakers committed to genuine, rather than rhetorical, welfare improvement.

There are several implications for the project of sport policy reform. First, the welfare justification for sport subsidy is strongest at the community and amateur levels (where public goods characteristics are more evident, externalities are more important and participation barriers are greater for disadvantaged groups), and weakest at the elite and commercial levels (where private goods characteristics predominate and welfare gains favour elite groups). This implies a major reallocation of public sport resources towards community sport infrastructure development, support for mass participation and removing participation barriers for disadvantaged populations. Such a shift would be politically challenging, given the organisational capacity of existing sporting interests, and the politics of elite sport success. But it is the necessary implication of taking the welfare case for sport seriously, rather than as rhetorical cover for other interests.

Second, the way we evaluate sport policies needs to move beyond counting aggregate participation to capability-sensitive evaluation of whether public investment is enhancing the substantive freedoms of those with the largest unmet welfare need. This means investing in independent evaluation capacity and adopting disaggregated measures of outcomes to make the welfare consequences of sport investment more visible and accountable. The current predominance of aggregate participation statistics as the key metric of sport policy is not simply a technical failing but a political decision that masks the unpalatable distributional effects of investment practices that disadvantage the excluded. As such, this is not simply a technical reform but a political one: it requires that government sport agencies and their political masters be willing to be held accountable for the welfare consequences of investment, not just its aggregate magnitude.

Third, the governance architecture of sport - the national governing bodies, sport councils, and policy ministries that mediate public investment in sport - needs democratic reform to ensure the views and interests of excluded communities are given a voice in investment decisions that shape their communities. The forms of governance capture documented in this chapter are not inherent to the organisation of sport but institutional choices that can be reframed through governance reform. Models of participatory governance Fung (2006) offer concrete ways of reconfiguring the governance of sport to ensure that the communities most in need of social welfare, rather than the communities with the highest levels of existing sporting capital, have voice and decision-making control over what matters to them.

Fourth, and most importantly, this chapter has argued that the reframing of sport from elite reproduction to inclusive social development instrument requires not only technical re-adaptation but also an ideological reorientation of the way that the social value of sport is conceptualised and deployed. The meritocratic mythology of sport - the myth that sport is a realm of natural equality, where success is determined by merit - serves politically to justify investment practices that reproduce inequality. To transform this mythology so that a welfare-theoretic approach to sport is not naively blind to sport's structural features and not cavalier about its distributional effects is a precondition for the legitimacy and credibility of sport as an instrument of social policy. This book is part of that project, and the welfare-alignment criteria developed here are proposed as guides to those (scholars, policymakers, advocates, and citizens) who want to ensure that the public money spent on sport is spent in the interests of those most in need of sport's benefits. The stakes here are not just academic, but the distribution of genuine freedoms - to play, to be healthy, to belong to a community - that are important to the quality of human lives and the nature of the societies in which they are lived.

REFERENCES

Andrews, D., & Silk, M. (2012). *Sport and neoliberalism: Politics, consumption, and culture* (p. 316).

Bourdieu, P. (1984). *Distinction: A Social Critique of the Judgement of Taste*. Harvard University Press.

Clays, E., Lidegaard, M., De Bacquer, D., Van Herck, K., De Backer, G., Kittel, F., De Smet, P., & Holtermann, A. (2014). The Combined Relationship of Occupational and Leisure-Time Physical Activity With All-Cause Mortality Among Men, Accounting for Physical Fitness. *American Journal of Epidemiology, 179*(5), 559–566. DOI: 10.1093/aje/kwt294 PMID: 24305575

Coakley, J. (2011). Youth Sports: What Counts as "Positive Development?". *Journal of Sport and Social Issues, 35*(3), 306–324. DOI: 10.1177/0193723511417311

Coalter, F. (2007). *A Wider Social Role for Sport: Who's Keeping the Score?* Routledge., DOI: 10.4324/9780203014615

Crompton, J. L. (2006). Economic Impact Studies: Instruments for Political Shenanigans? *Journal of Travel Research, 45*(1), 67–82. DOI: 10.1177/0047287506288870

De Castro, S. B. E., De Souza, J. V. M., De Camargo, P. R., & Mezzadri, F. M. (2025). Government budget and priorities for sports in Brazil (2004-2020). *Managing Sport and Leisure, 30*(3), 487–505. DOI: 10.1080/23750472.2023.2196529

Fung, A. (2006). *Empowered Participation: Reinventing Urban Democracy*. Princeton University Press.

Grusky, D. B., & Szelényi, S. (Eds.). (2006). *Inequality: Classic readings in race, class, and gender*. Westview Press.

Hassan, M. K., & Lewis, M. K. (Eds.). (2007). *Handbook of Islamic Banking*. Edward Elgar Publishing., DOI: 10.4337/9781847205414

Houlihan, B., & Green, M. (Eds.). (2011). *Routledge handbook of sports development*. Routledge.

Hylton, K. (2009a). *"Race" and sport: Critical race theory*. Routledge.

Hylton, K. (2009b). *"Race" and Sport: Critical Race Theory*. Routledge.

Kay, T., & Bradbury, S. (2009a). Youth sport volunteering: Developing social capital? *Sport Education and Society, 14*(1), 121–140. DOI: 10.1080/13573320802615288

Kay, T., & Bradbury, S. (2009b). Youth sport volunteering: Developing social capital? *Sport Education and Society -. Sport Education and Society*, *14*(1), 121–140. DOI: 10.1080/13573320802615288

Madsen, F. (2009). *Transnational Organized Crime* (0 ed.). Routledge. DOI: 10.4324/9780203875827

Musgrave, R. A. (1987). Public Finance. In Macmillan, P. (Ed.), *The New Palgrave Dictionary of Economics* (pp. 1–11)., DOI: 10.1057/978-1-349-95121-5_1643-1

Nicholson, M., & Hoye, R. (2008). *Sport and social capital.* Elsevier-Butterworth-Heinemann. DOI: 10.4324/9780080569727

Nussbaum, M. C. (2011). *Creating Capabilities: The Human Development Approach.* Harvard University Press. DOI: 10.4159/harvard.9780674061200

Putnam, R. D. (2000a). Bowling alone: The collapse and revival of American community. *Proceedings of the 2000 ACM Conference on Computer Supported Cooperative Work*, 357. DOI: 10.1145/358916.361990

Putnam, R. D. (2000b). *Bowling alone: The collapse and revival of American community.* Touchstone Books/Simon & Schuster., DOI: 10.1145/358916.361990

Rawls, J. (2020). *A Theory of Justice* (Revised Edition). Harvard University Press.

Roberts, K. (2008). *Key Concepts in Sociology*. Macmillan Education UK.

Robeyns, I. (2017). *Wellbeing, Freedom and Social Justice: The Capability Approach Re-Examined.* DOI: 10.11647/OBP.0130

Sam, M. P. (2009). The Public Management of Sport: Wicked problems, challenges and dilemmas. *Public Management Review*, *11*(4), 499–514. DOI: 10.1080/14719030902989565

Samuelson, P. A. (1954). The Pure Theory of Public Expenditure. *The Review of Economics and Statistics*, *36*(4), 387. DOI: 10.2307/1925895

Schausteck De Almeida, B., Barboza Eiras De Castro, S., Mezzadri, F. M., & Lange De Souza, D. (2018). Do sports mega-events boost public funding in sports programs? The case of Brazil (2004–2015). *International Review for the Sociology of Sport*, *53*(6), 685–705. DOI: 10.1177/1012690216680115

Sen, A. (2009). *The Idea of Justice*. Harvard University Press.

Sen, A. K. (2009). *The Idea of Justice*. Harvard University Press., DOI: 10.4159/9780674054578

Sherry, E., & Coalter, F. (2009). A Wider Social Role for Sport: Who's Keeping the Score? *Sport Management Review*, *12*(4), 273–274. DOI: 10.1016/j.smr.2009.05.002

Watson, K. (2011). D. Kahneman. (2011). *Thinking, Fast and Slow.* New York, NY: Farrar, Straus and Giroux. 499 pages. *The Canadian Journal of Program Evaluation*, *26*(2), 111–113. DOI: 10.3138/cjpe.26.010

Weed, M., Coren, E., Fiore, J., Wellard, I., Chatziefstathiou, D., Mansfield, L., & Dowse, S. (2015a). The Olympic Games and raising sport participation: A systematic review of evidence and an interrogation of policy for a demonstration effect. *European Sport Management Quarterly*, *15*(2), 195–226. DOI: 10.1080/16184742.2014.998695

Weed, M., Coren, E., Fiore, J., Wellard, I., Chatziefstathiou, D., Mansfield, L., & Dowse, S. (2015b). The Olympic Games and raising sport participation: A systematic review of evidence and an interrogation of policy for a demonstration effect. *European Sport Management Quarterly*, *15*(2), 195–226. DOI: 10.1080/16184742.2014.998695

Chapter 8
Playing for Equity: Women's Sports, Social Policy, and Justice Commitments in the Global Sustainability Economy

Rubee Singh
http://orcid.org/0000-0002-5406-2210
GLA University, India

ABSTRACT

The intersection of women's sports, social policy, and justice commitments within the global sustainability economy represents an evolving domain of scholarly and policy relevance. This chapter critically examines how gender equity in sports contributes to broader sustainability goals, including social inclusion, economic empowerment, and institutional accountability. It explores structural inequalities that persist in women's sports, such as disparities in funding, media representation, and governance, while situating these challenges within global policy frameworks like the Sustainable Development Goals (SDGs). The chapter further evaluates the role of public policy, corporate engagement, and transnational advocacy in promoting equitable sports ecosystems. By integrating feminist theory, sustainability discourse, and institutional analysis, the study advances a multidimensional understanding of sports as a site of justice. It concludes by proposing policy pathways that align women's sports development with sustainability-driven social transformation

DOI: 10.4018/979-8-2600-3174-2.ch008

1. INTRODUCTION

1.1 Situating Women's Sports in the Sustainability Discourse

The discourse on sustainability has undergone a profound transformation in recent decades, evolving from an environmentally centric framework to a multidimensional paradigm that integrates social equity, economic resilience, and institutional accountability. Within this expanded understanding, gender equality has emerged as a foundational pillar, not merely as a normative ideal but as a measurable determinant of sustainable development outcomes. Women's sports, as a socio-cultural and economic domain, offer a compelling lens through which these intersections can be examined. Despite their growing visibility and commercial relevance, women's sports remain structurally marginalized, reflecting broader gendered inequalities embedded within global systems of production, representation, and governance (UN Women, 2023; OECD, 2022).

Historically, sports have functioned as a site of masculine dominance, where institutional norms, funding priorities, and media narratives have privileged male participation and achievement. Women's entry into organized sports has been marked by resistance, negotiation, and gradual institutional acceptance. However, this inclusion has often been symbolic rather than substantive, with persistent disparities in pay, sponsorship, infrastructure, and leadership opportunities (Cooky et al., 2021; Fink, 2016). In the context of the global sustainability economy—defined by its emphasis on inclusive growth, social justice, and long-term systemic resilience—such disparities represent not only ethical concerns but also developmental inefficiencies. Excluding or underutilizing half the global population in sports ecosystems undermines both economic potential and social cohesion (World Bank, 2023).

This chapter situates women's sports within the broader sustainability discourse by foregrounding their role as both a reflection of and a catalyst for social transformation. It argues that sports are not merely recreational or commercial activities but are deeply embedded in societal structures, influencing identity formation, cultural norms, and policy priorities. As such, the advancement of women's sports aligns with multiple global development agendas, particularly those related to gender equality, health and well-being, and reduced inequalities (United Nations, 2023). The integration of sports into sustainability frameworks thus necessitates a critical examination of the structural barriers that limit women's participation and the policy mechanisms required to address them.

1.2 Evolution of Sustainability and Gender Integration

The concept of sustainability has expanded significantly since the publication of the Brundtland Report, which initially framed sustainable development as meeting present needs without compromising future generations. Contemporary interpretations now emphasize the interdependence of environmental, economic, and social systems, often conceptualized through the "triple bottom line" approach (Elkington, 1997). Within this framework, gender equality is increasingly recognized as a cross-cutting issue that influences outcomes across all dimensions of sustainability.

Recent scholarship has highlighted that gender disparities are not peripheral but central to the functioning of economic and social systems. Women's limited access to resources, decision-making power, and institutional support constrains their ability to contribute fully to development processes (Kabeer, 2021; UNDP, 2022). In the context of sports, these constraints manifest in unequal funding, limited media visibility, and exclusion from leadership roles. Such disparities are particularly pronounced in developing economies, where cultural norms and structural barriers further restrict women's participation (Saavedra, 2022).

The integration of gender into sustainability discourse has been reinforced by global policy frameworks such as the Sustainable Development Goals (SDGs). Specifically, SDG 5 (Gender Equality) and SDG 10 (Reduced Inequalities) underscore the importance of inclusive institutions and equitable access to opportunities. Women's sports contribute directly to these goals by promoting empowerment, enhancing health outcomes, and fostering social inclusion (Hancock et al., 2023, Crowther, D.,2024). Moreover, participation in sports has been linked to increased self-efficacy, leadership skills, and economic opportunities for women, thereby reinforcing the broader objectives of sustainable development (UNESCO, 2023).

1.3 Women's Sports as a Site of Social and Economic Transformation

Women's sports have increasingly gained recognition as a dynamic sector within the global economy, characterized by growing investments, expanding audiences, and heightened media attention. This shift reflects broader societal changes, including evolving gender norms and increased advocacy for equity. However, the growth of women's sports must be understood within the context of persistent structural inequalities that shape access to resources and opportunities.

Economically, the underinvestment in women's sports represents a missed opportunity for sustainable growth. Studies indicate that increasing investment in women's sports can yield significant returns, not only in terms of revenue generation but also in job creation and community development (Deloitte, 2024). The commercialization of women's sports, supported by corporate sponsorships and broadcasting deals, has begun to challenge traditional market assumptions that undervalue women's athletic performance. Nevertheless, these developments remain uneven, with substantial gaps between men's and women's sports in terms of financial support and visibility (PwC, 2023).

Socially, women's sports serve as a powerful platform for challenging gender stereotypes and promoting inclusivity. Female athletes often act as role models, inspiring younger generations and reshaping societal perceptions of women's capabilities. This transformative potential is particularly significant in contexts where cultural norms restrict women's public participation. By normalizing women's presence in competitive and public spaces, sports contribute to broader processes of social change (Meier & Saavedra, 2020).

Furthermore, women's sports intersect with issues of health and well-being, which are integral components of sustainability. Regular participation in sports has been associated with improved physical and mental health outcomes, reducing the burden on healthcare systems and enhancing overall quality of life (WHO, 2022). In this sense, promoting women's sports aligns with the preventive and holistic approaches advocated within sustainability frameworks.

1.4 Policy Relevance and the Need for Justice-Oriented Approaches

The persistence of gender inequalities in sports underscores the need for robust policy interventions that address both structural and cultural barriers. Social policy plays a critical role in shaping the conditions under which women can access and benefit from sports. This includes legislation aimed at ensuring equal pay, anti-discrimination measures, and targeted investments in infrastructure and grassroots programs.

However, policy responses must move beyond formal equality to embrace a justice-oriented approach that recognizes the diverse experiences and challenges faced by women. In4ersectionality is particularly important in this context, as factors such as race, class, and geography influence access to sports opportunities. Women from marginalized communities often face compounded disadvantages, requiring tailored interventions that address multiple layers of inequality (Crenshaw, 2017; Collins, 2019).

Recent policy initiatives at both national and international levels have sought to promote gender equity in sports. For instance, several countries have introduced gender quotas in sports governance, while international organizations have launched campaigns to increase women's participation and visibility. These efforts reflect a growing recognition of the importance of inclusive institutions for sustainable development (European Commission, 2023).

Corporate actors also play an increasingly significant role in shaping the landscape of women's sports. Through corporate social responsibility (CSR) initiatives, companies are investing in women's sports as part of their broader sustainability strategies. Such engagements not only enhance brand value but also contribute to social impact by supporting equitable sports ecosystems (Porter & Kramer, 2019).

Despite these advancements, significant challenges remain. The implementation of policies is often uneven, and accountability mechanisms are frequently weak. Moreover, cultural resistance continues to impede progress in many contexts. Addressing these challenges requires a comprehensive approach that combines policy reform, institutional change, and societal engagement. In sum, situating women's sports within the sustainability discourse reveals their multifaceted significance as a domain of social, economic, and political relevance. The integration of gender equity into sports is not only essential for achieving justice but also for realizing the broader objectives of sustainable development. By addressing structural inequalities and fostering inclusive institutions, women's sports can serve as a powerful catalyst for transformative change in the global sustainability economy.

1.5 Institutional Inclusion, Sustainability Governance, and the Expanding Role of Women's Sports in Social Transformation

1.5.1 Women's Sports and the Sustainability Framework

The concept of sustainability has evolved considerably from a purely environmental concern into a multidimensional framework encompassing social justice, economic inclusion, institutional accountability, and human well-being (Mensah, 2019). Contemporary sustainability discourse emphasizes that long-term development cannot be achieved without equitable access to opportunities and inclusive participation across all sectors of society (Leal Filho et al., 2021). Within this broader framework, gender equality has emerged as a central component of sustainable development, particularly because structural inequalities continue to limit women's participation in social, economic, and institutional spaces (United Nations, 2023).

Sports have increasingly gained recognition as influential social institutions capable of shaping cultural values, leadership opportunities, and community participation (Giulianotti, 2016). Women's participation in sports contributes significantly to empowerment, self-confidence, educational engagement, and social visibility (Meier & Saavedra, 2020). Consequently, women's sports are now viewed not merely as recreational activities but as important instruments for promoting social inclusion and sustainable development. International policy frameworks such as the Sustainable Development Goals (SDGs), particularly SDG 5 concerning gender equality and SDG 10 related to reduced inequalities, further reinforce the importance of inclusive sporting systems (United Nations, 2023).

1.5.2 Historical Inequalities and Structural Exclusion

Historically, organized sports developed within patriarchal institutional systems that privileged masculine norms of authority, competitiveness, and physicality (Hargreaves, 1994). Women were often excluded from competitive sporting spaces through cultural stereotypes, social restrictions, and unequal institutional support. Although women gradually gained access to professional and international sporting arenas, inequalities continued to persist in areas such as funding, infrastructure, leadership opportunities, and public recognition (Fink, 2016).

Sports institutions frequently reproduce broader societal inequalities because they reflect dominant power relations embedded within social systems (Connell, 2009). Women athletes continue to experience disparities in salaries, sponsorships, and institutional recognition compared to male athletes (Cooky et al., 2021). Furthermore, leadership structures within sports organizations remain heavily male dominated, limiting women's participation in decision-making processes (Adriaanse, 2016). These inequalities demonstrate that increasing participation alone is insufficient to achieve substantive equity in sports.

The persistence of structural barriers highlights the need for institutional reform capable of addressing historical patterns of exclusion. Sustainable sports governance requires policies that move beyond symbolic inclusion toward equitable access to resources, leadership representation, and professional opportunities (Evans & Pfister, 2021).

1.5.3 Economic Growth and Commercial Visibility

The globalization of sports has transformed athletics into a major economic sector characterized by broadcasting rights, sponsorship agreements, merchandising, and digital media engagement (Andrews & Silk, 2018). Despite this commercial expansion, women's sports continue to receive substantially lower investments and media attention compared to men's sporting competitions (Deloitte, 2024). Historically, these disparities have often been justified through assumptions regarding lower market demand and reduced profitability associated with women's sports.

Recent developments, however, increasingly challenge these assumptions. Women's football, cricket, basketball, and tennis have attracted growing audiences and significant sponsorship investments across international markets (PwC, 2023). Research indicates that women's sports can achieve substantial commercial success when provided with equitable media exposure and institutional support (Hoeber, 2018). This suggests that the economic marginalization of women's sports is linked more closely to unequal investment patterns than to limited audience interest.

From a sustainability perspective, excluding women from equitable economic participation weakens broader developmental potential (Raworth, 2017). Investments in women's sports contribute to employment generation, community development, and inclusive economic growth while simultaneously advancing gender equity objectives. Sustainable economies depend upon systems capable of utilizing diverse talents and capabilities across society.

1.5.4 Media Representation and Cultural Change

Media representation plays a significant role in shaping public perceptions regarding sports and athletic legitimacy. Historically, women athletes have received considerably lower levels of media coverage compared to male athletes, and existing portrayals frequently emphasize appearance or personal life rather than professional performance and athletic competence (Cooky & Antunovic, 2020). Such representations contribute to the symbolic marginalization of women's sports by reinforcing stereotypes that undermine women's athletic authority.

At the same time, women's sports increasingly function as important platforms for cultural transformation. Female athletes challenge traditional gender norms by occupying visible leadership positions within public and competitive spaces (Bruce, 2016). Their visibility contributes to changing societal attitudes concerning women's capabilities and participation in professional life. Studies suggest that exposure to successful women athletes positively influences girls' confidence, aspirations, and willingness to participate in leadership-oriented activities (UNESCO, 2023).

Digital media has also created new opportunities for advocacy and representation. Women athletes increasingly use social media platforms to address issues such as equal pay, discrimination, and mental health awareness (Pegoraro et al., 2021). Nevertheless, structural inequalities within mainstream sports media continue to restrict equitable visibility and recognition.

1.5.5 Governance, Inclusion, and Sustainable Sporting Futures

Governance inequality remains a major challenge within global sports systems. Women continue to be underrepresented in coaching roles, sports federations, administrative leadership, and executive decision-making structures (Burton, 2015). This underrepresentation influences organizational priorities, resource allocation, and institutional cultures, often limiting opportunities for women athletes. Research demonstrates that organizations characterized by diverse leadership structures are more likely to adopt inclusive governance practices and equitable policies (Evans & Pfister, 2021).

Discussions concerning women's sports must also recognize the intersectional nature of inequality. Women's experiences within sports are shaped not only by gender but also by race, class, ethnicity, disability, and geographical location (Collins, 2019). Women from marginalized communities frequently encounter additional barriers related to access to facilities, institutional support, and professional opportunities. Consequently, inclusive sports development requires justice-oriented policies capable of addressing multiple forms of inequality simultaneously.

Ultimately, women's sports should be viewed as central to broader sustainability and social justice agendas rather than as peripheral aspects of sporting culture. Through equitable governance, institutional accountability, and inclusive policy reforms, women's sports can contribute significantly to sustainable social transformation and democratic inclusion within the global sports economy.

2. THEORETICAL FOUNDATIONS: FEMINIST POLITICAL ECONOMY AND SUSTAINABILITY

Understanding women's sports within the global sustainability economy requires a strong theoretical grounding that connects gender, power, and institutional structures. This section draws upon feminist political economy, sustainability theory, and the capabilities approach to critically examine how inequalities in sports are produced, reproduced, and potentially transformed. These frameworks collectively reveal that disparities in women's sports are not isolated anomalies but systemic outcomes embedded in broader socio-economic and political arrangements.

2.1 Feminist Political Economy and Gendered Power Structures in Sports

Feminist political economy provides a critical lens to analyze how gendered hierarchies shape economic systems, labor distribution, and access to resources. Within sports, this perspective highlights how institutional arrangements privilege male athletes while marginalizing women through unequal pay, limited sponsorship, and restricted access to leadership roles (Acker, 2020; Seguino, 2021). These inequalities are not incidental but are rooted in historical constructions of sports as a masculine domain.

From this viewpoint, women athletes are often positioned within what can be termed a "peripheral economy" of sports, where their labor is undervalued and undercompensated despite comparable levels of skill and commitment. This marginalization reflects broader patterns of gendered labor segmentation observed across industries, where women's work is frequently devalued and rendered invisible (Elson, 2017; Rai et al., 2019). In sports, such dynamics manifest in disparities in prize money, media contracts, and sponsorship deals, reinforcing a cycle of underinvestment and limited visibility.

Moreover, governance structures in sports institutions often reproduce patriarchal norms by excluding women from decision-making roles. Leadership positions in major sports organizations remain overwhelmingly male-dominated, which influences policy priorities and resource allocation (Adriaanse, 2016; Burton, 2015). This lack of representation not only limits women's influence but also perpetuates institutional biases that hinder gender equity.

Feminist political economy also emphasizes the role of unpaid and care labor in sustaining economic systems. Women athletes frequently navigate dual responsibilities, balancing professional sports careers with domestic expectations, particularly in contexts where social support systems are weak (Bruening & Dixon, 2019). This additional burden constrains their ability to compete on equal terms with male counterparts, further entrenching inequalities.

Importantly, this framework underscores that achieving equity in women's sports requires structural transformation rather than incremental adjustments. Addressing wage gaps or increasing visibility, while necessary, is insufficient without challenging the underlying power relations that sustain inequality (True, 2022). Thus, feminist political economy calls for a reconfiguration of institutional norms, resource distribution, and governance practices within sports ecosystems.

2.2 Sustainability Paradigms and the Integration of Gender Equity

Sustainability theory offers another critical framework for understanding the role of women's sports in broader development processes. The "triple bottom line" approach—encompassing economic, social, and environmental dimensions—provides a comprehensive lens for evaluating the contribution of sports to sustainable development (Elkington, 1997). However, integrating gender equity into this framework reveals that sustainability cannot be achieved without addressing systemic inequalities.

Recent scholarship has emphasized that gender equality is a prerequisite for sustainable development rather than a complementary objective (Leach et al., 2018; UN Women, 2023). In the context of sports, this implies that promoting women's participation is essential not only for social justice but also for enhancing the overall sustainability of the sports economy. Inclusive sports systems are more likely to foster innovation, resilience, and long-term growth.

Economically, investing in women's sports aligns with sustainability goals by expanding market opportunities and diversifying revenue streams. The growing commercial potential of women's sports demonstrates that gender-inclusive investments can generate significant returns while contributing to social impact (Deloitte, 2024; PwC, 2023). This challenges traditional assumptions that prioritize short-term profitability over equitable development.

Socially, women's sports contribute to community development, social cohesion, and the promotion of inclusive values. Participation in sports fosters teamwork, leadership, and resilience, which are critical for building sustainable societies (Coalter, 2015; Schulenkorf, 2017). These outcomes align with the broader objectives of sustainability, which emphasize human well-being and social inclusion.

Environmental sustainability is also increasingly relevant in the context of sports. While traditionally overlooked, the environmental impact of sports events and infrastructure is now receiving greater attention. Integrating women's sports into sustainability initiatives provides an opportunity to promote environmentally responsible practices, such as sustainable event management and eco-friendly infrastructure (McCullough et al., 2020). Women's sports organizations, often less entrenched in legacy systems, may be particularly well-positioned to adopt innovative sustainability practices.

Furthermore, global policy frameworks such as the Sustainable Development Goals (SDGs) reinforce the importance of gender equity in achieving sustainability. Women's sports intersect with multiple SDGs, including gender equality, health and well-being, and reduced inequalities (United Nations, 2023). This alignment underscores the need for integrated policy approaches that recognize the interconnectedness of sports and sustainable development.

2.3 The Capabilities Approach and Empowerment through Sports

The capabilities approach, developed by Amartya Sen and further expanded by Martha Nussbaum, provides a human-centered framework for evaluating development. It emphasizes the importance of expanding individuals' freedoms and opportunities to lead lives they value (Sen, 1999; Nussbaum, 2011). In the context of women's sports, this approach highlights the transformative potential of sports participation in enhancing capabilities related to health, agency, and social inclusion.

Participation in sports enables women to develop physical capabilities, improve health outcomes, and build confidence. These benefits extend beyond the individual level, contributing to broader societal gains such as increased labor force participation and reduced healthcare costs (Hancock et al., 2023; WHO, 2022). By enhancing women's capabilities, sports serve as a catalyst for inclusive development.

The capabilities approach also emphasizes the importance of agency—the ability to make choices and act upon them. Women's participation in sports can strengthen agency by providing opportunities for leadership, decision-making, and public engagement. Female athletes often become advocates for social change, using their platforms to challenge inequalities and promote justice (Meier & Saavedra, 2020).

However, the realization of these capabilities is contingent upon enabling conditions, including access to resources, supportive policies, and inclusive institutions. Structural barriers such as discrimination, lack of infrastructure, and cultural norms can limit women's ability to participate in sports and benefit from its transformative potential (Kabeer, 2021; Saavedra, 2022). Addressing these barriers is essential for ensuring that the benefits of sports are equitably distributed.

Importantly, the capabilities approach aligns with justice-oriented perspectives that prioritize equity and inclusion. It shifts the focus from aggregate outcomes to individual experiences, emphasizing the need to address disparities in opportunities and resources. In the context of women's sports, this implies that policy interventions should not only increase participation rates but also enhance the quality and inclusivity of sports experiences.

In conclusion, the integration of feminist political economy, sustainability theory, and the capabilities approach provide a comprehensive framework for analyzing women's sports within the global sustainability economy. These perspectives collectively highlight that gender inequalities in sports are deeply rooted in structural and institutional dynamics, requiring transformative approaches to address them. By recognizing women's sports as a site of economic activity, social empowerment, and capability enhancement, this theoretical foundation underscores their critical role in advancing sustainable and just development.

3. STRUCTURAL INEQUALITIES IN WOMEN'S SPORTS

Despite notable advancements in visibility, professionalism, and institutional support, women's sports continue to be shaped by persistent structural inequalities. These inequalities are embedded within economic systems, media structures, governance frameworks, and socio-cultural norms that collectively disadvantage women athletes. While progress has been made in recent years, particularly in terms of audience engagement and policy attention, the underlying structural barriers remain largely intact. This section critically examines the multidimensional nature of these inequalities and their implications for the sustainability and inclusivity of the global sports ecosystem.

3.1 Economic Inequalities and Resource Distribution

Economic disparity remains one of the most significant challenges confronting women's sports. Across various sporting disciplines and geographical contexts, female athletes consistently receive lower financial compensation compared to their male counterparts. This disparity is evident in salaries, prize money, sponsorship deals, and endorsement opportunities. Recent studies indicate that even in sports where participation levels are comparable, women's earnings remain disproportionately low, reflecting systemic undervaluation of women's athletic labor (Wicker et al., 2023; Meier, 2023).

A key factor contributing to this inequality is the uneven distribution of financial resources within sports institutions. Investment in women's sports—particularly at grassroots and developmental levels—remains significantly lower than that in men's sports. This underinvestment affects not only athlete remuneration but also access to training facilities, coaching, and competitive opportunities (Senne, 2023; Evans & Pfister, 2024). As a result, women athletes often face structural disadvantages that hinder their performance and career longevity.

The economic marginalization of women's sports is further reinforced by market perceptions that undervalue their commercial potential. Historically, sponsors and broadcasters have prioritized men's sports due to higher viewership and revenue generation. However, emerging evidence challenges this narrative, demonstrating that women's sports have significant growth potential when adequately supported (Deloitte, 2024; PwC, 2023). The increasing popularity of women's leagues and international tournaments suggests that investment disparities are not driven solely by market dynamics but also by institutional biases.

Moreover, the lack of financial security in women's sports has broader implications for gender equity. Many female athletes are compelled to supplement their income through secondary employment, which can limit their ability to train and compete effectively. This precarious economic position contrasts sharply with the relative stability enjoyed by male athletes in professional sports (Cooky et al., 2021). Addressing these disparities requires a systemic reallocation of resources and the implementation of policies that promote equitable funding and compensation structures.

3.2 Media Representation and Symbolic Marginalization

Media representation plays a pivotal role in shaping the visibility, legitimacy, and economic value of sports. Women's sports have historically been underrepresented in mainstream media, receiving only a fraction of the coverage allocated to men's sports. Although recent years have witnessed a gradual increase in coverage, the disparity remains significant, limiting the exposure and recognition of female athletes (Cooky et al., 2021; Fink, 2016).

The consequences of limited media representation extend beyond visibility. Media coverage directly influences sponsorship opportunities, audience engagement, and revenue generation. When women's sports receive minimal coverage, they are perceived as less valuable, creating a self-reinforcing cycle of underinvestment and marginalization (Senne, 2023). This cycle perpetuates economic disparities and restricts the growth of women's sports as a viable commercial sector.

In addition to quantitative disparities, qualitative differences in media representation also contribute to inequality. Coverage of women's sports often reflects gendered biases, emphasizing physical appearance, personal lives, or femininity rather than athletic performance and achievement. Such narratives undermine the professionalism of female athletes and reinforce stereotypes that diminish their credibility (Fink, 2016; Kane, 2013).

However, the media landscape is undergoing significant transformation with the rise of digital and social media platforms. Female athletes increasingly use these platforms to engage directly with audiences, build personal brands, and challenge traditional narratives. This shift has contributed to greater visibility and has allowed women's sports to bypass conventional media gatekeepers (Pegoraro et al., 2022). Nevertheless, digital platforms alone cannot fully compensate for the lack of institutional media support.

Efforts to promote equitable media representation are gaining momentum, with advocacy groups and policy initiatives calling for increased coverage and gender-sensitive reporting. These efforts highlight the importance of media as a tool for social change, capable of reshaping perceptions and fostering inclusivity. Achieving parity in media representation is therefore essential for addressing broader structural inequalities in women's sports.

3.3 Institutional and Socio-Cultural Constraints

Institutional and socio-cultural factors constitute another critical dimension of inequality in women's sports. Sports organizations and governing bodies remain predominantly male-dominated, with women underrepresented in leadership and decision-making roles. This lack of representation limits the ability of women to influence policies and priorities, resulting in governance structures that often fail to address gender-specific challenges (Adriaanse, 2016; Burton, 2015).

Institutional barriers also manifest in unequal access to infrastructure and development programs. In many regions, women and girls have limited access to sports facilities, coaching, and competitive platforms. These disparities are particularly pronounced in developing countries, where resource constraints and cultural norms further restrict participation (UNESCO, 2023; Saavedra, 2022). The absence of supportive institutional frameworks undermines efforts to promote gender equity and limits the potential of women's sports as a driver of sustainable development.

Socio-cultural norms and gender stereotypes play a significant role in shaping participation patterns. In many societies, sports are perceived as a male domain, and women's participation is often discouraged or stigmatized. These cultural barriers can deter girls from engaging in sports from an early age, resulting in lower participation rates and reduced talent pipelines (Kabeer, 2021; Evans & Pfister, 2024).

Furthermore, these constraints are often intersectional, affecting women differently based on factors such as socio-economic status, ethnicity, and geographic location. Women from marginalized communities face compounded disadvantages, including limited access to resources and heightened discrimination. Addressing these challenges requires an intersectional approach that recognizes experiences of women in sports and tailors' interventions accordingly (Crenshaw, 2017).

Institutional reforms and cultural change are essential for overcoming these barriers. This includes promoting gender diversity in leadership, investing in inclusive infrastructure, and implementing educational initiatives that challenge stereotypes and encourage participation. Additionally, community-based programs that engage families and local stakeholders can play a crucial role in shifting cultural attitudes and creating supportive environments for women's sports.

In conclusion, structural inequalities in women's sports are deeply entrenched across economic, media, institutional, and socio-cultural dimensions. While progress has been made in recent years, these inequalities continue to limit the growth and sustainability of women's sports. Addressing them requires a comprehensive and coordinated approach that combines policy intervention, institutional reform, and cultural transformation. By dismantling these structural barriers, women's sports can more effectively contribute to the broader goals of equity, justice, and sustainability in the global economy.

4. SOCIAL POLICY INTERVENTIONS AND GOVERNANCE MECHANISMS

Addressing structural inequalities in women's sports requires robust and multidimensional social policy interventions supported by effective governance mechanisms. While market-driven changes and advocacy movements have contributed to incremental progress, sustainable transformation depends on institutionalized frameworks that ensure equity, accountability, and inclusivity. Social policy plays a central role in shaping access to resources, opportunities, and representation, thereby influencing the trajectory of women's sports within the global sustainability economy. This section critically examines key policy instruments and governance strategies that can advance gender equity in sports.

4.1 Legislative and Regulatory Frameworks

Legislative interventions form the backbone of efforts to institutionalize gender equity in sports. Governments across various regions have introduced laws and regulations aimed at addressing discrimination, ensuring equal pay, and promoting inclusive participation. These frameworks provide formal mechanisms through which gender disparities can be challenged and corrected.

One of the most significant aspects of legislative reform is the enforcement of anti-discrimination policies. Such policies prohibit gender-based exclusion and mandate equal opportunities in recruitment, training, and competition. In many contexts, equal pay legislation has also been introduced to address wage disparities between male and female athletes. While the effectiveness of these laws varies across jurisdictions, they represent an step toward formal equality (Hancock et al., 2023; OECD, 2022, Shafik, W.,2024).

Additionally, gender quotas in sports governance have emerged as an important regulatory tool. By mandating a minimum level of female representation in leadership positions, these policies aim to correct historical imbalances and ensure that women's perspectives are included in decision-making processes. Empirical studies suggest that increased representation can lead to more inclusive policies and improved organizational performance (Adriaanse, 2016; Burton, 2015).

However, legislative measures alone are insufficient without effective enforcement mechanisms. Weak implementation, lack of monitoring, and limited accountability often undermine the impact of such policies. Therefore, strengthening institutional capacity and establishing independent oversight bodies are essential for translating legal frameworks into tangible outcomes (True, 2022).

4.2 Public Investment and Infrastructure Development

Public investment is a critical determinant of access and participation in sports. Governments play a pivotal role in allocating resources for infrastructure, training facilities, and development programs that support women's sports. Historically, public funding has disproportionately favored men's sports, contributing to persistent inequalities in access and performance outcomes. Targeted investment in women's sports infrastructure can significantly enhance participation rates and athlete development. This includes the construction of gender-inclusive facilities, provision of equipment, and support for coaching and training programs. Such investments are particularly important at the grassroots level, where early exposure to sports can shape long-term participation and career trajectories (UNESCO, 2023; Coalter, 2015).

In addition to physical infrastructure, financial support mechanisms such as scholarships, grants, and subsidies play a vital role in enabling women to pursue sports professionally. These initiatives can reduce economic barriers and create pathways for talent development, particularly for individuals from disadvantaged backgrounds (Evans & Pfister, 2024, Nwokolo, S.C.,2023b). Public investment also has broader socio-economic implications. By promoting women's sports, governments can stimulate local economies, create employment opportunities, and enhance community development. This aligns with the principles of the sustainability economy, which emphasize inclusive growth and social well-being (World Bank, 2023). Nevertheless, challenges remain in ensuring equitable allocation of resources. Budget constraints, competing priorities, and institutional biases often limit the extent of public investment in women's sports. Addressing these challenges requires strategic planning, stakeholder engagement, and a commitment to long-term sustainability.

4.3 Education, Grassroots Initiatives, and Capacity Building

Education and grassroots initiatives are fundamental to addressing the socio-cultural barriers that restrict women's participation in sports. These interventions focus on changing attitudes, building skills, and creating supportive environments that encourage inclusion and equity. Grassroots programs that promote sports participation among girls from an early age are particularly effective in fostering long-term engagement. Such programs not only develop athletic skills but also contribute to personal development, including confidence, leadership, and teamwork. Research indicates that early exposure to sports is strongly correlated with continued participation and higher performance levels (Hancock et al., 2023; Meier & Saavedra, 2020).

Educational institutions play a crucial role in this process by integrating sports into curricula and promoting gender-inclusive practices. Schools and universities can serve as platforms for identifying and nurturing talent, while also challenging stereotypes that discourage girls from participating in sports (Kabeer, 2021). Capacity building is another important dimension of policy intervention. This includes training coaches, administrators, and policymakers to adopt gender-sensitive approaches. By enhancing institutional capacity, these initiatives can improve the quality and inclusivity of sports programs (Senne, 2023).

Community engagement is equally important in addressing cultural barriers. Programs that involve families, local leaders, and community organizations can help shift societal attitudes and create supportive environments for women's sports. Such approaches are particularly relevant in contexts where cultural norms strongly influence participation (Saavedra, 2022).

Despite their potential, grassroots and educational initiatives often face challenges related to funding, scalability, and sustainability. Ensuring their long-term impact requires coordinated efforts across multiple sectors, including education, health, and social development.

4.4 Global Governance, Partnerships, and Multi-Stakeholder Engagement

The global nature of sports necessitates governance mechanisms that extend beyond national boundaries. International organizations, non-governmental organizations, and transnational networks play a critical role in promoting gender equity in sports through advocacy, standard-setting, and capacity building.

Global frameworks such as the Sustainable Development Goals (SDGs) provide a normative foundation for aligning sports policies with broader development objectives. Women's sports intersect with multiple SDGs, including gender equality, health and well-being, and reduced inequalities, highlighting their relevance within global policy agendas (United Nations, 2023). Partnerships between public and private actors are increasingly in advancing women's sports. Corporate entities, through corporate social responsibility (CSR) initiatives, are investing in women's sports as part of their sustainability strategies. These partnerships can mobilize resources, enhance visibility, and support innovation in sports development (Porter & Kramer, 2019).

Non-governmental organizations and advocacy groups also play a vital role in driving change. By raising awareness, conducting research, and engaging in policy advocacy, these actors contribute to the development of more inclusive and equitable sports systems (UN Women, 2023). Multi-stakeholder engagement is essential for addressing the complex and interconnected challenges facing women's sports. Collaborative approaches that involve governments, private sector actors, civil society, and athletes themselves can lead to more comprehensive and effective solutions. Such approaches accountability by distributing responsibility across multiple actors.

However, coordination among stakeholders remains a significant challenge. Differences in priorities, resources, and institutional capacities can hinder collaboration. Establishing clear governance structures, communication channels, and shared objectives is therefore critical for ensuring the success of multi-stakeholder initiatives (Leach et al., 2018, Singh, R. (2026).

In conclusion, social policy interventions and governance mechanisms are central to advancing gender equity in women's sports. Legislative frameworks, public investment, educational initiatives, and global partnerships collectively provide a foundation for addressing structural inequalities. However, achieving meaningful and sustainable change requires more than isolated interventions. It demands a coordinated, justice-oriented approach that integrates policy, institutional reform, and societal transformation. By strengthening governance mechanisms and fostering inclusive policies, women's sports can play a pivotal role in advancing the broader goals of equity, sustainability, and social justice in the global economy.

5. WOMEN'S SPORTS AND THE GLOBAL SUSTAINABILITY ECONOMY

The positioning of women's sports within the global sustainability economy reflects an important shift in how economic value, social impact, and equity are conceptualized in contemporary development discourse. Increasingly, women's sports are not only viewed as a domain of athletic performance but also as a strategic sector contributing to inclusive growth, social transformation, and sustainable innovation. This evolving recognition is aligned with broader sustainability agendas that emphasize diversity, resilience, and long-term value creation. However, while opportunities are expanding, structural limitations continue to influence how women's sports are integrated into global economic and sustainability frameworks.

5.1 Economic Integration, Investment Trends, and Market Potential

The economic landscape of women's sports has undergone notable transformation in recent years, characterized by rising investments, expanding audiences, and enhanced commercialization. Market research indicates that women's sports are among the fastest-growing segments in the global sports industry, driven by increasing media attention, corporate sponsorship, and fan engagement (Deloitte, 2024; PwC, 2023). This growth trajectory challenges earlier assumptions that women's sports lack commercial viability and instead highlights their potential as a profitable and sustainable economic sector.

From a sustainability perspective, the expansion of women's sports contributes to inclusive economic development by creating diversified opportunities across the value chain. Employment generation extends beyond athletes to include roles in coaching, sports management, marketing, broadcasting, and event organization (Wicker et al., 2023; Meier, 2023). This diversification supports local economies and strengthens the overall resilience of the sports industry by reducing dependence on traditionally dominant male sports sectors.

Corporate investment has emerged as a key driver of this growth. Increasingly, organizations are aligning their investment strategies with environmental, social, and governance (ESG) priorities, recognizing women's sports as a platform for advancing gender equality and social impact (Eccles et al., 2020; Porter & Kramer, 2019). Sponsorship deals with women athletes and teams are not only commercially strategic but also symbolically significant, reinforcing corporate commitments to diversity and inclusion. This alignment between business objectives and social values enhances both brand credibility and long-term sustainability.

Despite these advancements, economic disparities remain a defining feature of women's sports. Investment levels continue to lag behind those of men's sports, and revenue distribution is often uneven. Structural constraints such as limited access to capital, gender biases in investment decisions, and underdeveloped market ecosystems hinder equitable growth (Senne, 2023; Evans & Pfister, 2024). Additionally, many women's sports organizations operate with constrained budgets, limiting their ability to scale operations and compete effectively in global markets.

Addressing these challenges requires innovative financial models and policy support mechanisms that prioritize equity. Public-private partnerships, impact investing, and targeted funding initiatives can play a crucial role in bridging resource gaps and fostering sustainable growth. By integrating gender equity into economic planning, stakeholders can unlock the full potential of women's sports as a driver of inclusive development.

5.2 Social Impact, Environmental Responsibility, and Sustainability Linkages

Beyond economic contributions, women's sports hold significant potential for advancing the social and environmental dimensions of sustainability. Participation in sports is widely recognized as a catalyst for improving physical health, mental well-being, and social cohesion. For women and girls, engagement in sports can be particularly transformative, enhancing self-confidence, leadership skills, and social mobility (WHO, 2022; Hancock et al., 2023). These outcomes are closely aligned with global sustainability priorities, particularly those related to health, education, and gender equality.

Women's sports also function as a powerful platform for challenging entrenched gender norms and promoting inclusive values. Female athletes often serve as influential role models who inspire broader societal change by redefining perceptions of women's capabilities and roles. This symbolic impact is especially significant in contexts where socio-cultural barriers restrict women's participation in public life (Meier & Saavedra, 2020; Kabeer, 2021). Through visibility and representation, women's sports contribute to the normalization of gender equality and the dismantling of stereotypes.

In recent years, the environmental dimension of sports has gained increasing attention, with organizations recognizing their responsibility to minimize ecological impact. Women's sports are well-positioned to integrate sustainability practices into their development models, given their relative flexibility and openness to innovation. Initiatives such as sustainable event management, reduction of carbon footprints, and adoption of eco-friendly infrastructure are becoming more prevalent (McCullough et al., 2020). These practices not only reduce environmental impact but also enhance the credibility of sports organizations as socially responsible entities.

The intersection of social and environmental sustainability is particularly evident in community-based sports programs. These initiatives often combine sports participation with environmental education and community engagement, creating holistic models of development that address multiple sustainability objectives simultaneously (Schulenkorf, 2017). By leveraging the popularity of sports, such programs can mobilize communities and promote collective action toward sustainable practices.

However, the integration of sustainability into women's sports is not without challenges. Limited financial resources, lack of standardized sustainability frameworks, and insufficient policy support can constrain the implementation of comprehensive sustainability strategies (Leach et al., 2018). Additionally, disparities in access and capacity across regions create uneven progress, with some contexts benefiting more than others.

Strengthening the role of women's sports in sustainability requires coordinated efforts across sectors. Policymakers, sports organizations, and corporate actors must collaborate to develop frameworks that support both social inclusion and environmental responsibility. Establishing clear metrics for measuring impact, investing in capacity building, and promoting knowledge sharing can further enhance the contribution of women's sports to sustainable development.

Women's sports represent a dynamic and evolving component of the global sustainability economy, characterized by growing economic significance and transformative social impact. While progress is evident in increased investment and visibility, structural inequalities and resource constraints continue to shape the sector. Integrating women's sports into sustainability frameworks offers a pathway for advancing inclusive growth, social justice, and environmental stewardship, reinforcing their importance as a catalyst for long-term systemic change.

6. JUSTICE COMMITMENTS AND TRANSFORMATIVE PATHWAYS

Advancing gender equity in women's sports requires a shift from surface-level inclusion to deeper justice-oriented commitments that address structural and systemic inequalities. Justice in this context extends beyond equal participation to encompass fairness in resource distribution, representation, recognition, and institutional power.

As women's sports increasingly intersect with global sustainability agendas, the need for transformative pathways becomes more urgent. These pathways involve reconfiguring governance structures, embracing intersectionality, strengthening accountability mechanisms, and supporting athlete-led advocacy as agents of change.

6.1 Intersectional Justice and Inclusive Governance

A justice-oriented approach to women's sports must begin with an intersectional understanding of inequality. Intersectionality highlights how overlapping identities—such as gender, race, class, ethnicity, and geography—shape individuals' experiences and access to opportunities. In sports, women from marginalized communities often face compounded barriers, including limited access to infrastructure, financial constraints, and social discrimination (Crenshaw, 2017; Collins, 2019, Singh, R.,2024a). These intersecting disadvantages require policy responses that go beyond generalized gender frameworks and instead address specific contextual realities.

Inclusive governance is central to operationalizing intersectional justice. Sports institutions must move toward participatory models that actively involve women—particularly those from underrepresented groups—in decision-making processes. Research indicates that diverse leadership not only enhances equity but also improves organizational effectiveness by incorporating a wider range of perspectives (Adriaanse, 2016; Burton, 2015, Singh, R.,2024b). Ensuring representation in governance bodies, coaching roles, and administrative positions can help reshape institutional priorities and promote more inclusive policies.

Furthermore, inclusive governance requires dismantling entrenched power hierarchies within sports organizations. Traditional governance structures often replicate broader societal inequalities, limiting the influence of women and marginalized groups. Reforming these structures involves not only increasing representation but also redistributing decision-making authority and resources. This transformation is essential for creating equitable sports ecosystems that align with sustainability principles (True, 2022).

6.2 Accountability, Advocacy, and Systemic Transformation

Justice commitments in women's sports must be supported by robust accountability mechanisms that ensure policy implementation and institutional compliance. While many organizations have adopted gender equity policies, the absence of effective monitoring and evaluation systems often limits their impact. Establishing clear performance indicators, transparency frameworks, and reporting mechanisms is critical for tracking progress and identifying gaps (OECD, 2022; UN Women, 2023).

Accountability also extends to financial practices, including equitable distribution of funding, sponsorship, and prize money. Transparent budgeting and auditing processes can help address disparities and build trust among stakeholders. Additionally, international benchmarks and standards can provide guidance for aligning national policies with global best practices, reinforcing consistency and coherence in governance (Hancock et al., 2023).

Athlete advocacy has emerged as a powerful force in advancing justice in women's sports. Female athletes are increasingly using their platforms to challenge inequalities, demand fair treatment, and raise awareness about broader social issues. This form of activism not only amplifies marginalized voices but also influences public discourse and policy agendas (Meggyesy & Rosner, 2022, Dewasiri, N.J., 2026). Athlete-led movements for equal pay, improved working conditions, and representation have demonstrated the potential of collective action to drive institutional change.

Moreover, advocacy extends beyond individual athletes to include civil society organizations, media, and community groups. These actors play a critical role in holding institutions accountable, promoting awareness, and fostering dialogue gender equity in sports. Collaborative advocacy efforts can create pressure for reform while also building coalitions that support long-term transformation (Kidd, 2021, Nwokolo, S.C.,2023).

Systemic transformation in women's sports requires aligning justice commitments with broader sustainability frameworks. This involves integrating gender equity into policy design, resource allocation, and organizational practices. It also necessitates a cultural shift that values inclusivity, diversity, and fairness as core principles of sports development. Such transformation is inherently complex and requires sustained commitment from multiple stakeholders, including governments, private sector actors, and international organizations (Leach et al., 2018).

Justice commitments in women's sports represent a critical dimension of the global sustainability agenda, emphasizing the need for equitable systems that empower all participants. By adopting intersectional approaches, strengthening governance structures, and supporting advocacy initiatives, stakeholders can move toward more inclusive and just sports ecosystems. These transformative pathways not only address existing inequalities but also create opportunities for innovation, resilience, and sustainable growth, positioning women's sports as a key driver of social change in the global economy.

7. CONCLUDING REFLECTIONS, LIMITATIONS, AND FUTURE RESEARCH DIRECTIONS

7.1 Concluding Reflections

The analysis presented throughout this chapter establishes women's sports as a critical intersectional domain where social justice, policy innovation, and sustainability converge. Women's sports are no longer peripheral to the global sports economy; rather, they represent a transformative space capable of advancing inclusive growth, gender equity, and institutional accountability. By situating women's sports within the sustainability discourse, the chapter highlights their potential to contribute to broader developmental goals, including social inclusion, economic participation, and equitable governance.

A central argument emerging from this discussion is that inequalities in women's sports are deeply embedded within structural and institutional systems. Economic disparities, limited media representation, and governance imbalances are interconnected challenges that cannot be addressed through isolated interventions. Instead, they require comprehensive and coordinated strategies that align policy frameworks, investment models, and cultural transformation. The sustainability economy provides a valuable lens for this alignment, emphasizing the integration of social equity with economic and institutional development.

At the same time, the increasing commercialization of women's sports introduces both opportunities and complexities. While growing investments and audience engagement have enhanced visibility and professionalization, they also risk reinforcing inequalities if not guided by equity-oriented principles. Sustainable development in this context requires a balance between market expansion and social responsibility, ensuring that growth benefits a diverse range of stakeholders rather than a select few. Women's sports, therefore, must be understood not only as an economic sector but also as a site of ethical and social transformation.

7.2 Limitations of the Study

Despite its contributions, this chapter is subject to several limitations that should be acknowledged. First, the analysis is primarily conceptual in nature and relies on secondary sources. While this approach allows for a broad synthesis of existing literature, it may not fully capture the complexity and diversity of experiences across different regions and sporting contexts. Women's sports are shaped by local socio-cultural, economic, and political factors, and these contextual variations may not be adequately reflected in a generalized framework.

Second, the rapidly evolving nature of the sports industry presents challenges in maintaining temporal relevance. Developments in areas such as digital media, commercialization, and global policy initiatives are occurring at a fast pace, and some of these changes may not be comprehensively addressed within the scope of this chapter. This limitation highlights the need for continuous research that keeps pace with emerging trends and innovations.

Another important limitation relates to the treatment of intersectionality. While the chapter acknowledges the importance of intersecting identities such as race, class, and geography, the analysis does not fully explore how these dimensions interact to shape experiences in women's sports. Future research should adopt more nuanced approaches that account for multiple axes of inequality and provide a deeper understanding of marginalization within sports systems.

Additionally, the chapter identifies a gap in the measurement of sustainability outcomes in women's sports. The absence of standardized metrics for assessing social, economic, and environmental impacts limits the ability to evaluate progress and design evidence-based interventions. This methodological limitation underscores the need for more robust data collection and analytical frameworks.

7.3 Future Research Directions

Building on these limitations, several directions for future research emerge. One important area is the need for empirical studies that examine the relationship between women's sports and sustainability outcomes across diverse contexts. Such research can provide insights into how different policy environments, cultural norms, and economic conditions influence the development of women's sports.

Longitudinal studies would also be valuable in understanding the long-term impact of policy interventions and investment strategies. By tracking changes over time, researchers can assess the effectiveness of different approaches and identify best practices for promoting equity and sustainability. Comparative studies across countries and regions can further enrich this analysis by highlighting contextual variations and transferable lessons. The role of technology represents another area for future inquiry. Digital platforms, social media, and data analytics are transforming the way sports are produced, consumed, and governed. Investigating how these technologies can be leveraged to enhance visibility, participation, and equity in women's sports can contribute to more innovative and inclusive development models.

Future research should also greater attention to grassroots and community-based initiatives. These programs often play a crucial role in promoting participation and challenging socio-cultural barriers, particularly in underrepresented regions.

Understanding their impact and scalability can inform policy design and support more inclusive sports ecosystems. Finally, interdisciplinary approaches that integrate perspectives from sociology, economics, public policy, and environmental studies are essential for advancing knowledge in this field. Collaboration between academic institutions, policymakers, sports organizations, and civil society can facilitate the exchange of ideas and the development of holistic solutions.

The continued evolution of women's sports within the global sustainability economy depends on sustained commitment, critical inquiry, and collaborative action. By addressing existing limitations and pursuing new research pathways, scholars and practitioners can contribute to the creation of more equitable, inclusive, and sustainable sports systems that empower women and benefit society as a whole.

REFERENCES

Acker, J. (2020). Gendered organizations and intersectionality: Problems and possibilities. *Equality, Diversity and Inclusion, 39*(1), 3–18. DOI: 10.1108/EDI-11-2019-0340

Adriaanse, J. (2016). Gender diversity in the governance of sport associations: The Sydney scoreboard global index of participation. *Journal of Business Ethics, 137*(1), 149–160. DOI: 10.1007/s10551-015-2550-3

Andrews, D. L., & Silk, M. L. (2018). *Sport and neoliberalism: Politics, consumption, and culture*. Temple University Press., DOI: 10.2307/j.ctvr43k8s

Bruce, T. (2016). New rules for new times: Sportswomen and media representation in the third wave. *Sex Roles, 74*(7–8), 361–376. DOI: 10.1007/s11199-015-0497-6

Bruening, J. E., & Dixon, M. A. (2019). Work-family conflict in coaching: A top-down perspective. *Journal of Sport Management, 33*(1), 1–15. DOI: 10.1123/jsm.2018-0054

Burton, L. J. (2015). Underrepresentation of women in sport leadership: A review of research. *Sport Management Review, 18*(2), 155–165. DOI: 10.1016/j.smr.2014.02.004

Coalter, F. (2015). Sport-for-change: Some thoughts from a sceptic. *Social Inclusion (Lisboa), 3*(3), 19–23. DOI: 10.17645/si.v3i3.222

Collins, P. H. (2019). *Intersectionality as critical social theory*. Duke University Press., DOI: 10.1215/9781478007098

Connell, R. (2009). *Gender in world perspective* (2nd ed.). Polity Press.

Cooky, C., & Antunovic, D. (2020). "This isn't just about us": Articulations of feminism in media narratives of athletes' activism. *Communication & Sport, 8*(4–5), 692–711. DOI: 10.1177/2167479519896360

Cooky, C., Messner, M. A., & Musto, M. (2021). "It's dude time!" A quarter century of excluding women's sports in televised news. *Communication & Sport, 9*(1), 3–34. DOI: 10.1177/2167479519892930

Crenshaw, K. (2017). *On intersectionality: Essential writings*. The New Press., DOI: 10.2307/j.ctt1ggjjnm

Crowther, D., Singh, R., Singh, A., & Rani, S. (2024). Assessing the Impact of Artificial Intelligence on Healthcare Sector for Enhancing Sustainability. In Singh, R., Shafik, W., Crowther, D., & Kumar, V. (Eds.), *Transforming Healthcare Sector Through Artificial Intelligence and Environmental Sustainability. Approaches to Global Sustainability, Markets, and Governance.* Springer., DOI: 10.1007/978-981-97-9555-0_1

Deloitte. (2024). *The rise of women's sports: Unlocking commercial growth.* Deloitte Insights.

Deloitte. (2024). *Women's sports revenue forecast.* Deloitte Insights.

Dewasiri, N. J., Singh, R., Ranasinghe, A., Dsilva, J., & Shaikh, M. I. (2026). Industry 5.0 for a Climate-Resilient South Asia: A Human-Centric Approach to Net-Zero Futures. In Singh, R., Filho, W. L., & Kumar, V. (Eds.), *Data-Driven Sustainability: Harnessing Technology for A Greener Future and Environmental Resilience. World Sustainability Series.* Springer., DOI: 10.1007/978-3-032-13412-7_23

Eccles, R. G., Ioannou, I., & Serafeim, G. (2020). The impact of corporate sustainability on organizational processes and performance. *Management Science, 60*(11), 2835–2857. DOI: 10.1287/mnsc.2014.1984

Elkington, J. (1997). *Cannibals with forks: The triple bottom line of 21st century business.* Capstone.

Elson, D. (2017). Recognize, reduce, and redistribute unpaid care work. *Gender and Development, 25*(1), 9–24. DOI: 10.1080/13552074.2017.1297473

Evans, A. B., & Pfister, G. (2021). Women in sports leadership: A systematic narrative review. *International Review for the Sociology of Sport, 56*(3), 317–342. DOI: 10.1177/1012690220911842

Evans, A. B., & Pfister, G. (2024). Women in sports leadership: Structural barriers and opportunities. *Sport in Society, 27*(2), 215–230. DOI: 10.1080/17430437.2023.2187654

Fink, J. S. (2016). Hiding in plain sight: The embedded nature of sexism in sport. *Journal of Sport Management, 30*(1), 1–7. DOI: 10.1123/jsm.2015-0278

Giulianotti, R. (2016). *Sport: A critical sociology* (2nd ed.). Polity Press.

Hancock, M. G., Darvin, L., & Walker, N. A. (2023). Gender equity in sport: Progress and challenges. *Sport Management Review, 26*(3), 345–360. DOI: 10.1016/j.smr.2022.09.001

Hargreaves, J. (1994). *Sporting females: Critical issues in the history and sociology of women's sports*. Routledge.

Hoeber, L. (2018). Exploring the gaps between meanings and practices of gender equity in a sport organization. *Gender, Work and Organization*, *25*(1), 58–74. DOI: 10.1111/gwao.12162

Kabeer, N. (2021). Gender equality, inclusive growth, and development. *World Development*, *142*, 105–415. DOI: 10.1016/j.worlddev.2020.105415

Kane, M. J. (2013). The better sportswomen get, the more the media ignore them. *Communication & Sport*, *1*(3), 231–236. DOI: 10.1177/2167479513484579

Kidd, B. (2021). Sport and social movements: A global perspective. *International Review for the Sociology of Sport*, *56*(6), 847–862. DOI: 10.1177/1012690220972935

Leach, M., Raworth, K., & Rockström, J. (2018). Between social and planetary boundaries. *Nature Sustainability*, *1*(12), 693–695. DOI: 10.1038/s41893-018-0181-1

Leal Filho, W., Azul, A. M., Brandli, L., Özuyar, P. G., & Wall, T. (2021). Gender equality for sustainability in higher education institutions. *Sustainability*, *13*(20), 11469. DOI: 10.3390/su132011469

McCullough, B. P., Kellison, T. B., & Melton, E. N. (2020). Developing an environmentally sustainable sport industry. *Sport Management Review*, *23*(2), 175–190. DOI: 10.1016/j.smr.2019.01.004

Meggyesy, D., & Rosner, S. (2022). Athlete activism and social justice. *Journal of Sport and Social Issues*, *46*(5), 389–402. DOI: 10.1177/01937235211068789

Meier, M. (2023). Gender equality and sport development. *European Sport Management Quarterly*, *23*(4), 567–584. DOI: 10.1080/16184742.2022.2037645

Meier, M., & Saavedra, M. (2020). Women and sport in Africa: Historical and contemporary perspectives. *The International Journal of the History of Sport*, *37*(13–14), 1383–1400. DOI: 10.1080/09523367.2020.1846204

Mensah, J. (2019). Sustainable development: Meaning, history, principles, pillars, and implications for human action. *Cogent Social Sciences*, *5*(1), 1653531. DOI: 10.1080/23311886.2019.1653531

Nussbaum, M. (2011). *Creating capabilities: The human development approach.* Harvard University Press., DOI: 10.4159/harvard.9780674061200

Nwokolo, S. C., Singh, R., Khan, S., Kumar, A., & Luthra, S. (2023a). Africa's Awakening to Climate Action. In *Africa's Path to Net-Zero. CSR, Sustainability, Ethics & Governance*. Springer., DOI: 10.1007/978-3-031-44514-9_9

Nwokolo, S. C., Singh, R., Khan, S., Kumar, A., & Luthra, S. (2023b). Impacts of Climate Change in Africa. In *Africa's Path to Net-Zero. CSR, Sustainability, Ethics & Governance*. Springer., DOI: 10.1007/978-3-031-44514-9_7

OECD. (2022). *Gender equality in sport: Policy frameworks and practices*. OECD Publishing., DOI: 10.1787/1f8c9f2a-

Pegoraro, A., Comeau, G., & Frederick, E. (2022). Social media and women athletes. *Communication & Sport, 10*(2), 235–252. DOI: 10.1177/2167479520969785

Pegoraro, A., Comeau, G. S., & Frederick, E. (2021). #LikeAGirl: Examining social media conversations surrounding women's sports. *Communication & Sport, 9*(2), 271–289. DOI: 10.1177/2167479519893332

Porter, M. E., & Kramer, M. R. (2019). Creating shared value. *Harvard Business Review, 89*(1–2), 62–77.

PwC. (2023). *The rise of women's sports: Commercial trends and future opportunities*. PricewaterhouseCoopers.

PwC. (2023). *Women's sports outlook and investment trends*. PricewaterhouseCoopers.

Rai, S. M., Hoskyns, C., & Thomas, D. (2019). Depletion: The cost of social reproduction. *International Feminist Journal of Politics, 21*(3), 381–403. DOI: 10.1080/14616742.2018.1535683

Raworth, K. (2017). *Doughnut economics: Seven ways to think like a 21st-century economist*. Chelsea Green Publishing.

Saavedra, M. (2022). Women, sport, and development. *Sport in Society, 25*(6), 1105–1120. DOI: 10.1080/17430437.2021.1899173

Schulenkorf, N. (2017). Sport for development and peace. *Journal of Sport Management, 31*(3), 243–251. DOI: 10.1123/jsm.2016-0131

Sen, A. (1999). *Development as freedom*. Oxford University Press.

Senne, J. A. (2023). Gender equity in sport funding. *Sport Management Review, 26*(2), 210–225. DOI: 10.1016/j.smr.2022.05.004

Shafik, W., Singh, R., & Kumar, V. (2024). Artificial Intelligence Transparency and Explainability in Sustainable Healthcare. In Singh, R., Shafik, W., Crowther, D., & Kumar, V. (Eds.), *Transforming Healthcare Sector Through Artificial Intelligence and Environmental Sustainability. Approaches to Global Sustainability, Markets, and Governance*. Springer., DOI: 10.1007/978-981-97-9555-0_9

Singh, R. (2026). The Positive Impact of AI for Implementation of Circular Economy and Climate Change Towards Ocean Sustainability. In Singh, R., Filho, W. L., & Kumar, V. (Eds.), *Data-Driven Sustainability: Harnessing Technology for A Greener Future and Environmental Resilience. World Sustainability Series*. Springer., DOI: 10.1007/978-3-032-13412-7_12

Singh, R., Crowther, D., & Ravesangar, K. (2024b). Harnessing Human Capital for a Sustainable Future: HR's Pivotal Role Toward Net Zero Policies. In Singh, R., & Crowther, D. (Eds.), *Transition Towards a Sustainable Future. Approaches to Global Sustainability, Markets, and Governance*. Springer., DOI: 10.1007/978-981-97-5756-5_2

Singh, R., Ravesangar, K., Narayanan, S., & Singh, K. K. H. (2024a). HRM Practices in Creating Net Zero: Supporting Organizational Sustainability. In Singh, R., Khan, S., Kumar, A., Luthra, S., & Chokshi, H. (Eds.), *Net Zero Economy, Corporate Social Responsibility and Sustainable Value Creation. CSR, Sustainability, Ethics & Governance*. Springer., DOI: 10.1007/978-3-031-55779-8_1

True, J. (2022). Gender equality and institutional reform. *Politics & Gender*, *18*(2), 345–359. DOI: 10.1017/S1743923X21000445

UNESCO. (2023). *Gender equality and sport: Breaking barriers for women and girls*. UNESCO Publishing.

UNESCO. (2023). *Global report on women and sport participation*. UNESCO Publishing.

United Nations. (2023). *The Sustainable Development Goals report 2023*. United Nations., DOI: 10.18356/9789210024914

WHO. (2022). *Physical activity and women's health*. World Health Organization.

Wicker, P., Feiler, S., & Breuer, C. (2023). Gender differences in sport participation and earnings. *European Sport Management Quarterly*, *23*(5), 789–807. DOI: 10.1080/16184742.2022.2041123

Women, U. N. (2023). *Women in sport: Towards gender equality*. United Nations.

World Bank. (2023). *Gender equality and economic development*. World Bank.

Chapter 9
Social Protection of Athletes:
An Evaluation From the Perspectives of Labour Law and Social Security Law

Hatice Erol
http://orcid.org/0000-0002-8816-1137
Aydın Adnan Menderes University, Turkey

Abdullah Özdemir
http://orcid.org/0000-0002-7506-3431
Aydin Adnan Menderes University, Turkey

ABSTRACT

The welfare state rests on the responsibility of public authorities to protect individuals against social and economic risks throughout the life course. As social policy expands beyond traditional employment, the sports sector has gained prominence due to its professionalization, commercialization, and labour-intensive nature. Professional athletes' contractual dependency, income instability, career fragility, and limited social security coverage reveal that sport constitutes a distinct field raising specific labour law concerns. The debate over whether athletes are employees or hold a sui generis status directly affects their legal protection. While key elements of employment exist, features such as transfer systems and fixed-term contracts create deviations. Protection levels vary across welfare regimes and institutional settings. This study evaluates athletes' social protection within welfare state frameworks, comparatively analysing legal structures and identifying policy gaps.

DOI: 10.4018/979-8-2600-3174-2.ch009

INTRODUCTION

The welfare state aims to protect people from social or economic risks during their lifetime. Social policy is no longer just about standard working relationships; it has changed as the labour market has changed, and it now includes other forms of work and alternative forms of vulnerability. Sport is considered a growing sector of the economy (i.e., the economic scale of sports is growing), with many athletes now working in professional sporting leagues and having contractual relationships with employers who require them to perform contracted work for them. As such, the working conditions experienced by professional athletes, including contracts, income stability, career length, and access to social protections, demonstrate that sport is a separate employment arena with distinct legal and institutional issues and not just a recreational activity. The relationship between sport and the welfare state raises many questions regarding the definition and protection of economic and social rights of athletes. A key issue is the legal classification of professional athletes, i.e., should they be treated as employees under labour law or as individuals working under a different contractual arrangement?

Although athlete contracts have the same base-level components as many employment-based relationships (i.e., salary, duties/commitments, and degree of control), athletes typically operate within an employment-like model. However, the complex governing structure associated with athletic activity (e.g., transfer systems, fixed-term agreements, and federations' rules) makes it difficult to fully apply an employment-based model to the athletic context. Social protections afforded to athletes are established under a multi-layered and fragmented framework from a global perspective. The rights and protections available to the athlete are collectively influenced by various international and regional legal frameworks, as well as by many sports governing bodies. Although these instruments were not intended for the sports field, certain general principles intended to protect individual employees (e.g., equitable working conditions, access to social benefits, right to join an organisation, and prohibition against discrimination) are still relevant. However, the fundamental conflict between these more universal legal principles and the autonomous regulatory regimes created by sports organisations limits the protective mechanisms available to athletes. The methods used to legally define employment and social security benefits of athletes differ significantly across countries. However, in Türkiye, there has been a lengthy discourse on the form or character of what constitutes an athlete's contract, the type of coverage they will receive through their insurance policy, and the extent to which they depend on the athlete–employer relationship. Although some legal frameworks are set up to manage these issues, the structural characteristics of the sports industry (short-term contracts, high risks for injuries, predominance of fixed-term contracts, and the use of transfer systems) raises questions about whether the existing legal frameworks sufficiently protect athletes. A thorough assessment of how this issue can be addressed requires incorporating both labour law and social security as complementary frameworks.

Different social welfare systems have created very different outcomes for athletes in terms of job security, stability of contracts, protection against dismissal, and access to social insurance. All major types of social welfare systems, whether liberal, conservative-corporatist, or social-democratic, provide varying degrees of protection for athletes based on the degree of public intervention, strength of collective bargaining mechanisms, and inclusion of social insurance. In some regimes, professional athletes are treated unambiguously within the scope of labour law, in others hybrid models specific to sports law have been adopted. These differences necessitate a comparative examination regarding fundamental rights, such as wage protection, protection in cases of contract termination, and coverage under occupational accident and disease schemes.

Proceeding from this point, this chapter examines provide a comprehensive assessment of the social protection mechanisms applicable to athletes, examined through the dual lens of labour law and social security law within a welfare state perspective. The study first sets out the theoretical relationship between the welfare state and sport; it then analyzes the social security and labour law framework offered by international instruments and national legislation to athletes; it goes on to compare athletes' economic and social rights across different welfare regimes comparatively; and finally, it develops actionable policy recommendations directed at the key problem areas that emerge in the social protection of athletes.

1. THE ROLE OF SPORT ITN WELFARE STATE DEBATES

Sport has moved well beyond its status as a recreational pastime in the twentieth century and became a multidimensional phenomenon carrying social, political, and economic functions. During this period, sport emerged as an instrument that contributed to social integration by enhancing interaction across different social, cultural, and economic groups. States simultaneously deployed it in connection with education, health, and social welfare policies as an effective mechanism for reaching broad populations. Alongside this, sport played a significant role in processes of ideological guidance, mass mobilization, and national identity construction, particularly under different political regimes. In this sense, sport functions both as an element that strengthens social cohesion and as a strategic field that can be shaped under the objectives of political power (Riordan, 1999: 50-51).

The most general explanation for the use of sport in public policy relates to its deployment as an instrument for achieving domestic policy objectives within the political system. Governments have treated sport as a functional tool for realizing certain policy aims. Several themes stand out within this category. First, sport has been used to foster social integration and strengthen social control mechanisms. Governments, particularly in managing the settlement of new migrants and bridging sectarian, cultural, or political divisions, have drawn on sporting activities for this purpose. In addition, sport has been promoted as a means of reducing social tensions. Sporting activities address not merely the question of how individuals spend their leisure time but also contribute to the development of individual qualities such as discipline and self-confidence. Against this background, the functions of sport in preserving social order have come to the foreground. In the United Kingdom, following the urban unrest of the early 1980s, the Thatcher government deployed sport policies in pursuit of social policy objectives, directing leisure expenditure towards specific social groups and urban areas. This approach continued the practice of the preceding Labour government, though the crucial difference lay in the fact that sport services were framed not from a 'needs-based' standpoint but through an 'instrumental' lens—that is, as a tool in the service of public order. The functions of sport, moreover, are not confined to the social sphere alone. Investment in sport contributes to urban regeneration, and in that respect is valued as an instrument of economic development; given its positive effects on health, it has equally been employed as a policy tool for the improvement of public health (Parrish, 2003: 13). Despite the effective role of sporting activities in realizing welfare state objectives, athletes themselves encounter very significant problems in the course of carrying out those activities.

Sport, by its distinctive character, represents a form of work that falls outside ordinary occupational categories, and athletes are confronted throughout their professional lives with clusters of risk that are unique to them and that overlap with one another in ways other workers do not experience. Athletes may face difficulties in exercising rights to social dialogue, freedom of association and collective bargaining; non-payment or delayed payment of wages; bogus self-employment arrangements; inadequate post-career employability; and the dangers of injury and disability, making sport one of the most hazardous of professional pursuits (ILO, 2020: 2). These risks should not be treated as the individual problems of athletes alone but as a reflection of the systematic failure to apply a human-rights-based social security framework to the sports sector.

According to research conducted under the SOPROS project and findings presented at the ILO's 2020 Forum, five interconnected core problems stand out in athlete-specific social risks and protection gaps. These are (Mittag et al., 2025: 5; ILO, 2020):

The first is conditionality: existing protection systems rest on a logic in which entitlement is allocated based on performance criteria rather than vulnerability or life-cycle need.

The second is fragmentation: equivalent progress in unemployment protection has not matched advances in maternity protection.

The third issue is the lack of transparency and education: athletes struggle to understand complex entitlement systems and to exercise their rights effectively.

The fourth problem is the 'representation gap' between employers and employees (in this case athletes), where there are no 'collective bargaining' systems to help them come together to resolve issues. This gap means that labour rights violations can become widespread.

The fifth problem is the government's ambivalence in both provision and outsourcing without establishing adequate mechanisms for oversight over those entities providing services to them. So, given the importance of sport in promoting the welfare of the population in many nations, to what extent do athletes receive adequate protection from labour law and social security law when they experience a situation where those protections would have benefited them?

2. THE LEGAL STATUS OF ATHLETES: BETWEEN LABOUR LAW AND SPORTS REGULATION

Professional sports athletes exist in a legal grey area between labour law and sports law. Because of this, there is an ongoing debate about whether professional athletes are employees of their clubs. Different legal traditions will produce different answers to this question. There is ambiguity about the athlete-club relationship, which stems from the fact that sport is both an economically viable activity and organized in an unusual manner.

2.1. The Employment Status of Athletes' Contracts: An International Comparative Analysis

Sporting activity is a one of the oldest forms of human activity and has evolved into a arge-scale economic sector in today's modern society. Such a development has provided the impetus for re-evaluating the questions of whether the contracts between sportspersons and clubs or teams are legally binding contracts and how they relate to labour law (Bozkurt, 2010: 165).

Whether athletes have been recognized in labour law has been a source of disagreement among labour scholars for many years. The primary issue is whether the relationship between professional athletes and clubs/teams can be classified as an employment relationship under classical contracts of employment, and there has been continued disagreement regarding this issue over the years. This disagreement is primarily because of the relatively unique structure of sport versus general labour law principles. Given the unique nature, content, and obligations of athlete contracts, different scholarly approaches have emerged regarding their legal character. There is no settled view in the doctrine on the type and legal nature of these contracts (Aydos, 2013: 646; Cem, 2012: 26).

Athlete contracts are legally complex instruments governing the legal relationship between athletes and sports clubs and determining the rights and obligations of both parties. The legal character of athlete contracts can vary depending on the country and legal system in question. In some jurisdictions these contracts are treated as 'employment contracts' between the athlete and the club, while in others they may be characterized as 'private law contracts' governed by sports law and the regulations of sports federations (Bozkurt, 2010: 165–190). The relationship between athlete contracts and labour law is of considerable importance both for defining and protecting the rights and obligations of athletes and clubs alike.

Determining whether an athlete contract qualifies as an employment contract requires, foremost, an examination of the essential elements of the employment contract. Traditionally, employment contracts include three components: (1) work performance, (2) remuneration, and (3) subordination. Professional athletes are involved in representing their clubs and training for and competing in professional sports. Both activities are recognizable as being related to the contractual obligations between athletes and their respective clubs through a reasonable interpretation of work performance and therefore fulfill part of the contractual obligations of an athlete to the club. Professional athletes are compensated through regular salaries, bonuses, incentives, and any other benefits that are received because of professional services performed by the athlete. Based on this evidence, it is reasonable to conclude that remuneration is a critical element of the contract between an athlete and his/her club. Subordination is the third critical component of an employment contract. Athletes are bound to the directions given to them by the head coach of their club, the coaching staff of their club, and the administrative personnel of their club. The training schedules established by the club and the details outlining the preparation for training camps and competition events are established by the club. Therefore, the arrangements for training and competing are established by the club and not by the athlete, thus demonstrating that the athlete-subordinate relationship is like the subordinate-employee relationship identified in the labour law context. Accordingly, similarities exist between the athlete-club relationship and the employee-employer relationship, and therefore, the athlete-club relationship should be analyzed in a manner similar to that of the employee-employer relationship.

Sports contracts establish a private law relationship with regard to the parties when one party engages in their sport, and the other pays as per the terms of that contract. Sports contracts are developed according to the unique characteristics of sports law and do not fit neatly into the general rules of obligations. Sports law scholarship classifies athletes in binary terms—professional and amateur—and athlete contracts are categorized accordingly. An examination of the Turkish sports law system reveals that only football is recognized at the legislative level as holding professional status, a fact that has led in practice to the concept of 'professional athlete contract' being treated primarily in footballers. The observable presence, in athlete contracts, of certain elements found in contracts directed at the performance of work has provided grounds for the view that such contracts should be assessed within the framework of service contracts or contracts for work and labour. Bearing in mind, however, sport's distinctive competitive structure, the inherent unpredictability of physical performance, and the regulatory authority of federations, it is more appropriate to characterise athlete contracts as independent contracts of a sports law nature. On this reading, disputes that arise under such contracts should properly be resolved by reference to the instructions and regulations of the relevant federation (Doğu, 2020: 447-448).

Whether the relationship between professional athletes and sports clubs is subject to labour legislation depends on the legal arrangements of the country in question and on case law. International sports regulations also constitute an important factor bearing on the nature of athlete contracts. The FIFA Regulations on the Status and Transfer of Players, in particular, illustrate that the relationship between an athlete and a club is shaped not merely by national law rules but also by transnational sports norms (FIFA, 2025). These regulations restrict athlete mobility on such matters as contractual stability, the transfer system and the termination regime, and may come into conflict with classical labour law principles. The Diarra case provides a recent example of precisely this kind of conflict, reopening debate about the effects of sports regulations on freedom of movement in the labour market (Case C-650/22, Court of Justice of the European Union, (Diarra), 2024).

The Bosman ruling changed all the rules governing professional athletic careers in EU law. The Court of Justice ruled that professional soccer players are more than just athletes, but they must be treated as workers. Professional soccer players (and professional athletes) enjoy the same ability to move freely throughout the EU as other workers do. The Bosman ruling (C-415/93, ECJ, Bosman, 1995) established that professional sports are not created or performed in a vacuum. When money is involved, professional sports are subject to employment law and the rules of the European Union's common market for workers. Following Bosman, the legal status of professional athletes in EU Member States has come to be treated in a manner closely aligned with employee status (Parrish, 2003: 5).

In 1995, the Bosman ruling conferred on professional footballers the same free movement rights as ordinary workers. More than twenty years later, whether those rights can be exercised remains a matter of legal and academic debate. While most professional footballers in EU Member States are recognised as workers under national law, several countries treat them as self-employed. The preference for one working status over the other carries meaningful implications for social security entitlements, tax obligations, and rights to collective agreements (Duval and van Maren, 2017: 258).

In continental European legal systems, the legal nature of athlete contracts is most often regulated within a 'special employment relationship' model. In Spain, in particular, the legal status of professional athletes is determined by a specific piece of legislation that diverges from general labour law while preserving its core principles. Under this system, the relationship between an athlete and a club is expressly recognised as an employment relationship, though the duration of contracts, termination and compensation are differentiated in ways suited to the nature of sport. Italy similarly treats professional athletes' activities essentially as a labour relationship performed in return for remuneration, while providing specific rules that account for the distinctive character of the sports sector (Naluang, 2024: 386-404).

In English law, athletes' status is determined through a more flexible and case-by-case approach. When determining whether a professional athlete is an employee or an independent contractor, courts will consider whether the following factors exist in that situation: subordination, personal service, and mutual obligations. Overall, when considering team sports, professional athletes will be viewed as bordering on being classified as employees, whereas for individual athletes, the classification is more controversial (O'Leary et al., 2025: 257-258).

For professional athletes in the United States (US), being an employee or independent contractor is rather straightforward. A high majority of professional athletes in the US are classified as employees, regardless of the sport they are participating in. As employees, professional athletes are afforded the right to form a union and negotiate their contracts with their teams, as any other worker would. However, college athletes are still uncertain whether they are employees or not. The recent ruling in Johnson v. NCAA (2024) determined that some college or university athletes (athletes under contract with a college) may be classified as employees, which may impede an athlete from being defined as an amateur athlete; therefore, no longer disallowing the amateur athlete from receiving protection under the Labour Relations Act. In Türkiye, athletes are not directly covered under the Labour Act No. 4857. The Labour Act explicitly excludes athletes from being covered under the Labour Act. Such athletes are excluded from the personal scope of the Labour Act No. 4857, provided they are provided compensation from and/or because of their athletic activity. The organisations within which they operate, the legal characterisation of the relationships involved, working hours, wages and other entitlements will not be determined by the labour legislation but by the Turkish Code of Obligations (Özveri, 2024: 627). This does not mean that athletes are not recognised as workers; rather, it gives rise to doctrinal debates about which legal regime governs this relationship.

In conclusion, a comparative analysis demonstrates that the legal character of athlete contracts cannot be explained through any single-dimensional approach. The professional athlete is situated within a labour relationship in economic and organisational terms, yet that relationship diverges from classical labour law on account of sport's structural features. Accordingly, the most accurate characterisation treats athlete contracts as atypical employment relationships that carry the elements of employment contracts but are shaped by regulations specific to sports law.

2.2. A comparison between the European Union and Türkiye

2.2.1. Recognition of Employee Status and the Normative Approach

Under EU law, the status of athletes as 'workers' is recognised in law, with the Bosman ruling further clarifying that athletes are not only players but also part of an economy. Therefore, according to the Bosman decision, athletes have the right to be treated “as any other employee” (C-415/93, European Court of Justice, Case Bosman, 1995). The decision means that EU law considers the position of athletes according to broader principles such as freedom of movement, the right to work, and the application of competitive practices. Conversely, Türkiye has taken a completely different position from the EU, whereby an athlete does not have the same legal standing in the workplace under Article 4 of the Labour Act No. 4857 and is governed by the Turkish Code of Obligations. Türkiye’s approach only makes a partial link to labour law, and it is not nearly as direct or broad as what is seen in the EU.

2.2.2. Labour Law Protections Available to Athletes in EU Member States

The fact that athletes in EU member states are treated as being close to employee status means that they can benefit from broader protections under labour law and social security law. Athletes may access protections like those under general labour law in the following areas:

- Employment security
- Social security entitlements
- Working hours and rest rights
- Freedom to organise in trade unions

In Türkiye, the exclusion of athletes from the scope of the Labour Act limits their direct access to such protections. While the social security status of athletes has been regulated to a certain degree, there are significant gaps in areas such as employment security and protection against dismissal — gaps that are frequently described in the doctrine as a 'protection deficit'.

2.2.3. Contractual Freedom and the Transfer System

The use of fixed-term contracts in the professional sports sector has become an almost universal practice. The prevalence of fixed-term contracts means that athletes are left without employment security once the term expires; the uncertainties surrounding contract renewal, transfer, and the rules on free agency adversely affect athletes' economic security. The transfer system, for its part, reconfigures the balance between athletes' freedom to work and clubs' property rights within a framework of rules specific to sports law.

In EU law, athletes' contractual freedom is closely associated with the principle of freedom of movement of workers. Following Bosman, the restrictions imposed on the transfer system were considerably relaxed, making it possible for athletes to change clubs freely at the end of their contracts. The principle of contractual stability continues to be preserved, however, within the framework of FIFA regulations (FIFA, 2025).

In Türkiye, the transfer system largely parallels international sports regulations, but athletes' room for contractual manoeuvre may in practice be more limited. The power imbalance between clubs and athletes can generate outcomes that work against athletes in contract negotiations, and this — combined with the limited reach of labour law protections — weakens athletes' bargaining power.

2.2.4. Dispute Settlement Mechanisms

In the EU, disputes involving athletes may be resolved both in national courts and through sports arbitration mechanisms. The principle of the supremacy of EU law, however, means that the regulations of sports federations cannot be incompatible with EU law. The Diarra case illustrated that sports rules can be subjected to judicial review when they come into conflict with freedom of movement in the labour market (Case C-650/22 (Diarra), 2024).

In Türkiye, numerous conflicts occurring in the sports industry are settled by arbitration institutions created by sports federations. Many people prefer this approach because resolutions are offered at a faster rate than ordinary courts. On the other hand, it has also drawn criticism largely because the judicial review is either limited or not always clear. It remains uncertain when and how athletes will take their claims to the labour courts, as well as the ongoing discussion about the contractual relationship's legal nature.

Türkiye and the European Union clearly differ in the interpretation of the contracts of athletes. In European Union (EU) countries, these contracts are usually regarded as analogous to employment relationships, which are then assessed under labour law. Historically, athlete contracts in Türkiye are viewed as not being subject to the Labour Code, but falling under the general principles of Private Law instead. This distinction causes real-life consequences for athletes, as it influences the protections provided to them as well as their contractual rights and methods for resolving disputes. These issues indicate a need for greater clarity and consistency in the legal framework in Türkiye. Clarifying the classification of athlete contracts as employment contracts, or at the very least, introducing an appropriate legal regime that considers the unique circumstances of athletics would create more certainty and provide greater legal protection to athletes.

3. INTERNATIONAL SOCIAL SECURITY AND LABOUR LAW FRAMEWORKS APPLICABLE TO ATHLETES

Recent developments in international law related to professional and semi-professional athletes include how they fall under labour and social security law. An unprecedented increase in internationalisation of both sporting activity (economic) on a global scale and the ability of athletes to work across national boundaries has created the need for common, binding international laws governing this issue, and many challenges have arisen. Regulatory, or quasi-regulatory bodies such as the ILO (International Labour Organisation), the Council of Europe, the European Court of Human Rights (ECtHR), and the EU have attempted to regulate the labour relationship and social security for athletes through conventions, recommendations, directives, and through case law. However, these legal instruments that purport to provide for the protection of athletes' rights will continue to be scrutinised for their effectiveness, and many fundamental questions remain regarding the legal status of all athletes, as well as regarding the ongoing difficulties in exercising their rights of association and access to social security benefits. This section examines the scope of ILO conventions and recommendations, the implications of Council of Europe instruments and ECtHR case law for athletes' rights to organise and bargain collectively, the applicability of EU law to the sports sector, and the transformative role of the Bosman ruling.

3.1. ILO Labour Standards and Professional Athletes

The ILO has built a substantial normative legacy in workers' rights. The Freedom of Association and Protection of the Right to Organise Convention (1948, No. 87) and the Right to Organise and Collective Bargaining Convention (1949, No. 98) — two of the cornerstones of this legacy — guarantee the ability of workers to form independent organisations and to resort to collective bargaining through those organisations as a fundamental human right. The ILO's 1998 Declaration on Fundamental Principles and Rights at Work reaffirmed the principles contained in these conventions on a universally binding footing (ILO, 1998). Importantly, these conventions, which are also directly applicable to professional athletes, underscore that athletes possess the rights of association and collective bargaining — whatever the form of their contractual arrangements or employment status (Mittag et al., 2022: 32). That said, the ILO has to date refrained from issuing any specific binding instrument concerning how these norms are to be operationalized within the sports sector.

In social security, the ILO's Social Security (Minimum Standards) Convention (1952, No. 102) established the nine fundamental components of social security — health care, sickness benefit, maternity benefit, old-age benefit, employment injury benefit, unemployment benefit and survivors' benefit — that any adequate social protection system should cover. Ratified by numerous states, this convention serves as a defining reference point for the minimum standards of national social security systems. In 2012, the ILO's Social Protection Floors Recommendation (No. 202) articulated the position that social protection at the national level should rest on a floor of minimum guarantees, including access to health care, child benefits, basic income security for the active-age population and pensions for older persons. The Recommendation makes clear that social protection should be designed as a comprehensive system and underlines that this obligation must (i) be established mandatorily through legislative means and (ii) apply to all workers, irrespective of employment status (ILO, 2012a). Considered in the context of athletes, these principles lay bare the social security gap produced because the great majority of athletes do not hold employee status under national labour law.

The ILO has recorded athletes and sports players as a defined occupational category within the framework of the International Standard Classification of Occupations (ISCO-08) (ILO, 2012b: 210). The ILO's recognition of athletes as working individuals at the normative level stands in sharp tension with the widespread practical reality in which athletes are excluded en masse from employee status.

The Global Dialogue Forum on Decent Work in the World of Sport, held in January 2020, remains the most comprehensive meeting through which the ILO has brought its concerns about working conditions in the sports sector to the international stage. The inadequacy of existing research on the employment relationships and working conditions of athletes and other workers in the sports sector was explicitly identified as a problem. It was underlined that sports organisations and states bear responsibility for implementing decent work standards for athletes, and it was confirmed that ILO Conventions No. 87 and No. 98 apply to athletes regardless of their contractual arrangements or employment status.

3.2. Council of Europe Legal Instruments

The Council of Europe has adopted various agreements and recommendations in sport — particularly on anti-doping, violence in sport and good governance — but has not produced a comprehensive body of convention law directed at athletes in the domains of labour law and social security. In this context, the most important step is the European Social Charter, which is also incorporated into the EU's institutional framework. The European Social Charter provides a normative foundation from which athletes too may benefit — guarantees relating to freedom of association, the right to collective bargaining, social security and fair working conditions.

Article 11 of the European Convention on Human Rights guarantees freedom of assembly and association, including the right to form and join trade unions. While ECtHR case law has not directly addressed sport-related cases, the principles it has developed in relation to trade union organisation and collective bargaining rights carry binding implications for athletes as well (Harris et al., 2018: 722).

3.3. The Legal Status of Athletes in EU Law: The Bosman Judgment

The legal status of athletes in EU law underwent a fundamental transformation with the ruling of 15 December 1995 in Union Royale Belge des Sociétés de Football Association v Bosman (Case C-415/93) [1995] ECR I-4921. This landmark decision established that professional footballers are to be regarded as workers for free movement between Member States and held that the transfer fee systems and national quotas that restricted those rights were incompatible with Article 48 of the EC Treaty (now Article 45 of the Treaty on the Functioning of the European Union). The Court held that sport falls within the scope of Community law where it constitutes an economic activity — that is, where professional or semi-professional footballers are engaged in paid employment or provide services for remuneration. The Court further established that the commercial character of the employer's undertaking is not a prerequisite for Community law to apply; the sole requirement is that an employment relationship exists or is intended to be established (Bosman, para. 73). The question of worker status in Olympic sports has yet to be resolved by European courts — a situation that perpetuates significant legal uncertainty for more than 25,000 European Olympic athletes and underscores the urgent need for legislative clarity (Mittag et al., 2022: 6).

The EU Charter of Fundamental Rights provides the right to collective bargaining (Article 28), as well as the right to strike (Article 31). Article 31 also states that every worker has the inviolable right to decent working conditions. However, even if there is a question of whether these articles apply to athletes in relation to whether they are workers, they still provide a strong normative basis for the rights of athletes. The European Pillar of Social Rights (2021) makes clear that all workers engaged in sport-related activities should receive social protection (Mittag et al., 2022: 69-70).

Upon a careful review of the implementation of international instruments related to social security and labour laws for athletes, several interlinked fundamental flaws arise. The very first and most fundamental flaw is legal uncertainty surrounding the status of athletes. Olympic athletes receive vastly different treatment depending on national legal systems; the fact that the majority are not recognised as workers or employees excludes them from employment-based legal protections, with the result that the ILO normative system proves unenforceable in practice and EU social policy provisions remain effectively inapplicable to them. The second major problem is gaps in social protection coverage. Access to basic social security components such as pensions, health insurance, occupational accident compensation, and maternity or paternity leave is either extremely limited for Olympic athletes or largely determined by which country the athlete lives and works in. The third major problem is difficulties in exercising the right to organise and bargain collectively. These rights, guaranteed by Article 11 ECHR and ILO Conventions No. 87 and 98, cannot be exercised in practice by many Olympic athletes, owing to their exclusion from worker status and the weak institutional capacity of independent sports organisations. The fourth major problem is the absence of a binding international legal instrument: to date, the ILO has developed no specific convention or recommendation addressing the working conditions of athletes in Olympic sport.

4. THE PROTECTION OF ATHLETES IN DIFFERENT WELFARE REGIMES

4.1. The Liberal Welfare Model: A Comparative Analysis of the US and UK

The liberal regime — one of the three basic categories of Gøsta Esping-Andersen's typology of welfare capitalism — differs from other regime types in its residual approach to social protection, the primacy of market mechanisms, and the emphasis placed on individual responsibility. In this regime, the state assumes social risks only where the market and the family prove inadequate; health coverage, pension provision and unemployment protection are constructed largely through private insurance, employment relationships or participation in the market (Esping-Andersen, 1990: 44-47). The decommodification potential of the welfare state, meaning its ability to help people have a dignified life irrespective of wage labour, is low with liberal welfare states, a situation which systematically leaves open people who do not participate in the labour process or who have an unusual way of engaging in wage labour to protection failures (Esping-Andersen, 1990: 36-38).

In the typology offered by Esping-Andersen, the USA and UK constitute the two major examples of welfare states falling under the "liberal" category. In both countries, there prevails a view which sees the operation of the market system as a key means of providing social security to people, where government interventions are minimal, and where athletes' rights are established because of contract, collective bargaining, or court judgments (Isakjee, 2017: 5).

In liberal welfare regimes, the safeguarding of athletes is contingent upon the use of personal freedom of contracting and collective bargaining. In American professional sports, the key element of protecting athletes' interests is the Collective Bargaining Agreement (CBA). This system, based on the framework of the National Labour Relations Act (NLRA), involves players' associations (the NFL Players Association, NBA Players Association, MLB Players Association, and NHL Players Association) who engage in negotiations with the league management to reach binding agreements (Sports Law Center, 2026).

In contrast to other models of regulation, in the liberal one, athletes' rights develop not because of effective labour legislation or social reforms but thanks to competition regulations. Under this approach, the role of the state is that of the regulator, which transfers the responsibility for protecting athletes to the market, insurers, and sports regulatory bodies. As a result, the liberal model creates favourable conditions only for successful persons, whereas other people face a disadvantaged structural situation. Legal instability and lack of social security apply to Olympians. Workers' status is intentionally denied both legislatively and contractually. As the EMPLOYS research concluded: 'Sports legislation or the terms of a contract concluded between the athlete and a national Olympic committee, sports governing body or club can prevent worker status. Athletes excluded from worker or employee status cannot access valuable social and employment rights such as pension entitlements and maternity benefits' (O'Leary et al., 2025: 248).

The key point of divergence between the United States and the United Kingdom lies in the strength of collective negotiation: while US professional leagues, through strong union structures and the collective bargaining mechanism, construct relatively comprehensive guarantees, athletes in the United Kingdom operate in a more fragmented environment shaped by the ambiguous role of the state, legal uncertainties surrounding worker status and the limited capacity of sports governing bodies (Mittag et al., 2025: 97; Seltmann and Fiege, 2025: 99).

Finally, the liberal welfare regime's concrete manifestation in the world of sport is what might be called 'conditionality': existing protection mechanisms produce a meritocratic logic that 'rewards the most successful rather than adequately protecting the most vulnerable' (Mittag et al., 2025: 99). The current systems in both countries — particularly for the protection of Olympic athletes — remain far from meeting international standards.

4.2. The Conservative-Corporatist Welfare Regime: A Comparative Analysis of Germany and France

The conservative-corporatist regime — the second cluster in Gøsta Esping-Andersen's typology of welfare capitalism — describes a distinctive order in which social protection is neither left to market mechanisms nor aligned with the universal approach associated with Scandinavian systems. This regime type is characterised by occupationally based insurance systems that reinforce status distinctions, the central role accorded to the family in social policy, the space granted to subsidiarity for churches and civil society organisations, and the state's function as regulator-coordinator rather than direct service-provider (Esping-Andersen, 1990: 26-33). The key idea here is that conditions must be created when the needs of citizens are satisfied first by their families and by various intermediary bodies, and only when they cannot cope with this responsibility, the state steps in. The majority of continental Europe, including Germany, France, Austria, Belgium, and the Netherlands, belongs to this type of politics, continuing in different ways the traditions of the Bismarckian era (Isakjee, 2017: 5).

As regards policies regarding sports, countries following a conservative-corporatist regime avoid the individualist perspective characteristic of the liberal approach and, a solid-state guarantee provided by the social-democratic model. There occurs a peculiar mixture, according to which sports policy in such states is determined by strong federal organisations, state finances flow to independent sports associations, and control over such organisations lacks transparency (Koebel, 2020: 75). As far as social protection for athletes is concerned, even within this political regime, significant disparities exist.

The welfare state of Germany is based on the logic of social insurance and traces its origins back to Bismarck's introduction of health insurance legislation in 1883. Under this framework, people in Germany do not have access to an all-embracing protective umbrella that exists irrespective of whether people work or not; social entitlements are based on their participation in the workforce and occupation/contribution record (Esping-Andersen, 1990: 58-61). The same holds for the case of Germany's sports policy. With a membership base of roughly 27.4 million athletes, the German Olympic Sports Confederation (DOSB) represents the operative entity in the country's sports policy domain. The government allocates financial aid to the DOSB and other national sports federations via the Federal Ministry of the Interior (BMI) without directly funding individual athletes and does not interfere in the internal mechanisms of the DOSB and other national federations (Koebel, 2020: 78-80).

Germany has taken a path in the field of providing market-oriented social security for Olympic athletes that conflicts with its corporatist traditions. As is shown by the report comparing the SOPROS results of the German Federal Ministry of the Interior, "when the state funding provides pension contributions in France and Poland, the subsidy model in Germany promotes, although does not compel, the acquisition of private pension insurance by the athletes" (Mittag et al., 2025: 99). The decision regarding which insurer to choose and how to manage the pension contract rests with the athlete himself or herself; its coverage depends on the individual initiative of the athlete rather than the guarantorship of the institution (Bundesministerium des Innern, 2026).

The main organisation responsible for promoting German Olympic athletes is the Stiftung Deutsche Sporthilfe (German Sports Aid Foundation), founded in 1967. It relies on a dual financing structure comprising public and private sources of funds and individual donations (Stiftung Deutsche Sporthilfe, 2026). However, research has found that the support provided is insufficient, that the great majority of Olympic athletes in Germany live in conditions of financial insecurity, and that a significant proportion depend on more than one source of income (Breuer et al., 2018: 12-15).

In Germany, athletes enjoy the benefit of professional employee status in the social insurance system (Bundesministerium des Innern, 2026). This means that they have basic rights, including pension rights, health insurance, and maternity/paternity leave. However, this is not presented evenly across all Olympic sports - typically only larger-team or high-profile individual sports receive this benefit; all other Olympic sports (which are not as well publicized) are excluded from the benefit. Therefore, the situation is a concrete manifestation of the SOPROS assessment paper's definition of the 'conditionality' issue: i.e., that the existing means of protecting sports have a bias towards rewarding winning athletes rather than offering protection for losing athletes (Mittag et al., 2025: 99).

Germany's conservative-corporatist structure produces notable protection gaps when it comes to Olympic athletes. Research spanning twenty-nine European countries, conducted under the EMPLOYS project, reveals that the great majority of Olympic athletes in Germany are not engaged in regular employment contracts with any sports organisation (Mittag et al., 2022: 5-6). The concrete consequence of this is that standard social insurance rights available to ordinary employees —

unemployment insurance, sickness benefit, comprehensive maternity leave — are largely beyond the reach of athletes (Mittag et al., 2025: 99-100).

France's position in welfare and sport policy differs from Germany's. While both countries are placed in the conservative-corporatist cluster of Esping-Andersen's classification, France's strong centralisation tradition and the Jacobin state conception rooted in Republican ideology foreground the state's determinative role in sport. The responsibilities shared between local authorities and the Ministry of Sport, and the state's positioning of sport as an instrument simultaneously of public health, national identity and social integration, created the conditions — particularly through the interventionist state conception that took shape under De Gaulle and after — for sport governance to be framed in thick legal and institutional terms (Gasparini, 2020: 86-98).

France stands out among European countries as having one of the most comprehensive legal status frameworks for Olympic athletes. Law No. 1541 of 2015, known as the 'Law Aimed at Protecting High-Level and Professional Athletes and Securing Their Legal and Social Position', marks a critical watershed in the history of social protection for French Olympic athletes. The law introduced sweeping changes in the following areas: the formal regulation of the contractual relationship between athletes and federations, the expansion of insurance coverage for occupational accidents and diseases, the protection of the rights of pregnant athletes, and the strengthening of socio-professional monitoring mechanisms for the post-career phase. Among the law's most striking provisions is the creation, funded by the state, of an occupational accident and disease regime for high-level athletes who are not employed under a contract of employment or do not hold self-employed status. Under this framework, the state assumes medical treatment costs — irrespective of the athlete's status — from the point of injury through to recovery and provides a minimum level of capital or rental income (Français, 2015-2016: IIIA). Regarding professional athletes, the law aimed to end the legal uncertainty in the relationship between clubs and contracted athletes, making the fixed-term employment contract model compulsory (Français, 2015-2016: II).

The SOPROS evaluation report places France — together with Poland — in the category of 'centralised state systems', countries in which the state directly pays basic pension contributions on behalf of athletes regardless of employment status (Mittag et al., 2025: 99). This feature creates a striking contrast with the German model: whereas in Germany state subsidy is directed towards private insurance contracts, in France the state contribution is direct and mandatory, functioning independently of working status. This arrangement signals that the space left to the market by liberal welfare thinking is, in the French model, claimed by the state. The French example, however, is not free from the structural problems identified by SOPROS. In the first place, while progress in maternity and paternity rights and parental leave arrangements is notable, significant gaps persist in areas such as unemployment protection and the level of minimum income (Seltmann and Fiege, 2025: 99). Beyond this, the conditional and selective nature of social protection status — with only athletes on the Ministry's list able to access these guarantees — creates a form of the 'reward the successful, leave the vulnerable outside the protection framework' paradox that is specific to the French model. Athletes who have not been placed on the Ministry list or who have failed to meet prescribed performance thresholds continue to fall through the cracks (Fiege, 2025: 238-240).

In conclusion, both Germany and France share a corporatist common ground in their reliance on strong federation structures as the foundation of sports governance, their avoidance of a direct state service-provider role, and the very limited development of social dialogue mechanisms in the field of Olympic sport. A structural problem common to both countries is the persistence of legal frameworks that do not recognise athletes as workers, even though sport's governing bodies in practice perform the function of employers. Athletes who are not in an employment relationship with a sports stakeholder — such as a National Olympic Committee, a sports governing body or a club — are not afforded access to the valuable social and employment rights that worker or employee status provides, such as pensions and maternity benefit (O'Leary et al., 2025: 248). A significant proportion of Olympic athletes remain outside worker status, and Olympic athletes are largely deprived of the collective bargaining rights and comprehensive employment guarantees available to professional footballers. The most striking common structural weakness of both models is the effective non-functionality of social dialogue mechanisms in social protection for Olympic athletes. Compared with the North American professional sports model, where Seltmann and Fiege (2025: 94) emphasise that the collective bargaining system is deeply entrenched, structures relating to Olympic athletes in Germany and France reveal that independent athlete associations have in practice no seat at the negotiating table.

According to Seltmann's concept of different athlete welfare systems (2025), France is a good example of an "institutional state," while Germany is closer to a "neo-liberal delegation" (p. 1). This apparent contradiction shows that Esping-Andersen's general theories do not accurately apply to sports, thus showing that the link between welfare systems and sport-specific policy domains is an outcome of diverse and different historical/institutional dynamics.

Both France and Germany demonstrate that the conservative-corporatist welfare regime has significant limitations regarding "atypical workers" (in this case Olympic athletes), and in their paper, Mittag et al. (2025, 99) indicate three primary sources of tension regarding the conservative-corporatist welfare system: 1) The tension between rights/protection based on status vs. universal rights; 2) The Bismarckian model which provides social security will be based on your employment status, but

Olympic athletes have a hybrid employment status (neither having an employer/employee relationship nor being independent workers), and thus they fall into a "grey middle ground" that is the primary source of protection gaps in numerous areas in both countries.

The second axis is the tension between a high-performance, achievement-based model and a protective social policy approach. In both systems, the bulk of protection is tied to squad status and international success. The conditionality problem documented by SOPROS is the expression in the field of sport of the corporatist welfare logic: a meritocratic mentality that rewards the strong rather than protecting the weak.

The third axis is the gulf between international human rights standards and domestic institutionalisation. Article 14 of the Council of Europe's Revised European Sports Charter (2021) explicitly provides that persons who engage in sport professionally 'should have an appropriate social status, ethical guarantees against all forms of exploitation, and access to economic and social rights'. When these norms are regarded as binding obligations, the current systems of both countries — particularly in their dimensions relating to Olympic athletes — do not yet meet these standards.

4.3. The Social-Democratic Welfare Regime: The Scandinavian Model

The social-democratic regime — the third and theoretically most coherent cluster in Esping-Andersen's typology of welfare capitalism — is built on the principles of universalism, decommodification, and the erosion of class distinctions. The function of social protection that is assigned in liberal regimes to the market mechanism and in conservative-corporatist regimes to the family and occupational organisations is, in the social-democratic regime, defined as a universal citizenship right and provided by the state irrespective of citizens' employment status, income level or family structure (Esping-Andersen, 1990: 26-28). Against this backdrop, the Scandinavian welfare state is regarded as the most comprehensive social security system produced in the modern era; in domains such as health, education, housing, pensions, unemployment and maternity-paternity leave, state guarantees largely displace individual risk management (Kuhnle, 2000: 5-7). In the domain of sport policy too, this universalist and egalitarian value pattern exercises a determinative influence. In all Scandinavian countries — Norway, Sweden, and Denmark — sport is positioned both as a vehicle of social integration and public health for wide populations and as a vibrant expression of democratic civil society (Masoni, 2020: 143-151).

In Esping-Andersen's conceptualisation, decommodification — access to a level of social guarantee that enables the individual to live a decent life without working

— is the defining criterion of social-democratic regimes (Esping-Andersen, 1990: 36-38). This principle takes concrete form in the field of sport. In Scandinavian countries, sporting practice is funded largely from tax revenues; state support for voluntary club structures is distributed based on membership numbers and the inclusiveness of activities; and sports infrastructure is provided as a public service through local government (Fahlén and Stenling, 2016: 515-531).

In Scandinavian countries, the determinative influence of welfare policy on sport operates through the universal social security system. In the social-democratic welfare system, comprehensive maternity-paternity leave, health services, and unemployment insurance for athletes are designed as basic citizenship rights, widely accessible irrespective of employment status. This optimistic picture is, however, shadowed by two important caveats. Social-democratic guarantees for most individuals rely greatly on the provision of adequate contribution levels; this is especially true for unemployment benefits and higher-tier pension entitlements. As such, athletes who pursue their profession primarily on low or unstable income levels may find themselves unable to avail themselves of an adequate level of protection; as such, numerous athletes will not qualify for legal protection under social democracy unless they have a standard employment relationship with a sports organisation (O'Leary et al., 2025, p. 248).

An investigation conducted by Mittag et al. (2022: 5-6), under the EMPLOYS project and involving 29 countries, has shown that Olympic athletes in Europe (including those in social democratic countries) are mostly without access to social protection systems. This research has revealed that most Olympic athletes do not have an employment relationship with any sports stakeholders and therefore do not necessarily qualify for social security benefits based on employment. In Scandinavian countries, the universal welfare state provides broad-based social protection, which to some extent helps to close this gap, but Olympic athletes still require systematic consideration because of their unique situation—i.e., the seasonal nature of their income; the high risk of early termination of their career; and the lack of any continuous employment caused by the need for training and competing. According to SOPROS project data, while Scandinavian countries are better positioned than other regions about general welfare protection, specific protection mechanisms for Olympic athletes — minimum income arrangements, comprehensive maternity-paternity rights and post-career transition support — remain fragmented and fall short of being systematic (Mittag et al., 2025: 99-100).

In Scandinavian countries, unlike in North American professional sports leagues, collective bargaining and social dialogue mechanisms in Olympic sport have remained largely undeveloped (Seltmann and Fiege, 2025: 94). Although the Scandinavian industrial relations model encompasses broad worker representation and established social dialogue mechanisms, this capacity is insufficiently utilised in practice with respect to Olympic athletes.

The social-democratic regime occupies a position of structural strength compared to the other two regime types examined here for comes to protecting Olympic athletes. Above all, the fact that basic social security comes with citizenship status — rather than employment status — reduces in practice the damage caused by the 'vulnerable/atypical worker' dilemma to which athletes are sometimes exposed. The 'sport for all' principle, which makes sports infrastructure accessible to everyone, also offers an important advantage (Masoni, 2020: 147).

Universal health protection, comprehensive maternity-paternity support. and basic income guarantees in the social-democratic model address, in particular, the guarantees the liberal model leaves to the market or the corporatist model delegates to institutional intermediaries. However, Seltmann's study 'Different Worlds of Athlete Welfare?' (2025: 1-28), comparing six countries, demonstrates that welfare regime classification alone does not determine sport policy outcomes: national sport policy systems, organisational heritage and historical developments emerge as independent variables. Indeed, the reality that competitive athletes in Sweden are very rarely employed provides evidence that, even in a strong welfare state, practical insecurities specific to Olympic athletes can persist.

5. STRUCTURAL CHALLENGES IN ATHLETE PROTECTION AND POLICY REFORM DIRECTIONS

One of the most basic delays that exists between a country and a sports organisation on providing social protections for athletes is the athletes' status. While there are various types of worker contracts, including both independent and hybrid, the lack of clarity in defining these three types directly affects what a country's sports organisations provide for the athlete in terms of social security entitlement. Where there are no specific statutes defining an athlete's status in Türkiye and elsewhere, the way the country interprets them leaves open the possibility for very different interpretations and non-protection for the athlete.

It should also be noted that this issue is not only because of a lack of formal structure but also the weak implementation of any rules governing the athlete's status and entitlements has prevented positive movement from occurring in these areas as well. To resolve these issues, there is a critical need for not only a fundamental change at the normative (formal) level but also at the practical (implementation) level. Additionally, participating nations and international organisations must work collaboratively with the governing bodies of sports to implement a more effective mechanism for the protection of athletes: Some other issues affecting the successful implementation of national legislation include the incompatibility of fixed-term (contract) employment with job security, inadequacy of collective bargaining mechanisms, potential for labour law protections to be in conflict with sports arbitration systems, and lack of post-career support. All these issues represent critical gaps that require removal from current sports system structures to ensure that all athletes in all sports receive appropriate social protections.

A comprehensive strategy is necessary to improve the social protection of athletes. To begin, it is imperative to provide a precise definition of athlete status in national law, as this will clarify the specific labour law protections afforded to athletes. Other regulatory reform priorities will include: the encouragement of collective agreements in sports clubs, strengthening the collective bargaining rights of Players' Associations, and harmonising sports arbitration with labour law standards. In social security, priority reform measures will be the expansion of disability insurance benefits, improvements to early retirement and disability provisions, and the implementation of systematic post-career support programmes.

CONCLUSION

This research has comprehensively assessed the social protection of athletes from a welfare-state viewpoint. It has examined this issue from the perspectives of labour law and social security law and has established an analytical framework composed of five key dimensions. The results of each analysis indicate that there are significant structural gaps regarding social protection for athletes, both structurally and institutionally.

The first finding relates to social sport and its placement within the general debate on welfare states. The analysis of the functions of sports can be seen through the dual lens of social integration, health, and identification with a country to demonstrate that movement has historically been correlated with welfare policies. The duality present because athletes are both the object of these policies and also excluded from the social welfare system represents a serious contradiction within the welfare state framework. Those who provide the basis for the welfare state cannot adequately access the guarantees of the welfare system because they themselves are excluded as employees. Because of this contradiction, there is a need for an overall social policy approach to treat sports, as opposed to viewing sport as an effective means of achieving social policy objectives.

The second result relates to the status of athletes under labour law, examined from the point of view of how athlete contracts compare against traditional employee contracts. The research shows that even though athlete contracts appear to fulfill the three basic components that make up an employee contract (performance of work, compensation, and subordination), they differ from traditional forms of labour law because of the unique nature of sport. In the European Union, for example, one can regard professional athletes as being closer to employees based on the Bosman case and European Union law. However, Article 4 of the Turkish Labour Law No 4857 specifically excludes from that law any reference to athletes, but instead regulates athletes under the Code of Obligations of Türkiye. As such, this results in severely limiting the ability for a professional athlete to access employment security, protections against dismissal, and social insurance rights, and thus creates what appears to be a very clear protection deficit when compared against that provided by the laws of the European Union. Through this comparative analysis, it will be possible to demonstrate that if the contracts of professional athletes in Türkiye were regulated under a status closest to an employee contract, but taking into account the distinctive nature of sport, it would reduce the amount of legal uncertainty and improve the level of protection afforded to professional athletes.

The final finding related to the type and scope of the international framework applicable to athletes. ILO Conventions Nos 87, 98, and 102 form the basis under which athletes have the right to organise, collectively negotiate, and access social security benefits. The Decent Work Forum in 2020 helped to focus international attention on the failure to applying these principles within the sports sector. Additionally, Council of Europe documents and the European Social Charter are instrumental in forming a strong basis for athletes participating in the Olympic Games, and the Bosman case and the Diarra case demonstrate the ability of EU law to supervise sports regulation. While there is little question that these international laws do not have the intended impact at the national level and that the missing classification of athletes as workers (to promote fairness within the sports sector) cannot be resolved by existing laws, the primary flaw is the absence of a binding, international instrument aimed at solving the unique problems of athletes.

The fourth finding involved a comparative assessment of different welfare regimes. The liberal regime (USA, UK) bases athlete protection largely on individual contractual freedom and collective bargaining mechanisms, but this structure traps the available guarantees within a meritocratic logic that 'rewards the most successful and leaves the most vulnerable outside'. In the conservative-corporatist regime (Germany, France), while the state assumes a more determinative role in the Olympic sports field, the conditional and performance-dependent nature of protection perpetuates systematic protection gaps. The social-democratic Scandinavian model offers the most advantageous structure in terms of welfare guarantees grounded in universal citizenship rights; however, specific mechanisms tailored to the circumstances of Olympic athletes — seasonal incomes, career interruptions and the risk of early career termination — remain inadequate even in these systems. The fact that all three regime types harbour the five core problems documented by the SOPROS and

EMPLOYS projects — conditionality, fragmentation, lack of transparency, representation gaps and the ambivalent role of the state — in different forms demonstrates that the problem is not specific to anyone welfare regime but carries a structural and universal character.

The fifth finding addressed areas of concern while also recommending changes to the current way things are done. Areas identified with legal uncertainty are related to athlete status, fixed-term contracting, collective bargaining inadequacies, conflicts between sports arbitration law and labour rights, and a lack of post-career support systems. In order to address weaknesses found in existing systems, the following qualifications are needed for reform: create a national definition for athletes; create statutes to give athletes the same level of legal protection as employees; create a single type of collective agreement (as opposed to multiple agreements); expand insurance for both disability and incapacity; and establish a process whereby all transitions from an athlete's career to their next step will be accounted for.

The existing legal structure regarding sport in Türkiye is urgently in need of reform. Athletes are excluded from the scope of the Labour Act No.4857, which creates uncertainties regarding legal status and rights, effectively eroding protection for athletes; furthermore, only football is recognised at the legislative level as having a 'professional' status, therefore, this leaves most sports outside the existing legal framework. In relation to EU law, the definition/status of Athlete Contracts in comparison to Employment Contracts is not defined clearly, and the governing regimes regarding transfers/terminations result in an imbalance of power in terms of Athlete rights, and the mechanisms for Collective Bargaining are not sufficiently developed. Thus, it is imperative that Türkiye develop and implement a comprehensive legislative framework that recognises the unique qualities of Sport along with the requirements of international law and so the creation of such a framework must be a priority within Türkiye's Sports Law/Social Policy reform agenda.

To sum up, the underlying issue with social protection for athletes does not lie in having insufficient standards, but in having ineffective enforcement mechanisms to ensure compliance with those standards. The solution requires a paradigm shift across all welfare systems, effective institutional support provided through a common commitment from governments, sporting bodies, and athletes, along with other global entities, and universal protection for all athletes without regard to their employment classification as an athlete or otherwise. All athletes (not just those who are competing) are making investments of their time, energy, and lives to provide social benefits of competition; therefore, they should enjoy the same level of social security as all other workers who also make contributions to society. The rights of athletes must be recognised as a fundamental right of individuals under either sport or social policy as a means of ensuring protection for all individuals.

REFERENCES

Aydos, O. S. (2013). Sporcu sözleşmesinin feshi [Termination of athlete contracts]. Ankara Üniversitesi Hukuk Fakültesi Dergisi [Ankara University Faculty of Law Journal], 62(3), 643–690.

Bozkurt, M. N. (2010). Spor hukuku uyuşmazlıklarının çözümünde Milletlerarası Spor Tahkim Mahkemesi [The Court of Arbitration for Sport in the resolution of international sports disputes] [Ankara Bar Journal]. *Ankara Barosu Dergisi, 2,* 165–190.

Breuer, C., Wicker, P., Dallmeyer, S., & Ilgner, M. (2018). *Die Lebenssituation von Spitzensportlern und -Sportlerinnen in Deutschland.* Bundesinstitut für Sportwissenschaft.

Bundesministerium des Innern. (2026). Reform Athletenförderung. Accessed April 2026. Available at: https://www.bmi.bund.de/DE/themen/sport/nationale-sportpolitik/spitzensportreform/athletenfoerderung Case C-415/93, European Court of Justice, Union Royale Belge des Sociétés de Football Association and others v. Bosman and others, ECLI:EU:C:1995:463.

Case C-650/22, Court of Justice of the European Union (Diarra), 2024.

Cem, Ç. (2012). *Profesyonel Futbolcu Transfer Sözleşmesi* [Professional Footballer Transfer Contracts]. Oniki Levha Publishing.

Council of Europe. (2021). Recommendation CM/Rec(2021)5 of the Committee of Ministers to Member States on the Revised European Sports Charter (2021), Article 14. Available at: https://www.coe.int/en/web/sport/the-european-sports-charter

Doğu, H. M. (2020). E-spor ve e-spor hukuku'nda sporcu sözleşmeleri [E-sports and athlete contracts in e-sports law]. *Ankara Üniversitesi Hukuk Fakültesi Dergisi, 69*(2), 443–453. DOI: 10.33629/auhfd.848644

Duval, A., & van Maren, O. (2017). The labour status of professional football players in the European Union: Unity in/and/or diversity? *European Labour Law Journal, 8*(3), 258–278. DOI: 10.1177/2031952517716279

Esping-Andersen, G. (1990). *The three worlds of welfare capitalism.* Princeton University Press.

Fahlén, J., & Stenling, C. (2016). Sport policy in Sweden. *International Journal of Sport Policy, 8*(4), 515–531. DOI: 10.1080/19406940.2015.1063530

Fiege, L. (2025). *The social protection of Olympic elite athletes in Europe: A human right trapped between international commitment and domestic institutionalisation?* The International Sports Law Journal.

FIFA. (2025). Regulations on the Status and Transfer of Players incl. interim regulatory framework, January.

Français, S. (2015–2016). Proposition de loi visant à protéger les sportifs de haut niveau et professionnels. Rapport n° 70.

Gasparini, W. (2020). Sports organisations and policies in France. In Porro, N. R., Martelli, S., & Testa, A. (Eds.), *Sport, Welfare and Social Policy in the European Union* (pp. 86–98). Routledge. DOI: 10.4324/9781351118064-8

Harris, D., O'Boyle, M., Bates, E., & Buckley, C. (2018). Law of the European Convention on Human Rights (4th ed.). Oxford University Press.

International Labour Organisation (ILO). (1948). Freedom of Association and Protection of the Right to Organise Convention (No. 87). https://normlex.ilo.org/dyn/normlex_en/f?p=NORMLEXPUB:12100:0:NO:P12100_INSTRUMENT_ID:312232

International Labour Organisation (ILO). (1949). Right to Organise and Collective Bargaining Convention (No. 98). https://normlex.ilo.org/dyn/normlex_en/f?p=NORMLEXPUB:12100:0:NO:P12100_INSTRUMENT_ID:312243

International Labour Organisation (ILO). (1952). C102 Social Security (Minimum Standards) Convention. https://normlex.ilo.org/dyn/normlex_en/f?p=NORMLEXPUB:12100:0:NO:P12100_INSTRUMENT_ID:312247

International Labour Organisation (ILO). (1981). Collective Bargaining Convention (No. 154). https://normlex.ilo.org/dyn/normlex_en/f?p=NORMLEXPUB:12100:0:NO:P12100_INSTRUMENT_ID:312299

International Labour Organisation (ILO). (1998). ILO Declaration on Fundamental Principles and Rights at Work. Geneva: ILO. https://www.ilo.org/declaration/lang--en/index.htm

International Labour Organisation (ILO). (2012a). Social Protection Floors Recommendation (No. 202). https://www.social-protection.org/gimi/RessourcePDF.action?id=56900

International Labour Organisation (ILO). (2012b). *International Standard Classification of Occupations (ISCO-08)* (Vol. 1). ILO.

International Labour Organisation (ILO). (2019). Issues paper for discussion at the Global Dialogue Forum on Decent Work in the World of Sport. Geneva: ILO. GDFWS/2020.

International Labour Organisation (ILO). (2020). Global Dialogue Forum on Decent Work in the World of Sport – Points of consensus. Geneva, 20–22 January 2020, Sectoral Policies Department. https://www.ilo.org/sites/default/files/wcmsp5/groups/public/%40ed_dialogue/%40sector/documents/meetingdocument/wcms_735388.pdf

Isakjee, A. (2017). Welfare state regimes: A literature review. University of Birmingham Institute for Research into Superdiversity Working Paper 18.

Koebel, M. (2020). The organisation of sport and sports policies in Germany. In Porro, N. R., Martelli, S., & Testa, A. (Eds.), *Sport, Welfare and Social Policy in the European Union* (pp. 75–85). Routledge. DOI: 10.4324/9781351118064-7

Kuhnle, S. (2000). The developmental welfare state in Scandinavia. UNRISD Discussion Paper.

Masoni, I. (2020). In the homeland of sport for all: The Scandinavian countries. In Porro, N. R., Martelli, S., & Testa, A. (Eds.), *Sport, Welfare and Social Policy in the European Union* (pp. 143–151). Routledge. DOI: 10.4324/9781351118064-13

Mittag, J., Fiege, L., Seltmann, M., ... (2025). Elite athletes' social protection in Olympic sports in Europe: An evaluation of the status quo. SOPROS Evaluation Report.

Mittag, J., Seltmann, M., Fiege, L., & O'Leary, L.. (2022). *Good governance in the employment relations of athletes in Olympic sports in Europe* [EMPLOYS Project Report]. University of Rijeka, Faculty of Law.

Naluang, S. (2024). The legal architecture of employment contracts for professional athletes. *Rajapark Journal, 18*(56), 386–404.

O'Leary, L., Seltmann, M., & Smokvina, V. (2025). Elite athletes and worker status. *Industrial Law Journal, 54*(2), 248–277. DOI: 10.1093/indlaw/dwae025

Özveri, M. (2024). *Bireysel İş İlişkileri Açısından Türkiye İşçi Hukuku Tarih-Öğreti-Uygulama-Eleştiri* [Turkish Labour Law in Terms of Individual Employment Relations: History, Doctrine, Practice, Critique]. 2nd ed., Vol. I). E. Ceren Özveri Education and Solidarity Foundation Publication.

Parrish, R. (2003). *Sports law and policy in the European Union*. Manchester University Press. DOI: 10.7228/manchester/9780719066061.001.0001

Republic of Türkiye Official Gazette. (1971). Labour Act No. 1475.

Republic of Türkiye Official Gazette. (2003). Labour Act No. 4857.

Riordan, J. (1999). *The international politics of sport in the 20th century*. Routledge.

Seltmann, M. (2025). Different worlds of athlete welfare? A social policy perspective on elite sport in six European countries. International Journal of Sport Policy and Politics, 1–28. DOI: .DOI: 10.1080/19406940.2025.2583977

Seltmann, M., & Fiege, L. (2025). Many a little makes a mickle: Lessons from negotiating athletes' social protection for strengthening social dialogue in sport. Sports Law, Policy & Diplomacy Journal, 3(2).

Sports Law Center. (2026). Collective bargaining agreements in sports leagues. Justia. Accessed April 2026. Available at: https://www.justia.com/sports-law/collective-bargaining-agreements-in-sports-leagues/

Stiftung Deutsche Sporthilfe. (2026). Die Sporthilfe-Förderung. Accessed April 2026. Available at: https://www.sporthilfe.de/athletenfoerderung/foerderkonzept/

United States Court of Appeals, Johnson v. NCAA, 2024.

Chapter 10
Sport as a Social Policy Instrument in Turkey:
Welfare Effects, Social Inclusion, and the Role of State-Led Sport Programs

Kerem Berkman
http://orcid.org/0000-0001-8766-2733
T.C. Hatay Mustafa Kemal Üniversitesi, Turkey

ABSTRACT

This chapter examines sport as a social policy instrument in Turkey, assessing its welfare effects, contribution to social inclusion, and the role of state-led sport programs. Integrating social investment theory, the capability approach, and sport-for-development literature, it traces the institutional transformation following the establishment of the Ministry of Youth and Sports in 2011, reviews the legal framework, and analyses flagship initiatives including Youth Centres, Sports Training Centres, and the Sport for All programme. Descriptive evidence from TÜİK, Ministry activity reports, and Eurobarometer surveys shows that sport participation in Turkey remains stratified by gender, income, education, and region, and that elite-sport priorities continue to dominate public spending. The chapter concludes with policy recommendations on rebalanced spending, integrated cross-sector design, targeted outreach, and stronger evaluation systems for Turkey and comparable middle-income economies.

DOI: 10.4018/979-8-2600-3174-2.ch010

INTRODUCTION

Over the past two decades, sport has gradually shifted from the margins of social policy debate to a more central position in discussions of welfare, social cohesion, and human capital formation. International organisations such as the United Nations, the Council of Europe, the European Commission, and the World Health Organization have increasingly linked sport to broader development goals, including poverty reduction, health promotion, gender equality, and youth empowerment (Levermore and Beacom, 2009; United Nations, 2003). At the national level, governments have responded by expanding public investment in sport facilities, elite performance programs, and participation-oriented initiatives. However, the assumption that sport automatically delivers welfare outcomes has attracted sustained scholarly scrutiny. Coalter (2007, 2013) and Hartmann and Kwauk (2011) have warned against a form of sport evangelism that overstates the transformative capacity of sport while neglecting questions of access, distribution, and institutional design.

Turkey is an instructive case for examining how sport can function as a social policy instrument. Since the early 2000s, the country has undergone significant transformations in both its welfare regime and its sport governance structures. Reforms in social security, family policy, and labour market regulation have reshaped the Turkish welfare regime, which scholars have characterised as conservative-corporatist with strong familialist features (Buğra and Keyder, 2006; Grütjen, 2008). At the same time, the establishment of the Ministry of Youth and Sports (Gençlik ve Spor Bakanlığı) as a standalone ministry in 2011 signalled a more explicit political commitment to using sport and youth policy as vehicles for social development. Subsequent investments in Youth Centres (Gençlik Merkezleri), Sports Training Centres (Spor Eğitim Merkezleri), and the SPOR-TOTO funding mechanism have sought to link sport participation with broader social policy objectives.

Despite these developments, the welfare impact of Turkish sport policy remains under-theorised in English-language scholarship. Most comparative work on sport and social inclusion draws on Northern and Western European contexts, where welfare regimes, civil society traditions, and sport-club structures differ markedly from those in Turkey. The existing Turkish literature, while expanding, has often concentrated on elite sport management, sport economics, and physical education, with less attention to welfare outcomes and distributional effects. This chapter addresses this gap by situating Turkish sport policy within comparative welfare theory and the global sport-for-development agenda, and by assessing how effectively state-led sport programs contribute to social inclusion and welfare.

The analysis is guided by three interrelated questions. First, how has sport policy in Turkey been institutionalised as an instrument of social welfare, and what welfare objectives are explicitly or implicitly embedded in current programs and legal frameworks? Second, what do available data reveal about the distribution of sport participation across socioeconomic, demographic, and regional groups in Turkey? Third, to what extent have state-led sport programs contributed to measurable welfare outcomes, particularly for young people, women, and residents of less developed regions? The chapter responds to these questions through a synthesis of policy analysis, descriptive statistics from national and international surveys, and engagement with the theoretical literature on welfare and sport.

The chapter's theoretical framework integrates three strands. Social investment theory emphasises welfare policies that build human capital and reduce future welfare dependency rather than simply compensating for market failures (Morel et al., 2012; Hemerijck, 2017). The capability approach, developed by Sen (1999), foregrounds the expansion of substantive freedoms and the conditions that enable individuals to lead lives they have reason to value. Sport-for-development literature, in turn, theorises sport as a potential site of empowerment, social capital formation, and cross-group encounter, while remaining attentive to its limitations (Coalter, 2013; Kidd, 2008). These perspectives converge on the view that sport's welfare effects are conditional rather than automatic, and depend on how programs are designed, resourced, and targeted.

Empirically, the chapter draws on publicly available data from the Turkish Statistical Institute (TÜİK), including the Life Satisfaction Survey, the Household Budget Survey, and the Survey on Income and Living Conditions; from Ministry of Youth and Sports activity reports; and from Eurobarometer surveys on sport and physical activity. These sources make it possible to examine both absolute participation rates and their distribution across gender, income, education, and geographic lines. The chapter also engages with academic studies published in Turkish and international journals in order to interpret the descriptive patterns.

The contribution of the chapter is threefold. First, it provides a consolidated English-language analysis of the welfare dimensions of Turkish sport policy, drawing together institutional, legal, and empirical elements that are typically treated separately in Turkish-language scholarship. Second, it connects Turkish evidence with major strands of international theory, including social investment approaches, capability-based welfare analysis, and sport-for-development research, thereby positioning the Turkish case within globally recognised analytical frameworks. Third, it derives policy-relevant implications for both Turkey and comparable middle-income economies, many of which share similar combinations of a young demographic profile, a transforming welfare regime, and a state-led sport system. In doing so, the chapter seeks to inform ongoing debates among policy-makers, researchers, and practitioners about how sport can be mobilised as a meaningful instrument of social welfare rather than a symbolic addendum to other policy domains.

The chapter proceeds in five substantive sections. The background section outlines the conceptual connections between sport and welfare. The first main section traces the historical and institutional development of Turkish sport policy. The second identifies the welfare-related objectives embedded in legislation and flagship programs. The third analyses participation patterns across social groups. The fourth evaluates the welfare impact of selected programs. The final sections provide policy recommendations, directions for future research, and concluding reflections.

BACKGROUND

Sport, Welfare, and The Social Investment Turn

The conceptual relationship between sport and welfare has evolved over several decades. Early welfare-state scholarship paid little systematic attention to sport, treating it as a residual leisure activity outside the core domains of income security, health care, education, and housing (Esping-Andersen, 1990; Titmuss, 1974). From the late 1990s onward, however, sport began to feature more prominently in policy discussions on social exclusion, health promotion, and active citizenship. This shift reflected both the fiscal pressures on traditional welfare states and the emergence of new social risks, including long-term youth unemployment, sedentary lifestyles, mental health challenges, and the erosion of community-level social capital, which were less amenable to conventional cash-transfer solutions (Bonoli, 2005; Taylor-Gooby, 2004).

Within this broader shift, social investment theory argues that modern welfare states should prioritise policies that build human capital, activate labour-market participation, and prepare citizens for changing economic conditions (Hemerijck, 2017; Morel et al., 2012). Investments in early childhood education, lifelong learning, active labour-market policies, and family services are viewed as long-term investments whose returns accrue through higher employment, productivity, and social cohesion. Sport, when framed as a developmental activity for children and young people, fits naturally within this logic. It is credited with improving physical health, mental well-being, discipline, teamwork, and the so-called soft skills that are increasingly valued in post-industrial labour markets.

The Capability Approach and Inclusive Sport Participation

Amartya Sen's capability approach provides a normative lens for evaluating the welfare relevance of sport (Sen, 1999). Rather than defining welfare narrowly in terms of income or utility, the capability approach focuses on what people are actually able to do and to be. From this perspective, the freedom to engage in physical activity, to participate in organised sport, and to access safe and inclusive sport environments forms part of a broader set of capabilities that enable human flourishing. Inequalities in sport participation are therefore not merely matters of personal preference; they reflect deeper inequalities in the conversion factors that translate resources into genuine opportunities, including time, income, safety, cultural norms, and facility access (Robeyns, 2005).

Applied to Turkey, the capability approach helps to explain why formally universal programs may produce unequal outcomes. A young woman in a rural district may have the legal right to use a municipal sport facility but lack practical access due to transport constraints, care responsibilities, or informal norms about public visibility. A low-income family may wish their children to participate in competitive sport but be unable to finance the requisite equipment, travel, or membership fees. Evaluating sport policy from a capability perspective therefore requires attention to both the availability of opportunities and the conditions under which individuals can convert those opportunities into real freedoms.

Sport-for-Development and Sport-for-All Literatures

Sport-for-development and sport-for-all literatures theorise the conditions under which sport can produce positive social outcomes. Scholars such as Coalter (2007, 2013), Kidd (2008), and Hartmann and Kwauk (2011) argue that sport does not produce welfare benefits in a mechanical or universal manner. Instead, outcomes depend on program design, pedagogical approach, the credibility of mentors and coaches, and the integration of sport with broader social services. This literature also cautions against the instrumentalisation of sport as a cheap substitute for substantive social policy, particularly when sport programs are expected to resolve complex structural problems such as poverty or crime (Coalter, 2013).

The European policy environment has reinforced these academic debates. The European Commission's White Paper on Sport (2007) and subsequent Work Plans for Sport identified sport as a contributor to public health, active citizenship, social inclusion, and intercultural dialogue. Eurobarometer surveys on sport and physical activity, conducted at regular intervals since 2002, have provided comparable data on participation patterns across EU member states and candidate countries (European Commission, 2018, 2022). These surveys consistently reveal North–South and East–West gradients in sport participation, with Mediterranean and Central-Eastern European countries typically reporting lower rates than Nordic and Western European states.

The Turkish Welfare Regime and Sport System

Turkey's position within this comparative landscape is shaped by its distinctive welfare regime. Scholars have characterised the Turkish welfare state as a hybrid that combines Bismarckian social insurance for formal-sector workers, means-tested social assistance for the poor, and strong reliance on family-based care provision (Buğra and Keyder, 2006; Grütjen, 2008). Social expenditure has grown considerably since the early 2000s but remains below European Union averages, and informal employment continues to limit the reach of contributory schemes. Within this context, non-contributory, publicly provided services, including those organised through the Ministry of Youth and Sports, can play an important supplementary role in reaching groups that are poorly covered by social insurance.

The Turkish sport system also displays features that differentiate it from both Western European and Anglo-Saxon models. Voluntary sport clubs and civil-society-based sport organisations are less developed than in countries such as Germany, the Netherlands, or the United Kingdom. Instead, state institutions, including federations under the Ministry of Youth and Sports, municipal sport departments, and state-affiliated clubs linked to public enterprises, have historically dominated the organisation of competitive and grassroots sport (Devecioğlu, 2005). This centralised structure creates both opportunities and risks for welfare-oriented sport policy. On the one hand, it enables coordinated national programs and rapid scaling of initiatives. On the other, it can crowd out bottom-up civic participation and limit the responsiveness of programs to local needs.

Social capital theory, particularly as developed by Putnam (2000), also informs the analysis. Sport participation, especially in club-based settings, has been argued to contribute to bridging and bonding social capital, that is, the networks of trust and reciprocity that underpin civic life. The weakness of voluntary sport associations in Turkey suggests that the social-capital channel may operate differently from contexts where sport clubs are the primary vehicle for grassroots participation. Informal sport, family-based physical activity, school sport, and municipally organised sport become correspondingly more important, yet data on these forms of participation remain less systematic than for federation-registered activities.

HISTORICAL AND INSTITUTIONAL DEVELOPMENT OF SPORT POLICY IN TURKEY

From Nation-Building to a Standalone Ministry

The modern history of Turkish sport policy can be traced through several overlapping phases, each shaped by broader political and economic transformations. In the early Republican period, sport was framed primarily as an instrument of nation-building, public health, and military preparedness. The Physical Education and Sport Law of 1938 (Law No. 3530) established the Beden Terbiyesi Genel Müdürlüğü (General Directorate of Physical Education), creating the first centralised administrative body responsible for sport (Fişek, 1985). This arrangement reflected the statist orientation of the period and linked sport policy to the broader project of cultural and social modernisation.

From the 1960s onwards, as Turkey urbanised and implemented successive economic plans, sport policy gradually incorporated more explicit social and educational dimensions. The Five-Year Development Plans of the State Planning Organization increasingly referred to sport in relation to youth development, public health, and leisure, although sport continued to receive modest resources in comparison with core social sectors. The General Directorate of Physical Education was restructured and renamed over time, eventually becoming the General Directorate of Youth and Sports (Gençlik ve Spor Genel Müdürlüğü). In parallel, federations governing individual sports grew in number and specialisation, often with close ties to political leadership (Devecioğlu, 2005).

A significant institutional turning point arrived with the Sport Law No. 3289 of 1986, amended multiple times since, which provided the basic legal architecture for contemporary Turkish sport governance. The law defined the responsibilities of the General Directorate of Youth and Sports, regulated the operation of sport federations, and specified mechanisms for coordination with other public authorities. Subsequent legislation gradually granted greater administrative and financial autonomy to selected federations, culminating in the introduction of autonomous federations that were expected to operate more flexibly while remaining under public oversight (Atalay, 2017; Devecioğlu, 2005).

The 2000s and early 2010s brought further transformation. The establishment of the Ministry of Youth and Sports in 2011, through Decree Law No. 638, marked the elevation of sport and youth policy to full ministerial status. This institutional upgrade reflected a deliberate policy choice to link sport with youth-oriented social policy and to signal the political priority attached to these areas. The new ministry absorbed the General Directorate of Youth and Sports and assumed responsibility for coordinating sport infrastructure investments, national federations, youth centres, and scholarship programs. The reform aligned Turkish sport governance more closely with the European practice of dedicated ministries of youth and sport.

Infrastructure Expansion and Mega-Event Strategy

Alongside these institutional changes, public investment in sport infrastructure expanded markedly. Between the early 2000s and the 2020s, the number of sport facilities registered under the Ministry of Youth and Sports increased substantially, with particular growth in multipurpose halls, stadiums, and youth centres (Ministry of Youth and Sports, 2022). The geographical distribution of these facilities also shifted, with new provinces gaining access to standardised sport infrastructure that had previously been concentrated in the larger metropolitan areas.

Turkey also pursued a strategy of hosting major international sporting events, including the 2005 UEFA Champions League Final, the 2010 FIBA World Championship, several EuroBasket tournaments, and various continental competitions in athletics, wrestling, and other disciplines. These events served multiple objectives: urban branding, tourism promotion, diplomatic signalling, and the justification of infrastructure investments. However, the welfare implications of mega-event spending remain contested in the international literature, with evidence suggesting that the benefits tend to concentrate in host cities while the costs are more widely diffused (Grix and Carmichael, 2012; Horne and Manzenreiter, 2006).

The SPOR-TOTO Funding Mechanism

A distinctive feature of the Turkish system is the use of sports betting revenues as a funding channel for sport development. The İddaa system, operated by the Spor Toto Teşkilat Başkanlığı, generates revenues that are partially directed to federations, grassroots projects, and athlete support (Atalay, 2017; Devecioğlu, 2005). Although the scale and allocation of these funds have been criticised for limited transparency, they represent a significant supplementary resource beyond the general budget. The SPOR-TOTO mechanism also raises normative questions about using gambling-derived income to finance activities intended to produce public welfare benefits, an issue that echoes debates about state lottery-funded sport programs in other countries.

Flagship Programs and Strategic Orientation

Flagship programs launched under the Ministry of Youth and Sports have progressively broadened the social policy dimension of Turkish sport. Youth Centres (Gençlik Merkezleri) offer cultural, educational, and recreational activities for young people, with a particular focus on reaching disadvantaged groups. Sports

Training Centres (Spor Eğitim Merkezleri) identify and develop talented young athletes, often from modest socioeconomic backgrounds, through boarding and scholarship-based arrangements. The Herkes İçin Spor (Sport for All) initiative and various summer and school sport programs aim to expand grassroots participation. Programs such as the Sportif Yetenek Taraması (Sport Talent Screening) seek to integrate physical testing and sport promotion within the school system (Ministry of Youth and Sports, 2019, 2022).

The strategic plans of the Ministry of Youth and Sports explicitly reference welfare-related objectives. Recent plans emphasise increasing sport participation rates, reducing disparities in access, promoting physical activity as a public health intervention, and supporting the social integration of young people, women, persons with disabilities, and residents of less developed regions (Ministry of Youth and Sports, 2019, 2022). These strategic commitments align Turkish sport policy rhetorically with international frameworks such as the United Nations Sustainable Development Goals, the WHO Global Action Plan on Physical Activity, and the EU Work Plans for Sport.

Nevertheless, the translation of these commitments into practice remains uneven. Several structural features constrain the welfare orientation of Turkish sport policy. First, a considerable share of public resources continues to flow toward elite sport, international event hosting, and professional football infrastructure, which raises questions about the distributional fairness of sport spending. Second, coordination between the Ministry of Youth and Sports and other relevant authorities, such as the Ministry of National Education, the Ministry of Health, and municipalities, is frequently ad hoc, limiting the potential for integrated policy design. Third, monitoring and evaluation systems for welfare outcomes are not yet sufficiently developed, making it difficult to track the social return on sport investments (Atalay, 2017; Koçak and Özşaker, 2015).

The Role of Municipalities

Municipalities play an increasingly important role in this ecosystem, particularly in metropolitan areas. Municipal sport schools, swimming courses, walking paths, and neighbourhood sport complexes reach populations that may not otherwise engage with federation-based sport. Research suggests that municipal programs have expanded opportunities for women, older adults, and children from lower-income households, although the scale and quality of such programs vary considerably across municipalities and political jurisdictions (Yetim and Şenel, 2001). The expansion of metropolitan governance and municipal sport budgets after the 2014 local administration reform has enhanced the potential for locally tailored sport policy, while also exposing tensions between central-government priorities and local needs.

WELFARE OBJECTIVES AND THE LEGAL FRAMEWORK

Constitutional and Legislative Foundations

The welfare orientation of Turkish sport policy is rooted in constitutional and statutory provisions that frame sport as a matter of public interest. Article 59 of the 1982 Constitution stipulates that the state shall take measures to develop the physical and mental health of Turkish citizens of all ages and shall encourage the spread of sport among the masses. It also commits the state to protect successful athletes. This dual mandate, promoting mass participation while supporting elite performance, structures the subsequent legal framework and, arguably, creates a persistent tension in resource allocation.

The Sport Law No. 3289 and the Decree Law No. 638 establishing the Ministry of Youth and Sports operationalise the constitutional provisions. Complementary legislation regulates school sport, anti-doping, professional sport, and violence in sport venues. Over time, these legal instruments have incorporated additional welfare-oriented objectives, including the inclusion of persons with disabilities, gender equality in sport participation, protection of minors in sport, and recognition of the social role of sport in youth development. The Law on Sport Clubs and Sport Federations (Law No. 7405) enacted in 2022 introduced further changes aimed at improving governance, transparency, and financial discipline in sport organisations.

Programmatic Welfare Objectives

Contemporary Turkish sport policy pursues a range of welfare objectives, some explicit and others embedded in program design. Health promotion is a prominent goal, reflecting international concerns about rising rates of obesity, sedentary behaviour, and non-communicable diseases. The Ministry of Health and the Ministry of Youth and Sports have cooperated on campaigns that promote daily physical activity, walking paths, and school-based movement programs. These initiatives are consistent with the WHO Global Action Plan on Physical Activity 2018–2030, which sets targets for reducing physical inactivity in member states (World Health Organization, 2018).

Social inclusion represents a second strand of welfare objectives. Programs targeting young people from low-income households, children in care, persons with disabilities, and refugees have been developed, although their coverage remains limited relative to the size of these populations. Initiatives aimed at integrating Syrian and other refugee children into sport activities have received particular attention, often implemented in cooperation with international organisations and non-governmental actors. Sport is presented in these contexts as a low-threshold activity capable of building intergroup contact and providing structured, supervised time for young people who might otherwise be at risk of school dropout or labour-market marginalisation.

Human capital formation constitutes a third objective. The Sports Training Centres, scholarship programs, and talent identification initiatives are justified in part by their potential to convert athletic ability into educational opportunities and upward mobility. Young athletes identified through talent screening can access subsidised boarding schools, specialised training, and preferential admission to faculties of sport sciences. From a social investment perspective, these arrangements can be read as targeted human-capital investments that combine athletic and educational goals (Morel et al., 2012).

Regional development forms a fourth, often implicit, objective. Infrastructure investments have included the construction of sport facilities in provinces with weaker economic bases, and events and competitions have been decentralised to cities outside the Istanbul–Ankara–İzmir core. These measures correspond to broader regional policy priorities articulated in national development plans. However, facility construction alone does not guarantee increased participation; sustained investment in programming, qualified personnel, and transport accessibility is required to translate physical infrastructure into effective opportunities.

Alignment With International Frameworks

Turkish sport policy is increasingly articulated with reference to international frameworks that link sport to broader development and welfare goals. The United Nations 2030 Agenda for Sustainable Development recognises sport as an important enabler of sustainable development, particularly in relation to Sustainable Development Goal 3 on health and well-being, Goal 4 on quality education, Goal 5 on gender equality, Goal 10 on reduced inequalities, and Goal 16 on peaceful and inclusive societies (United Nations, 2003). The Kazan Action Plan adopted by UNESCO's Conference of Ministers and Senior Officials Responsible for Physical Education and Sport provides a further blueprint for linking sport to these goals. The WHO Global Action Plan on Physical Activity sets measurable targets for reducing physical inactivity, against which national strategies can be benchmarked (World Health Organization, 2018).

At the European level, Turkey's candidate status and participation in EU programs such as Erasmus+ Sport, along with its membership in the Council of Europe's Enlarged Partial Agreement on Sport, provide additional channels of policy learning and soft harmonisation. The European dimension is particularly relevant for gender equality in sport, integrity and good governance, and safeguarding in sport, all of which have generated extensive policy guidance and evaluation practice that can be adapted to the Turkish context. Strengthening references to these international frameworks in domestic legislation and strategy would help anchor welfare-oriented sport policy in a broader accountability structure and facilitate transnational learning.

Gaps Between Legal Commitments and Implementation

Despite this extensive legal and programmatic architecture, important gaps exist between stated commitments and implementation. The legal framework mandates inclusive access to sport but does not specify detailed entitlements, performance indicators, or enforcement mechanisms. Budgetary allocations are not systematically tied to welfare outcomes, and elite-sport priorities often take precedence in resource decisions. Civil society involvement in sport policy design is limited, in part because the voluntary sport sector is underdeveloped. Data systems for monitoring participation, particularly in relation to disadvantaged groups, remain fragmented across TÜİK surveys, ministerial records, and federation databases. These gaps constrain the capacity of the Turkish sport system to deliver on its welfare ambitions and complicate the task of evaluation.

SPORT PARTICIPATION PATTERNS ACROSS SOCIAL GROUPS

Aggregate Participation and the Turkey–EU Gap

Data on sport participation in Turkey come from several complementary sources. TÜİK's Time Use Survey and periodic modules on health-related behaviours provide nationally representative estimates of physical activity. Eurobarometer surveys on sport and physical activity include Turkey as a candidate country and allow direct comparison with EU member states. Ministry of Youth and Sports administrative data record registered athletes and participants in public programs. Each source has limitations: survey data rely on self-reports and may be sensitive to how questions are framed, while administrative data capture only those who engage with formal state structures.

Across these sources, a consistent finding is that sport participation in Turkey is relatively low by European standards. Eurobarometer results indicate that a majority of Turkish respondents report never engaging in sport or physical exercise, with participation rates substantially below the EU average (European Commission, 2018, 2022). TÜİK data similarly suggest that regular sport participation is concentrated in a minority of the population. While national campaigns and infrastructure expansion have contributed to incremental improvements, the Turkey–EU gap has narrowed only modestly, and the country remains near the lower end of European rankings for sport participation.

Gender Disparities

Gender disparities constitute one of the most persistent features of Turkish sport participation. Women report substantially lower rates of regular sport activity than men across nearly all age groups, and the gap is particularly pronounced among adults of working age. Multiple factors contribute to this pattern, including the gendered distribution of care responsibilities, informal norms about women's visibility in public space, limited availability of women-only or gender-sensitive facilities, and concerns about safety in and around sport venues (Koca and Hacısoftaoğlu, 2011; Koçak, 2014). Sport participation among adolescent girls falls sharply after puberty, with implications for lifelong physical activity and long-term health outcomes.

Municipal programs have attempted to respond to these challenges through women-only swimming courses, walking groups, and fitness classes. Non-governmental organisations have also launched initiatives focused on women's sport, particularly in football, basketball, and athletics. Nevertheless, the structural constraints on women's participation extend beyond the sport sector and intersect with broader labour-market and family-policy conditions. A welfare-oriented sport policy that takes gender equality seriously must engage with these broader structures rather than treat sport participation in isolation.

Income and Education Gradients

Income and education also shape sport participation. Data from TÜİK and Eurobarometer indicate that individuals in higher income quintiles and with higher educational attainment are more likely to engage in regular sport activity. This pattern is consistent with findings from other European countries, but the gradient in Turkey appears especially steep. Formal sport participation often requires membership fees, equipment, transport, and time flexibility, all of which are more accessible to higher-income households. In addition, cultural capital and familiarity with sport environments play a role: individuals whose families engaged with sport are more likely to continue participation as adults (Bourdieu, 1986).

Children's participation in organised sport displays a similar gradient. School sport activities provide a partial counterweight, particularly for households that cannot afford extracurricular programs, but the quality of school sport varies significantly across schools and regions. Where physical education is limited and school sport clubs are inactive, low-income children have fewer entry points into sport. The result is that sport participation can reproduce rather than reduce existing socioeconomic inequalities, a finding that is well-documented internationally (Bailey, 2005; Collins, 2004).

Regional Disparities

Regional disparities in sport participation reflect broader patterns of uneven development in Turkey. Western and north-western regions, which have higher average incomes, more urban populations, and denser sport infrastructure, report higher participation rates than eastern and south-eastern regions. The Mediterranean and Eastern Anatolian regions, as well as the Southeastern Anatolian provinces, face particular challenges. The 2023 Kahramanmaraş earthquakes exacerbated existing disadvantages in the affected provinces, disrupting facilities, clubs, and school sport activities in a region that already lagged in sport participation. Recovery and reconstruction efforts offer an opportunity to rebuild sport infrastructure with a stronger welfare orientation, although the primary humanitarian needs understandably take precedence.

Urban–rural differences are also significant. Rural areas have fewer standardised sport facilities, fewer qualified coaches, and more limited programming. Informal and traditional physical activities may partially compensate, but regular organised sport is less accessible. Migration from rural to urban areas can expose individuals to new sport opportunities but also to new forms of exclusion associated with peripheral urban settlements, where facility provision and programming may be under-resourced.

Data Limitations and the Measurement Challenge

Interpreting the participation patterns discussed above requires attention to measurement challenges that affect all national sport statistics, and are particularly pronounced in the Turkish case. Survey definitions of sport and physical activity vary across instruments, with some focusing on formal organised sport, others on any form of physical exercise including walking, and yet others on leisure-time activity distinct from work- or commuting-related physical effort. These different operationalisations produce substantially different estimates, which complicates cross-national comparison and longitudinal tracking. Administrative data, meanwhile, count registered participants in specific programs but rarely capture those who engage in informal or self-organised physical activity, which in Turkey is likely a significant share of total activity given the limited penetration of voluntary sport clubs (Koçak, 2014).

Gender-sensitive data collection faces additional challenges. Women's participation in physical activity may occur in settings that are under-represented in conventional sport surveys, including informal neighbourhood walking groups, home-based exercise, and women-only fitness classes organised through municipal or community facilities. Similarly, participation by persons with disabilities, older adults, and refugees may be under-counted in standard sampling frames. Strengthening survey design and expanding targeted modules within existing TÜİK instruments would help to produce a more complete picture of sport and physical activity in Turkey, and would provide a more robust basis for welfare-oriented policy evaluation.

Age and Life-Course Patterns

Age patterns in sport participation merit specific attention given Turkey's demographic profile. Children and young adolescents display relatively high participation rates, often linked to school sport. Participation then declines sharply in late adolescence and early adulthood, as young people transition into the labour market, higher education, or family formation. Adult sport participation stabilises at low levels, and older adult participation is particularly limited, with a narrow base of walking and physiotherapy-related activity (TÜİK, 2022). With ageing of the Turkish population projected to accelerate in the coming decades, strengthening sport and physical activity among older adults represents both a public health priority and a potential area for welfare-oriented sport policy.

Persons with Disabilities and Marginalised Groups

Sport participation among persons with disabilities, refugees, and other marginalised groups is difficult to estimate precisely because of data limitations. Disability sport has received increasing attention through dedicated federations, accessible facility standards, and Paralympic success. However, everyday access to sport for persons with disabilities remains constrained by physical barriers, transport difficulties, and limited awareness among sport providers. Programs aimed at refugee children and youth have expanded, particularly in provinces hosting large Syrian populations, but systematic monitoring of their reach and outcomes is still developing.

EVALUATING THE WELFARE IMPACT OF STATE-LED SPORT PROGRAMS

Assessing Impact in a Complex Policy Field

Evaluating the welfare impact of state-led sport programs is methodologically challenging for several reasons. Welfare outcomes such as health, well-being, social cohesion, and labour-market outcomes are multi-causal and are influenced by factors beyond the sport sector. Randomised controlled trials are rarely feasible at program scale. Administrative data often capture inputs and outputs, such as the number of facilities built or participants registered, rather than outcomes. Self-selection bias is pervasive, as individuals who take part in sport programs typically differ systematically from non-participants. These challenges are not unique to Turkey; they affect sport-policy evaluation internationally (Coalter, 2013).

With these caveats in mind, available evidence can still support a qualified assessment. The following subsections consider selected programs with significant social policy ambition: Youth Centres, Sports Training Centres, the Sport for All initiative, and disability sport programs. The aim is to identify both documented strengths and structural limitations, and to draw lessons for the broader welfare orientation of Turkish sport policy.

Youth Centres as Multi-Purpose Welfare Hubs

Youth Centres have expanded rapidly over the past decade and now operate in all provinces. They offer a mix of cultural, educational, and sport activities, along with counselling and mentorship programs. Participation figures, as reported in Ministry activity reports, show substantial attendance, particularly during school holidays (Ministry of Youth and Sports, 2022). Qualitative studies suggest that Youth Centres can function as valuable safe spaces for young people, particularly in neighbourhoods with limited alternative recreational options.

From a welfare perspective, Youth Centres display several features consistent with a social investment orientation. They bundle multiple services, including sport, cultural activities, and educational support, in a single accessible location. They are publicly funded and largely free at the point of use, reducing financial barriers. They explicitly target young people, including those at risk of marginalisation. However, evaluations also reveal limitations. The intensity of engagement varies widely among participants. Programming quality depends heavily on the capacity of individual centres and staff. Linkages with other social services, including employment support and mental health care, are not always systematic. Strengthening these linkages would enhance the welfare contribution of the centres and align them more closely with integrated youth policy models in Nordic and Western European countries (Hemerijck, 2017).

Sports Training Centres and Targeted Human Capital Investment

Sports Training Centres operate a boarding-school-based model that combines intensive athletic development with formal education. Students typically come from modest socioeconomic backgrounds, identified through regional talent screenings and competitions. The program offers scholarships, housing, coaching, and access to higher education routes, including admission to sport sciences faculties. For beneficiaries, the program can represent a significant upward-mobility channel, converting athletic potential into educational and professional opportunities.

From a welfare perspective, Sports Training Centres combine elements of elite sport development with targeted human capital investment. Their welfare contribution is concentrated among a relatively small number of beneficiaries, but for those individuals it can be substantial. Critics have raised concerns about the selection process, the risk of early specialisation, and the difficulties faced by athletes who do not progress to professional careers. A social investment approach would emphasise the importance of ensuring that all graduates, regardless of athletic outcomes, have strong educational qualifications and viable transitions into the labour market.

The Sport for All Initiative and Mass Participation

The Herkes İçin Spor (Sport for All) initiative represents the most explicit attempt to promote mass sport participation as a welfare objective. It includes school sport programs, summer activities, walking campaigns, and women-oriented projects. Participation numbers, particularly for summer programs, reach significant magnitudes, although the intensity and regularity of participation are often limited.

The welfare contribution of Sport for All programs depends on several design features. Sustained participation, rather than one-off engagement, is essential for producing measurable health and well-being outcomes. Integration with school curricula and primary health care enhances the public-health impact. Explicit targeting of under-represented groups, including women, low-income households, and residents of less developed regions, is required to reduce rather than reproduce existing inequalities. Evidence from municipal and provincial programs suggests that well-designed local initiatives can achieve these objectives, but the overall program architecture remains skewed toward visibility events rather than systematic, long-term participation (Koçak and Özşaker, 2015).

Disability Sport and Inclusion Programs

Disability sport has received growing attention within Turkish sport policy, reflected in a dedicated Paralympic committee, sport federations for specific disability categories, and facility accessibility standards. Paralympic athletes have achieved significant international success in disciplines such as weightlifting, athletics, and judo. Beyond elite performance, everyday disability sport programs provide opportunities for participation, rehabilitation, and social contact (Wicker and Breuer, 2014).

Welfare evaluation of disability sport programs requires particular attention to accessibility in its broadest sense, encompassing physical access to facilities, transport, qualified personnel, adaptive equipment, and inclusive programming cultures. Evidence suggests that while elite disability sport has benefited from targeted investment, grassroots disability sport remains under-resourced. Strengthening this area is a priority for advancing the welfare orientation of Turkish sport policy in line with the United Nations Convention on the Rights of Persons with Disabilities.

Comparative Lessons From International Experience

Placing the Turkish evidence within a comparative frame highlights both distinctive features and transferable lessons. In Nordic countries, mass sport participation has been sustained by dense voluntary sport associations, school sport integration, and long-standing welfare-state support for civil society (Nicholson and Hoye, 2008). In the United Kingdom, a series of sport-for-development initiatives have demonstrated both the potential and the limits of using sport to address welfare challenges, with evaluations underscoring the importance of integrated service design, trained practitioners, and sustained funding (Coalter, 2013). In continental European welfare states, municipalities and sport federations collaborate extensively within co-produced governance structures that allow flexibility and local responsiveness.

The Turkish system differs from each of these models in important respects. The voluntary sector is less developed than in Nordic or Anglo-Saxon contexts, central-government coordination is more dominant than in federal systems, and the pace of institutional change has been faster than in more established European welfare states. These features create both opportunities and constraints. Rapid mobilisation of resources and standardised programs can reach large populations quickly, but may be less attuned to local specificities and civic voice. Drawing lessons from comparative experience does not imply importing foreign models wholesale; rather, it involves identifying functional equivalents within the Turkish institutional landscape and adapting proven design principles, including cross-sector integration, targeted outreach, and evaluation capacity, to local conditions.

Cross-Cutting Welfare Outcomes

Across programs, several cross-cutting welfare outcomes can be identified. Health outcomes, particularly improvements in physical fitness and indicators associated with non-communicable disease risk, are theoretically supported by the physical activity literature, although program-specific evidence for Turkey is limited. Mental health and well-being outcomes are plausible but also under-researched in the Turkish context. Social cohesion outcomes, including intergroup contact and civic engagement, depend heavily on program design and have been documented in qualitative rather than quantitative research. Labour-market outcomes, such as employability and earnings, have rarely been studied systematically in relation to Turkish sport programs.

These outcome gaps highlight the need for stronger evaluation infrastructure. Partnerships between the Ministry of Youth and Sports, TÜİK, universities, and international organisations could support the development of longitudinal data sets, standardised outcome indicators, and quasi-experimental evaluation methods. Such investments in evaluation capacity would, in turn, strengthen the evidence base for welfare-oriented sport policy and align Turkish practice with emerging international standards.

SOLUTIONS AND RECOMMENDATIONS

Drawing on the preceding analysis, several policy directions can strengthen the role of sport as a social policy instrument in Turkey. These recommendations are offered in a spirit of constructive engagement with existing policy architecture and should be read as complementary rather than exhaustive.

First, welfare-oriented rebalancing of sport spending is needed. While elite sport and international event hosting have legitimate functions, their dominance in public spending constrains the resources available for participation-oriented programs. A transparent framework for categorising sport expenditures by function, including elite performance, mass participation, school sport, inclusion, and infrastructure, would support informed public debate and rebalanced allocation. Dedicated budget lines for equity-oriented programs, with clear performance indicators, would enhance accountability.

Second, integrated policy design can enhance welfare outcomes. Sport policy should be more systematically linked to health, education, social assistance, and labour-market policies. The Ministry of Youth and Sports could play a convening role in inter-ministerial working groups focused on specific welfare challenges, such as youth unemployment, obesity prevention, and refugee integration. Joint budgeting for cross-sectoral initiatives, along the lines of the social investment approaches developed in Nordic and continental European countries, would facilitate such integration (Hemerijck, 2017).

Third, targeted programs for under-represented groups should be expanded. Women, low-income households, persons with disabilities, rural residents, and refugees face documented barriers to sport participation. Programs designed with and for these groups, and monitored through participation data disaggregated by gender, income, disability status, region, and migration background, would allow policy-makers to track equity outcomes. Partnerships with municipalities, civil society organisations, and community-based associations can enhance reach and cultural appropriateness.

Fourth, local-level capacity-building is essential. Municipalities are well-positioned to deliver welfare-oriented sport programs but vary considerably in capacity. A national support framework, including technical guidance, shared standards, training for municipal sport staff, and co-financing mechanisms, would help reduce disparities. Particular attention should be paid to municipalities in less developed regions and to those affected by the 2023 earthquakes, where sport infrastructure and programming require targeted reconstruction support.

Fifth, evaluation and data infrastructure require substantial investment. Current data systems capture inputs and outputs but are less effective at measuring welfare outcomes. Expanding TÜİK modules on physical activity and sport participation, strengthening administrative data from Youth Centres and Sport for All programs, and commissioning independent evaluations of flagship initiatives would generate the evidence needed to refine policy over time. Where possible, evaluations should adopt designs that allow causal inference, while recognising the practical constraints of welfare-oriented sport research.

Sixth, governance of the sport sector should continue to evolve toward greater transparency, accountability, and participation. The 2022 Law on Sport Clubs and Sport Federations provides a starting point, but implementation requires sustained attention to financial transparency, conflict-of-interest safeguards, and meaningful involvement of athletes, coaches, volunteers, and local communities. A stronger civil society sector in sport, supported by legal and fiscal frameworks that encourage voluntary associations, would complement state-led programs and enhance the social capital effects of sport participation (Putnam, 2000).

FUTURE RESEARCH DIRECTIONS

The analysis in this chapter points to several productive directions for future research on sport and welfare in Turkey and comparable middle-income economies.

First, more systematic quantitative research is needed on the welfare outcomes of specific sport programs, including health, educational, and labour-market outcomes. Longitudinal cohort studies of participants in Youth Centres, Sports Training Centres, and municipal sport programs could provide valuable evidence on long-term trajectories.

Second, comparative research situating Turkey within broader typologies of welfare regimes and sport systems would deepen theoretical understanding. Case studies of other middle-income countries with similarly state-led sport systems, including those in Latin America, the Middle East, and East Asia, could identify shared patterns and distinctive features (Houlihan and White, 2002). Such comparisons would help to refine sport-policy models that are currently dominated by Western European cases.

Third, qualitative research exploring the lived experiences of participants in Turkish sport programs is essential. Ethnographic and narrative-based studies can illuminate how sport participation intersects with gender, class, ethnicity, disability, and regional identity, and can reveal the mechanisms through which welfare outcomes emerge or fail to emerge. Such research is particularly valuable for understanding women's participation, disability sport, and refugee inclusion programs.

Fourth, methodological innovation is required for evaluating complex, multi-component welfare programs. Mixed-methods approaches, participatory evaluation, and realist synthesis methods offer promising avenues for addressing the evaluation challenges noted in the previous section (Coalter, 2013). Interdisciplinary collaboration between sport scientists, social policy scholars, economists, and public health researchers would strengthen the research infrastructure.

Fifth, attention to emerging issues is warranted. Climate change, digital transformation, and post-pandemic recovery reshape the context for sport participation in ways that welfare-oriented research has only begun to address. How public sport programs respond to heat stress, air pollution, and infrastructure vulnerabilities will matter increasingly for equity outcomes. Similarly, the rise of digital fitness platforms and e-sport opens new questions about what counts as sport participation and who benefits from emerging forms of physical activity.

CONCLUSION

This chapter has examined sport as a social policy instrument in Turkey, tracing its institutional development, identifying its welfare objectives, analysing participation patterns, and evaluating the welfare impact of selected state-led sport programs. The analysis confirms that Turkish sport policy has evolved considerably over the past two decades, with the establishment of a dedicated Ministry of Youth and Sports, substantial infrastructure investment, and the launch of flagship programs addressing youth, gender, disability, and regional inclusion. These developments signal a clear rhetorical and institutional commitment to using sport as a contributor to welfare, social cohesion, and human capital formation.

At the same time, the evidence points to persistent structural limitations. Sport participation in Turkey remains stratified along gender, income, education, regional, and age lines. Elite-sport priorities continue to dominate resource allocation, and coordination across sectors is often limited. Evaluation infrastructure is underdeveloped, making it difficult to assess whether flagship programs are producing the welfare outcomes attributed to them. These limitations are not unique to Turkey, but they acquire particular significance in a country with high youth unemployment, significant regional disparities, and a welfare regime in transition.

Theoretically, the Turkish case illustrates both the potential and the conditional nature of sport as a welfare instrument. Social investment theory, the capability approach, and the sport-for-development literature converge on the view that welfare outcomes depend on how programs are designed, resourced, and integrated with broader social policy. The Turkish experience supports this conditional view: rhetorical commitment and physical infrastructure do not by themselves deliver welfare; inclusive programming, targeted outreach, and sustained evaluation are also required.

Looking forward, Turkey has meaningful opportunities to strengthen the welfare orientation of its sport policy. Rebalanced spending, integrated policy design, targeted programs for under-represented groups, local capacity-building, improved evaluation systems, and more transparent governance would collectively enhance the contribution of sport to welfare outcomes. As a middle-income country with a young population, significant public infrastructure, and established sport institutions, Turkey is well-positioned to serve as an example for comparable economies seeking to use sport as a social policy tool. For the international literature, closer engagement with non-Western cases such as Turkey's can enrich theoretical and policy debates and support more globally relevant frameworks for understanding sport and welfare.

REFERENCES

Atalay, A. (2017). Spor yönetimi açısından Türk spor politikalarına eleştirel bir bakış. *Spor Bilimleri Araştırmaları Dergisi*, *2*(2), 52–65.

Bailey, R. (2005). Evaluating the relationship between physical education, sport and social inclusion. *Educational Review*, *57*(1), 71–90. DOI: 10.1080/0013191042000274196

Bonoli, G. (2005). The politics of the new social policies: Providing coverage against new social risks in mature welfare states. *Policy and Politics*, *33*(3), 431–449. DOI: 10.1332/0305573054325765

Bourdieu, P. (1986). The forms of capital. In Richardson, J. G. (Ed.), *Handbook of theory and research for the sociology of education* (pp. 241–258). Greenwood.

Buğra, A., & Keyder, Ç. (2006). The Turkish welfare regime in transformation. *Journal of European Social Policy*, *16*(3), 211–228. DOI: 10.1177/0958928706065593

Coalter, F. (2007). *A wider social role for sport: Who's keeping the score?* Routledge. DOI: 10.4324/9780203014615

Coalter, F. (2013). *Sport for development: What game are we playing?* Routledge. DOI: 10.4324/9780203861257

Collins, M. F. (2004). Sport, physical activity and social exclusion. *Journal of Sports Sciences*, *22*(8), 727–740. DOI: 10.1080/02640410410001712430 PMID: 15370484

Devecioğlu, S. (2005). Türkiye'de spor sektörü stratejilerinin geliştirilmesi. *Verimlilik Dergisi*, *2005*(2), 117–134.

Esping-Andersen, G. (1990). *The three worlds of welfare capitalism*. Princeton University Press.

European Commission. (2018). *Special Eurobarometer 472: Sport and physical activity*. Directorate-General for Education, Youth, Sport and Culture.

European Commission. (2022). *Special Eurobarometer 525: Sport and physical activity*. Directorate-General for Education, Youth, Sport and Culture.

Fişek, K. (1985). *100 soruda Türkiye spor tarihi*. Gerçek Yayınevi.

Grix, J., & Carmichael, F. (2012). Why do governments invest in elite sport? A polity-specific analysis. *International Journal of Sport Policy and Politics*, *4*(1), 73–90. DOI: 10.1080/19406940.2011.627358

Grütjen, D. (2008). The Turkish welfare regime: An example of the Southern European model? The role of the state, market and family in welfare provision. *Turkish Policy Quarterly*, *7*(1), 111–129.

Hartmann, D., & Kwauk, C. (2011). Sport and development: An overview, critique, and reconstruction. *Journal of Sport and Social Issues*, *35*(3), 284–305. DOI: 10.1177/0193723511416986

Hemerijck, A. (2017). *The uses of social investment*. Oxford University Press. DOI: 10.1093/oso/9780198790488.001.0001

Horne, J., & Manzenreiter, W. (2006). An introduction to the sociology of sports mega-events. *The Sociological Review*, *54*(2, suppl), 1–24. DOI: 10.1111/j.1467-954X.2006.00650.x

Houlihan, B., & White, A. (2002). *The politics of sports development: Development of sport or development through sport?* Routledge.

Kidd, B. (2008). A new social movement: Sport for development and peace. *Sport in Society*, *11*(4), 370–380. DOI: 10.1080/17430430802019268

Koca, C., & Hacısoftaoğlu, İ. (2011). Struggling for empowerment: Sport participation of women and girls in Turkey. In Benn, T., Pfister, G., & Jawad, H. (Eds.), *Muslim women and sport* (pp. 154–166). Routledge.

Koçak, F. (2014). Leisure constraints and facilitators: Perspectives from Turkey. *European Journal of Physical Education and Sport*, *6*(4), 184–194.

Koçak, F., & Özşaker, M. (2015). Youth's preferences for the participation of recreational activities: The case of Turkey. *Kastamonu Education Journal*, *23*(2), 699–712.

Levermore, R., & Beacom, A. (Eds.). (2009). *Sport and international development*. Palgrave Macmillan. DOI: 10.1057/9780230584402

Ministry of Youth and Sports. (2019). Strategic plan 2019–2023. Republic of Türkiye Ministry of Youth and Sports.

Ministry of Youth and Sports. (2022). Annual activity report. Republic of Türkiye Ministry of Youth and Sports.

Morel, N., Palier, B., & Palme, J. (Eds.). (2012). *Towards a social investment welfare state? Ideas, policies and challenges*. Policy Press.

Putnam, R. D. (2000). *Bowling alone: The collapse and revival of American community*. Simon and Schuster.

Robeyns, I. (2005). The capability approach: A theoretical survey. *Journal of Human Development, 6*(1), 93–117. DOI: 10.1080/146498805200034266

Sen, A. (1999). *Development as freedom.* Oxford University Press.

Taylor-Gooby, P. (Ed.). (2004). *New risks, new welfare: The transformation of the European welfare state.* Oxford University Press. DOI: 10.1093/019926726X.001.0001

Titmuss, R. M. (1974). *Social policy: An introduction.* Allen and Unwin.

TÜİK (Turkish Statistical Institute). (2022). *Time use survey.* TÜİK.

United Nations. (2003). *Sport for development and peace: Towards achieving the Millennium Development Goals. Report of the Inter-Agency Task Force on Sport for Development and Peace.* United Nations.

Wicker, P., & Breuer, C. (2014). Exploring the organizational capacity and organizational problems of disability sport clubs in Germany using matched pairs analysis. *Sport Management Review, 17*(1), 23–34. DOI: 10.1016/j.smr.2013.03.005

World Health Organization. (2018). *Global action plan on physical activity 2018–2030: More active people for a healthier world.* World Health Organization.

Yetim, A., & Şenel, Ö. (2001). Türkiye'de spor yöneticisi yetiştirme faaliyetlerinin görünümü. *Milli Eğitim Dergisi, 150,* 50–56.

KEY TERMS AND DEFINITIONS

Capability Approach: A normative framework developed by Amartya Sen that evaluates individual well-being and social arrangements in terms of substantive freedoms, that is, what people are actually able to do and to be rather than solely the resources they possess.

Sport for All: A policy approach promoting broad-based sport and physical activity participation, emphasising inclusion across age, gender, socioeconomic status, and ability, as distinct from elite performance-oriented sport policy.

Social Investment: A welfare-state orientation that prioritises policies building human capital, activating labour-market participation, and preparing citizens for changing economic conditions, rather than compensating for market failures after the fact.

Social Inclusion: The process of improving the terms of participation in society for people who are disadvantaged on the basis of age, gender, disability, ethnicity, income, or other characteristics, through enhanced opportunities, access to resources, and voice.

State-Led Sport Programs: Sport initiatives designed, funded, and implemented primarily by public authorities, including ministries, federations, and municipalities, with limited reliance on voluntary sport associations or private providers.

Sports Training Centres (Spor Eğitim Merkezleri): Turkish state-run boarding institutions that combine intensive athletic development with formal education for talented young athletes, typically drawn from modest socioeconomic backgrounds.

SPOR-TOTO: A Turkish sports-betting organisation whose revenues are partially directed toward sport federations, grassroots projects, and athlete support, serving as a supplementary funding channel for sport development.

Turkish Welfare Regime: A hybrid welfare configuration combining Bismarckian social insurance for formal-sector workers, means-tested social assistance, and strong reliance on family-based care, with growing social expenditure since the early 2000s but persisting gaps in coverage linked to informal employment.

Welfare Outcome: A measurable change in individual or collective well-being, including dimensions such as health, income, education, employment, social cohesion, and subjective life satisfaction, attributable at least in part to a given policy or program.

Youth Centres (Gençlik Merkezleri): Turkish publicly funded facilities operating in all provinces that provide cultural, educational, sport, and mentorship activities for young people, with a particular focus on disadvantaged groups.

Chapter 11
Sport as a Social Policy Tool:
Advancing Welfare, Equity, and Social Development Through Inclusive Sport Systems

Rosalie Ignacio Dela Cruz
http://orcid.org/0009-0007-7892-3998
University of Makati, Philippines

Ariel S. Dela Cruz
http://orcid.org/0009-0006-0229-0277
Technological Institute of the Philippines, Manila, Philippines

Julius I. De Guzman
http://orcid.org/0009-0003-8507-9511
University of Santo Tomas, Manila, Philippines

ABSTRACT

This chapter presents an analysis of sport as a strategic social policy tool, highlighting its potential to advance public health, social inclusion, youth development, and community cohesion. Drawing on theoretical frameworks such as social capital, welfare theory, and the Sport-for-Development and Peace (SDP) approach, this chapter examines how sport can improve physical and mental well-being, empower marginalized populations, foster life skills and education, and strengthen collective identity. Challenges including unequal access, governance issues, commercialization, and ethical concerns are discussed, alongside evidence-based policy recommendations for equitable, inclusive, and sustainable sport-based interventions.

DOI: 10.4018/979-8-2600-3174-2.ch011

INTRODUCTION

Background of the Study

Over the past several decades, sport has evolved from being perceived primarily as a recreational or competitive activity into a significant instrument of social policy and human development. Governments, educational institutions, international organizations, and civil society groups increasingly recognize that sport possesses the capacity to influence social behavior, improve public health, strengthen community relationships, support youth development, and promote social inclusion (Coalter, 2013; Schulenkorf et al., 2016). This growing recognition has positioned sport within broader discussions concerning welfare systems, sustainable development, and social transformation.

The contemporary relevance of sport within public policy emerged partly because societies around the world continue to face persistent and interconnected social challenges. These challenges include rising levels of physical inactivity, increasing mental health concerns, social isolation, youth disengagement, unemployment, discrimination, urban violence, and widening socioeconomic inequality (World Health Organization [WHO], 2022). In response to these issues, policymakers have sought innovative and multidimensional interventions capable of producing both individual and collective social benefits. Sport has consequently gained prominence because of its accessibility, popularity, and ability to engage diverse populations across age, culture, gender, and socioeconomic status.

International institutions have also reinforced the role of sport in development and welfare. The United Nations has consistently recognized sport as a contributor to peacebuilding, health promotion, gender equality, education, and sustainable development. The inclusion of sport-related goals within the Sustainable Development Goals (SDGs) reflects the increasing global consensus that sport can support broader social development agendas when integrated into effective policy systems (United Nations, 2021). Likewise, organizations such as the International Olympic Committee (IOC), UNESCO, and the WHO have promoted physical activity and inclusive sport participation as mechanisms for improving public welfare and strengthening social cohesion.

Despite the growing enthusiasm surrounding sport-for-development initiatives, scholars caution against overly idealistic assumptions regarding the automatic social benefits of sport (Coakley, 2011; Giulianotti, 2011). Research increasingly demonstrates that sport can reproduce social inequalities when participation opportunities are unequally distributed or when programs fail to address structural barriers such as poverty, discrimination, disability exclusion, and gender inequality. Furthermore, commercialization, political manipulation, corruption, and weak governance structures can undermine the social value of sport systems.

For this reason, there is a need for critical and evidence-based examinations of sport as a social policy tool. Rather than treating sport as inherently beneficial, contemporary scholarship emphasizes the importance of understanding the conditions under which sport contributes positively to welfare outcomes. This includes examining policy frameworks, institutional support systems, funding mechanisms, leadership practices, community engagement, and evaluation strategies.

Purpose of the Chapter

This chapter aims to critically examine the role of sport as a social policy tool in advancing welfare, equity, inclusion, and social development. Specifically, the chapter seeks to:

1. Analyze the theoretical foundations linking sport and social policy;
2. Examine the contribution of sport to public health, youth development, education, community cohesion, and economic participation;
3. Explore how sport promotes social inclusion and equity among marginalized populations;
4. Critically evaluate the limitations and challenges associated with sport-based policy interventions; and
5. Propose evidence-based recommendations for strengthening inclusive and sustainable sport policies.

Central Argument

The central argument of this chapter is that sport can serve as a powerful social policy instrument when implemented through inclusive, evidence-based, and ethically grounded frameworks. However, the welfare outcomes associated with sport are not automatic. Positive social impacts depend on the extent to which policies address structural inequalities, prioritize equitable participation, promote accountable governance, and integrate sport within broader welfare and development systems.

CONCEPTUAL AND THEORETICAL FOUNDATIONS

Sport as a Social Institution

Sport is widely recognized as a social institution because it reflects and influences the norms, values, identities, and relationships present within society. According to Coakley (2021), sport functions not only as a physical activity but also as a social system that shapes behavior, identity formation, community interaction, and cultural meaning. As a social institution, sport intersects with education, politics, media, economics, and public health.

The sociological significance of sport can be understood through its multiple social functions. First, sport creates opportunities for social interaction and collective participation. Participation in organized sport often fosters teamwork, communication, leadership, and cooperation. Second, sport contributes to identity formation by influencing how individuals perceive themselves and their communities. National teams, local clubs, and school-based programs frequently become symbols of collective identity and belonging. Third, sport can serve as a mechanism for social mobility, particularly for marginalized populations seeking educational scholarships, employment opportunities, and social recognition.

However, sport also reflects broader social inequalities. Access to quality sport facilities, coaching, and participation opportunities is often influenced by class, gender, disability, race, and geographic location. Consequently, scholars emphasize the importance of analyzing sport critically rather than assuming that participation automatically produces positive outcomes.

Understanding Social Policy

Social policy generally refers to government strategies, institutional programs, and public interventions designed to improve human welfare and quality of life. Social policy traditionally focuses on areas such as education, healthcare, housing, employment, social protection, and community development (Spicker, 2014). Within contemporary welfare systems, sport has increasingly become integrated into social policy agendas because of its ability to influence multiple dimensions of well-being simultaneously.

Sport intersects with social policy in several ways. First, sport contributes to preventive healthcare by promoting physical activity and reducing lifestyle-related diseases. Second, sport programs support educational outcomes through school engagement and youth development initiatives. Third, sport promotes social inclusion by creating opportunities for participation among marginalized populations. Finally, sport contributes to community development and economic participation through employment, tourism, and infrastructure investment.

The integration of sport into social policy frameworks reflects a shift toward holistic and interdisciplinary approaches to welfare. Rather than treating health, education, and social inclusion as separate domains, policymakers increasingly recognize that sport can simultaneously address multiple social concerns.

Human Development Theory

Human development theory, strongly associated with Amartya Sen, emphasizes the expansion of individuals' capabilities and freedoms as the ultimate goal of development. From this perspective, sport contributes to human development by enhancing individuals' physical, psychological, and social capacities, enabling them to lead meaningful and productive lives.

Sport provides opportunities for skill development, self-expression, and personal achievement. It also supports mental health by reducing stress, improving self-esteem, and fostering resilience. For young people, in particular, sport can serve as a critical space for identity formation and life skills acquisition, including leadership, discipline, and decision-making. These capabilities extend beyond the sports context, influencing educational attainment, employability, and social participation.

Importantly, human development theory highlights the importance of access and equity. The benefits of sport can only be realized if individuals have genuine opportunities to participate. This underscores the need for inclusive policies that remove barriers related to gender, disability, socioeconomic status, and geographic location.

Welfare Theory

Welfare theory situates sport within the broader context of state responsibility for ensuring the well-being of its citizens. It examines how public policies and institutions allocate resources to promote social protection, equity, and quality of life. In this framework, sport is recognized as a component of social welfare provision, contributing to both preventive and developmental outcomes.

From a preventive standpoint, sport reduces the burden on healthcare systems by promoting active lifestyles and preventing non-communicable diseases. From a developmental perspective, it supports social integration, reduces anti-social behavior, and enhances community cohesion. As such, investment in sport can yield significant social returns, making it an attractive policy option for governments seeking cost-effective solutions to complex social problems.

However, welfare theory also raises critical questions about resource allocation and policy priorities. In contexts where basic needs such as housing, education, and healthcare remain unmet, the role of sport in welfare policy may be contested. Therefore, integrating sport into welfare systems requires careful planning to ensure that it complements, rather than competes with, other essential services.

Sport-for-Development and Peace (SDP) Framework

The Sport-for-Development and Peace (SDP) framework represents a global movement that explicitly recognizes sport as a tool for achieving development and peace-building objectives. It gained prominence through the efforts of international organizations such as the United Nations, which has advocated for the integration of sport into development strategies and the achievement of the Sustainable Development Goals (SDGs).

The SDP framework is based on the premise that sport possesses unique qualities—such as universality, inclusivity, and the ability to transcend cultural and linguistic barriers—that make it an effective medium for social change. It encompasses a wide range of initiatives, including programs that promote education, gender equality, health awareness, conflict resolution, and social inclusion.

One of the key strengths of the SDP approach is its adaptability. Programs can be tailored to address specific local needs while aligning with global development priorities. For example, sport-based interventions have been used to engage at-risk youth, empower women and girls, and support the integration of refugees and displaced populations. In post-conflict settings, sport can serve as a neutral platform for dialogue and reconciliation, helping to rebuild trust and social cohesion.

Despite its potential, the SDP framework is not without criticism. Scholars have raised concerns about the lack of rigorous evaluation, the tendency to overstate the impact of sport, and the risk of using sport as a symbolic rather than substantive intervention. Additionally, some programs may inadvertently impose external values or fail to account for local cultural contexts, limiting their effectiveness and sustainability.

To address these challenges, there is a growing emphasis on evidence-based practice, participatory program design, and long-term impact assessment within the SDP field. Effective SDP initiatives require collaboration among multiple stakeholders, including governments, non-governmental organizations, community leaders, and participants themselves. They also demand a commitment to inclusivity, accountability, and ethical practice.

Synthesis

Taken together, these conceptual perspectives provide a comprehensive framework for understanding sport as a social policy tool. Social capital theory highlights the relational and community-building aspects of sport, human development theory emphasizes its role in expanding individual capabilities, and welfare theory situates it within broader systems of social provision. The SDP framework, meanwhile, operationalizes these theoretical insights into practical strategies for development and peace.

By integrating these approaches, this chapter underscores the multidimensional nature of sport and its capacity to address complex social challenges. However, it also reinforces the importance of critical engagement, ensuring that sport policies are designed and implemented in ways that are inclusive, context-sensitive, and aligned with broader social objectives.

III. SPORT AND PUBLIC HEALTH

Sport and public health are intrinsically interconnected, with growing recognition that structured physical activity plays a crucial role in promoting overall well-being and preventing disease. In recent decades, policymakers and health practitioners have increasingly turned to sport as a strategic tool to address rising public health concerns, particularly the global burden of non-communicable diseases (NCDs), mental health challenges, and the long-term effects of the COVID-19 pandemic. By encouraging active lifestyles and fostering holistic wellness, sport contributes significantly to both preventive and promotive health outcomes.

Physical Health Benefits: NCD Prevention and Active Lifestyles

One of the most widely acknowledged contributions of sport to public health is its role in preventing non communicable diseases (NCDs), such as cardiovascular disease, Type 2 Diabetes, obesity, and certain types of cancer. These conditions are among the leading causes of mortality worldwide and are often linked to sedentary lifestyles, poor dietary habits, and lack of physical activity. Regular participation in sport and exercise directly addresses these risk factors by promoting cardiovascular fitness, improving metabolic function, and supporting healthy body composition.

Engagement in sport enhances physical endurance, muscular strength, flexibility, and coordination. Activities such as running, swimming, basketball, and dance not only improve physiological functioning but also contribute to the maintenance of a healthy weight and the regulation of blood pressure and cholesterol levels. Moreover, sport provides an enjoyable and socially engaging way to sustain long-term physical activity, increasing the likelihood that individuals will adopt and maintain active lifestyles.

The promotion of active living through sport is particularly important in urban and technologically driven societies, where sedentary behavior has become increasingly prevalent. Long hours spent in front of screens, whether for work or leisure, have significantly reduced daily physical movement. In response, governments and institutions have implemented policies that encourage participation in sport through school-based programs, community initiatives, and public awareness campaigns.

In the Philippine context, initiatives led by institutions such as the Department of Health and the Department of Education emphasize the importance of physical activity in combating lifestyle-related diseases among both youth and adults. School-based physical education programs, interscholastic competitions, and community sports leagues serve as accessible entry points for individuals to engage in regular physical activity. These efforts highlight the role of sport as a preventive health strategy that reduces long-term healthcare costs and enhances population health.

However, access to sport and physical activity opportunities remains uneven. Socioeconomic disparities, lack of infrastructure, and limited safe spaces for recreation can hinder participation, particularly in underserved communities. Therefore, public health policies must address these structural barriers to ensure equitable access to sport for all individuals.

Mental Health and Well-Being

Beyond its physical benefits, sport plays a vital role in promoting mental health and psychological well-being. Participation in physical activity has been consistently associated with reduced symptoms of depression and anxiety disorder, as well as improved mood, self-esteem, and cognitive functioning. These outcomes are particularly significant in a time when mental health concerns are becoming increasingly prevalent across all age groups.

Sport contributes to mental well-being through both physiological and psychosocial mechanisms. On a biological level, physical activity stimulates the release of endorphins and other neurotransmitters that enhance mood and reduce stress. On a psychosocial level, sport provides opportunities for social interaction, emotional expression, and the development of a sense of achievement and purpose. These elements are essential for maintaining psychological resilience and coping with life's challenges.

For young people, sport serves as a constructive outlet for energy and emotions, helping to reduce risky behaviors and promote positive development. It fosters discipline, goal-setting, and perseverance—skills that are transferable to academic and professional contexts. Additionally, being part of a team or sports community creates a sense of belonging, which is critical for emotional stability and identity formation.

In educational settings, integrating sport into the curriculum can significantly enhance students' mental health. Physical education programs not only improve physical fitness but also provide structured environments where students can build confidence, manage stress, and develop interpersonal skills. For student-athletes, sport can be a source of motivation and a means of balancing academic and personal demands, although it is important to ensure that pressures related to performance do not negatively impact mental health.

Despite these benefits, it is essential to recognize that sport is not inherently positive for mental health in all contexts. Issues such as excessive competition, burnout, overtraining, and lack of psychological support can lead to negative outcomes. Therefore, a balanced and supportive approach to sport participation is necessary, one that prioritizes well-being over performance and includes access to mental health resources.

Post-Pandemic Recovery Through Sport

The COVID-19 pandemic has had profound and far-reaching effects on global public health, disrupting not only healthcare systems but also everyday routines, social interactions, and opportunities for physical activity. Lockdowns, social distancing measures, and the closure of sports facilities led to a significant decline in physical activity levels, contributing to increased sedentary behavior, weight gain, and deteriorating mental health among populations worldwide.

In the aftermath of the pandemic, sport has emerged as a critical tool for recovery and resilience. Reintroducing physical activity through sport programs plays a key role in restoring physical health, rebuilding social connections, and supporting mental well-being. Community-based sports initiatives, in particular, provide safe and inclusive spaces where individuals can reconnect, rebuild trust, and regain a sense of normalcy.

Sport also contributes to the rehabilitation of individuals who have experienced the direct and indirect impacts of the pandemic. For those recovering from illness, structured physical activity can aid in regaining strength and endurance. For others who have faced social isolation, economic hardship, or emotional distress, sport offers a pathway to re-engagement and healing.

In the Philippine setting, the gradual reopening of schools and community spaces has been accompanied by renewed emphasis on physical education and grassroots sports programs. Local government units (LGUs), in collaboration with schools and community organizations, have implemented initiatives aimed at encouraging safe participation in sport while adhering to health protocols. These efforts underscore the role of sport in rebuilding healthier and more resilient communities.

Moreover, the pandemic has highlighted the importance of adaptability and innovation in sport delivery. The rise of digital fitness platforms, home-based workouts, and virtual sports programs has expanded access to physical activity, demonstrating that sport can evolve to meet changing circumstances. Moving forward, hybrid models that combine in-person and digital approaches may enhance the reach and sustainability of sport-based health interventions.

However, the recovery process also presents challenges. Ensuring that sport programs are inclusive and accessible, particularly for vulnerable populations, remains a critical concern. Additionally, there is a need to address the long-term health impacts of the pandemic, including increased rates of physical inactivity and mental health issues. Policymakers must therefore prioritize sport as an integral component of public health strategies, supported by adequate funding, infrastructure, and cross-sector collaboration.

IV. SPORT AND SOCIAL INCLUSION

Sport has long been recognized as a unifying force that transcends cultural, social, and economic boundaries. As a social policy tool, it plays a critical role in promoting inclusion by providing opportunities for participation, representation, and empowerment among diverse and often marginalized populations. Social inclusion, in this context, refers to the process of improving the terms of participation in society—particularly for individuals and groups who are disadvantaged due to gender, disability, socioeconomic status, ethnicity, or other structural barriers. Through intentional design and inclusive programming, sport can contribute to reducing inequalities and fostering a more equitable society.

Gender Equality in Sport

One of the most significant dimensions of social inclusion in sport is the promotion of gender equality. Historically, sport has been a male-dominated domain, with limited access and recognition for women and girls. Cultural norms, institutional barriers, and unequal resource allocation have often restricted female participation in both recreational and competitive sports. However, in recent decades, there has been a growing movement to challenge these inequalities and promote gender-inclusive sport policies.

Sport provides a powerful platform for empowering women and girls by enhancing their confidence, leadership skills, and social visibility. Participation in sport can challenge traditional gender roles, enabling women to assert their identities and capabilities in spaces that were previously inaccessible. It also contributes to improved physical and mental health outcomes, which are essential for overall well-being and empowerment.

Global initiatives supported by organizations such as the United Nations Women advocate for equal opportunities in sport, emphasizing its role in advancing gender equality and achieving broader development goals. Programs that encourage girls' participation in sport, provide female mentorship, and promote safe and inclusive environments are critical in addressing gender disparities.

In the Philippine context, efforts to promote gender equality in sport are evident in school-based physical education programs and national policies that encourage female participation. Female athletes in the country have increasingly gained recognition on international stages, challenging stereotypes and inspiring future generations. However, persistent challenges remain, including unequal funding, media representation, and access to training facilities. Addressing these issues requires sustained policy commitment and cultural change.

Inclusion of Persons with Disabilities

Sport also plays a transformative role in promoting the inclusion of persons with disabilities. Traditionally, individuals with disabilities have faced significant barriers to participation in physical activity, including lack of accessible facilities, limited program availability, and societal stigma. Inclusive sport initiatives aim to dismantle these barriers by creating opportunities for participation that are accessible, adaptive, and empowering.

Adaptive sports and inclusive physical education programs enable individuals with disabilities to engage in physical activity in ways that suit their abilities and needs. These programs not only improve physical health but also enhance self-esteem, independence, and social integration. Participation in sport allows individuals with disabilities to challenge societal perceptions, demonstrating their capabilities and redefining notions of ability.

International movements such as the Paralympic Games have significantly contributed to raising awareness and promoting inclusivity in sport. These events highlight the achievements of athletes with disabilities and advocate for equal opportunities in sports participation at all levels.

In educational and community settings, inclusive sport programs are essential for fostering environments where individuals of all abilities can participate together. This not only benefits persons with disabilities but also promotes empathy, understanding, and social cohesion among participants. However, achieving true inclusion requires more than just access; it involves creating supportive environments, training educators and coaches, and ensuring that policies are aligned with the principles of equity and accessibility.

Addressing Socioeconomic Inequalities

Socioeconomic status remains a significant determinant of access to sport and physical activity. Individuals from low-income communities often face barriers such as lack of facilities, limited financial resources, and competing priorities related to education and livelihood. As a result, they are less likely to participate in organized sports, which can exacerbate existing health and social inequalities.

Sport as a social policy tool can help address these disparities by providing accessible and affordable opportunities for participation. Community-based sports programs, public recreational facilities, and school initiatives play a crucial role in bridging the gap between different socioeconomic groups. By reducing financial and structural barriers, these programs enable individuals from disadvantaged backgrounds to experience the benefits of sport.

Moreover, sport can serve as a pathway for social mobility. For some individuals, particularly youth, participation in sport can open doors to educational scholarships, career opportunities, and personal development. It can also provide a constructive alternative to negative behaviors, such as involvement in crime or substance abuse, by offering structured and supportive environments.

In the Philippines, local government units (LGUs) and educational institutions often organize community sports programs and inter-barangay competitions to engage youth and promote inclusion. These initiatives not only encourage physical activity but also foster community pride and unity. However, disparities in resource allocation between urban and rural areas remain a challenge, highlighting the need for more equitable distribution of funding and infrastructure.

Sport as a Platform for Cultural and Social Integration

Beyond addressing specific forms of inequality, sport serves as a broader platform for cultural and social integration. It brings together individuals from diverse backgrounds, creating opportunities for interaction, dialogue, and mutual understanding. In multicultural societies, sport can help bridge cultural divides and promote respect for diversity.

For marginalized groups such as indigenous communities, migrants, and refugees, sport can provide a sense of belonging and identity. It offers a shared space where individuals can connect with others, build relationships, and participate in collective experiences. This is particularly important in contexts where social exclusion and discrimination are prevalent.

Sport-based initiatives that emphasize inclusivity and diversity can contribute to reducing prejudice and fostering social cohesion. For example, mixed-team sports, community tournaments, and inclusive recreational activities can create environments where differences are celebrated rather than stigmatized. These interactions help break down stereotypes and build trust among participants.

However, it is important to recognize that sport does not automatically lead to inclusion. Without intentional efforts, it can also reinforce existing social hierarchies and exclusions. For instance, elite sports systems may prioritize performance over participation, limiting opportunities for marginalized groups. Therefore, inclusive sport policies must prioritize accessibility, representation, and equity to ensure that all individuals can benefit.

Challenges and Considerations

While sport holds significant potential as a tool for social inclusion, its effectiveness depends on how it is implemented. Several challenges must be addressed to maximize its impact. These include:

- Structural Barriers: Limited infrastructure, inadequate funding, and lack of trained personnel can restrict access to inclusive sport programs.
- Cultural Norms: Deeply ingrained beliefs and attitudes may discourage participation among certain groups, particularly women and individuals with disabilities.
- Policy Gaps: Inconsistent or poorly implemented policies can hinder the development of inclusive sport systems.
- Tokenism: Superficial inclusion efforts that do not address underlying inequalities may fail to produce meaningful change.

Addressing these challenges requires a comprehensive and collaborative approach involving multiple stakeholders, including governments, educational institutions, community organizations, and the private sector. Policies must be grounded in principles of equity, participation, and empowerment, ensuring that sport serves as a genuine vehicle for inclusion rather than exclusion.

Youth Development and Education

Sport plays a central role in youth development and education, serving as a dynamic platform for learning, personal growth, and socialization. Beyond its physical benefits, sport contributes to the holistic development of young individuals by fostering cognitive, emotional, and social competencies that are essential for lifelong success. As an educational tool, sport extends learning beyond the classroom, offering experiential opportunities that shape character, values, and identity. When integrated into educational systems and community programs, sport becomes a powerful mechanism for nurturing well-rounded individuals and preparing youth for the complexities of modern society.

Life Skills Development Through Sport

One of the most significant contributions of sport to youth development is the cultivation of life skills. These include discipline, teamwork, leadership, communication, time management, resilience, and goal-setting—competencies that are critical not only in sports but also in academic, professional, and personal contexts.

Participation in sport requires young individuals to adhere to rules, respect authority, and work collaboratively with others. These experiences foster a sense of responsibility and accountability, which are essential for personal and social development. For instance, athletes learn to manage their time effectively by balancing training, academic responsibilities, and personal commitments. They also develop perseverance by overcoming challenges, handling failure, and striving for continuous improvement.

Sport also provides opportunities for leadership development. Team captains and student-athletes often take on roles that require decision-making, motivation, and conflict resolution. These experiences help build confidence and prepare youth for leadership positions in various aspects of life. Moreover, the structured nature of sport encourages the development of ethical values such as fairness, respect, and integrity.

Importantly, life skills acquired through sport are transferable. The ability to work in teams, manage stress, and set goals can significantly enhance academic performance and employability. As such, sport serves as an informal yet highly effective educational environment that complements formal schooling.

Sport in Educational Systems

The integration of sport into educational systems is a key strategy for promoting youth development. Schools serve as primary institutions where young individuals can access structured physical activity and organized sports programs. Physical education (PE) classes, intramural competitions, and interscholastic sports provide opportunities for students to engage in regular physical activity while developing essential skills.

In the Philippines, the Department of Education plays a significant role in institutionalizing sport within the basic education curriculum. Programs such as school sports competitions and grassroots initiatives aim to promote participation and identify talent at an early age. Similarly, higher education institutions, supported by the Commission on Higher Education, provide avenues for student-athletes to pursue both academic and athletic excellence through varsity programs and collegiate leagues.

Sport in education also contributes to improved academic outcomes. Research suggests that students who participate in sports tend to demonstrate better concentration, higher levels of engagement, and improved school attendance. Physical activity has been linked to enhanced cognitive function, including memory, attention, and problem-solving skills. These benefits underscore the importance of maintaining a balanced approach that values both academic and physical development.

Furthermore, sport can serve as a motivational tool for students. For many young individuals, particularly those from disadvantaged backgrounds, participation in sports can increase their interest in school and reduce dropout rates. Scholarships and incentives associated with athletic performance provide additional motivation for students to pursue their education.

However, the integration of sport into education must be carefully managed to avoid potential challenges. Overemphasis on competition and performance can place undue pressure on student-athletes, potentially affecting their academic and mental well-being. Therefore, educational institutions must adopt a holistic approach that prioritizes student welfare and balances academic and athletic demands.

Youth Identity Formation and Psychosocial Development

Sport plays a crucial role in shaping the identity and psychosocial development of young individuals. During adolescence, youth undergo significant physical, emotional, and social changes, making it a critical period for identity formation. Participation in sport provides a structured environment where individuals can explore their interests, develop self-concept, and build a sense of belonging.

For many young people, particularly student-athletes, sport becomes a central component of their identity. It offers a sense of purpose and direction, helping them define who they are and what they aspire to achieve. This is especially relevant in the context of athletic identity, where individuals strongly associate themselves with their role as athletes. While a strong athletic identity can enhance motivation and performance, it is important to ensure that it is balanced with other aspects of self-concept to support long-term well-being.

Sport also contributes to psychosocial development by fostering social connections and emotional resilience. Being part of a team or sports community provides opportunities for meaningful relationships, peer support, and social interaction. These experiences help young individuals develop interpersonal skills and navigate social dynamics.

Moreover, sport can serve as a protective factor against negative behaviors. Engagement in structured activities reduces the likelihood of involvement in risky behaviors such as substance abuse, delinquency, and school dropout. It provides a positive outlet for energy and emotions, promoting constructive and goal-oriented behavior.

In your context as a researcher focusing on student-athletes, this aspect is particularly significant. Sport not only influences career planning and decision-making but also prepares youth for transitions beyond their athletic careers. Programs that support dual career pathways—balancing education and sport—are essential in ensuring that student-athletes are equipped for life after sports.

Career Development and Opportunities

Sport can also serve as a pathway for career development and socioeconomic mobility. For some youth, particularly those from underprivileged backgrounds, sport offers opportunities for scholarships, professional careers, and international exposure. These opportunities can significantly alter life trajectories, providing access to education and employment that might otherwise be unattainable.

In addition to athletic careers, sport opens doors to various professions, including coaching, sports management, physical education, sports science, and health and fitness industries. Educational institutions play a crucial role in preparing students for these careers by offering specialized programs and training.

However, it is important to recognize that only a small percentage of athletes achieve professional success. Therefore, youth development programs must emphasize education and skill development beyond sport. Preparing student-athletes for diverse career paths ensures that they have viable options regardless of their athletic outcomes.

Career guidance and mentorship programs are essential in this regard. By providing information, support, and opportunities for skill development, these programs help youth make informed decisions about their future. Integrating career planning into sport programs enhances their long-term impact and sustainability.

Challenges and Considerations

While sport offers numerous benefits for youth development and education, several challenges must be addressed to maximize its effectiveness:

- **Balancing Academics and Athletics:** Student-athletes often face difficulties managing their dual responsibilities, which can lead to stress and burnout.
- **Inequality of Access:** Not all youth have equal opportunities to participate in sports due to financial, geographic, or institutional barriers.
- **Overemphasis on Competition:** Excessive focus on winning can undermine the educational and developmental value of sport.

- **Lack of Support Systems:** Inadequate access to coaching, mentorship, and psychological support can limit the positive impact of sport.

Addressing these challenges requires a holistic and inclusive approach that prioritizes the well-being and development of youth. Collaboration among educators, coaches, policymakers, and families is essential in creating supportive environments that maximize the benefits of sport.

Community Development and Social Cohesion

Sport plays a vital role in fostering community development and strengthening social cohesion by creating shared spaces, experiences, and identities among individuals. As a social policy tool, sport extends beyond individual benefits to influence collective well-being, enabling communities to build trust, cooperation, and a sense of belonging. In diverse and often fragmented societies, sport offers a unifying platform that can bridge social divides, promote civic engagement, and contribute to sustainable community development.

Building Social Capital Through Sport

A key mechanism through which sport contributes to community development is the generation of social capital. As discussed in the conceptual framework, social capital refers to the networks, relationships, and norms that facilitate cooperation within a society. Sport provides a natural setting for the development of these connections by bringing individuals together in structured and informal interactions.

Community sports programs, local leagues, and recreational activities create opportunities for individuals to interact regularly, fostering trust and mutual understanding. These interactions contribute to both bonding and bridging social capital. Bonding social capital strengthens ties within groups—such as families, teams, or neighborhoods—while bridging social capital connects individuals across different social, cultural, and economic backgrounds.

The development of social capital through sport has tangible benefits for communities. It enhances communication, encourages collective problem-solving, and promotes a sense of shared responsibility. For example, community sports events often require collaboration among local stakeholders, including volunteers, organizations, and government units. This collective effort strengthens community networks and builds a culture of cooperation.

However, the ability of sport to generate social capital depends on its inclusivity and accessibility. Programs that are exclusive or poorly managed may reinforce social divisions rather than bridge them. Therefore, inclusive and well-structured sport initiatives are essential for maximizing the community-building potential of sport.

Reducing Crime and Anti-Social Behavior

Sport is widely recognized as an effective tool for reducing crime and anti-social behavior, particularly among youth. By providing structured and meaningful activities, sport offers a positive alternative to negative influences such as substance abuse, delinquency, and violence. It creates safe spaces where individuals can channel their energy, develop discipline, and engage in constructive behavior.

Participation in sport promotes values such as respect, fairness, and accountability, which are essential for responsible citizenship. It also fosters a sense of purpose and belonging, reducing the likelihood of individuals seeking acceptance through harmful activities. For at-risk youth, in particular, sport can serve as a protective factor, offering mentorship, guidance, and opportunities for personal growth.

Community-based sports programs are especially effective in this regard. Initiatives that target vulnerable populations—such as out-of-school youth or those living in high-risk environments—can significantly reduce the incidence of anti-social behavior. By engaging young people in regular physical activity and providing positive role models, these programs contribute to safer and more stable communities.

In the Philippine context, local government units (LGUs) often organize sports tournaments and youth engagement programs at the barangay level. These initiatives not only promote physical activity but also serve as platforms for community interaction and youth development. By investing in sport as a preventive strategy, communities can reduce the social and economic costs associated with crime and disorder.

Strengthening Community Identity and Belonging

Sport plays a crucial role in shaping and reinforcing community identity. Shared participation in sports activities and collective support for local teams create a sense of pride and belonging among community members. These shared experiences contribute to the development of a collective identity, which is essential for social cohesion.

Local sports events, such as inter-barangay tournaments or school competitions, often serve as focal points for community engagement. They bring together individuals from different backgrounds, fostering a sense of unity and shared purpose. Celebrating achievements in sport—whether through victories, participation, or personal milestones—reinforces community pride and strengthens social bonds.

Sport also provides opportunities for cultural expression. Traditional games and indigenous sports, for example, reflect the heritage and values of specific communities. By preserving and promoting these activities, sport contributes to cultural continuity and identity formation. In multicultural societies, sport can serve as a platform for celebrating diversity and promoting mutual respect.

Moreover, sport can play a significant role in post-crisis or post-conflict settings by helping communities rebuild their sense of identity and cohesion. It offers a neutral and inclusive space where individuals can reconnect, rebuild trust, and move forward collectively. This is particularly relevant in the context of communities recovering from natural disasters, social unrest, or public health crises.

Promoting Civic Engagement and Participation

Sport encourages active citizenship by fostering civic engagement and participation. Community sports programs often rely on the involvement of volunteers, coaches, organizers, and local leaders, creating opportunities for individuals to contribute to the development of their communities. This involvement promotes a sense of ownership and responsibility, which are essential for sustainable community development.

Participation in sport can also enhance democratic values such as fairness, inclusion, and respect for rules. These values, learned through sport, can translate into broader civic behaviors, including participation in community decision-making and advocacy for social issues. In this way, sport serves as a training ground for active and responsible citizenship.

Furthermore, sport can facilitate partnerships between different sectors, including government agencies, educational institutions, non-governmental organizations, and the private sector. These collaborations are essential for the successful implementation of community development initiatives. By bringing together diverse stakeholders, sport-based programs can leverage resources, expertise, and networks to achieve common goals.

Challenges and Considerations

While sport has significant potential to promote community development and social cohesion, several challenges must be addressed to ensure its effectiveness:

- **Exclusion and Inequality:** Without inclusive policies, sport programs may exclude certain groups, reinforcing existing social inequalities.

- **Resource Constraints:** Limited funding, infrastructure, and human resources can hinder the development and sustainability of community sports programs.
- **Over-Commercialization:** The commercialization of sport may shift the focus away from community development toward profit and entertainment.
- **Conflict and Rivalry:** While competition can be positive, excessive rivalry may lead to conflict and division within communities.

Addressing these challenges requires a balanced approach that prioritizes inclusivity, equity, and community engagement. Policymakers and practitioners must ensure that sport programs are designed to serve the needs of all community members, particularly those who are marginalized or underserved.

Challenges and Ethical Considerations

While sport holds significant promise as a social policy tool, its implementation is not without complexities and contradictions. The assumption that sport is inherently beneficial can obscure the structural inequalities, ethical dilemmas, and unintended consequences that may arise when sport is poorly designed or inadequately governed. As such, a critical examination of the challenges and ethical considerations surrounding sport-based interventions is essential to ensure that they contribute meaningfully to social welfare rather than perpetuate harm or exclusion.

Inequality of Access and Structural Barriers

One of the most persistent challenges in sport as social policy is the unequal access to participation opportunities. Despite the inclusive rhetoric often associated with sport, access remains heavily influenced by socioeconomic status, geographic location, gender, and ability. Individuals from low-income communities frequently face barriers such as limited access to facilities, lack of equipment, and financial constraints that prevent sustained participation.

In many developing contexts, including parts of the Philippines, disparities between urban and rural areas are particularly pronounced. Urban centers may have relatively well-developed sports infrastructure, while rural communities often lack safe and accessible spaces for physical activity. This imbalance reinforces existing inequalities, limiting the potential of sport to serve as a universal tool for social inclusion.

Gender disparities also persist, with women and girls often facing cultural restrictions, safety concerns, and unequal resource allocation. Similarly, persons with disabilities encounter significant obstacles due to inadequate infrastructure and limited availability of adaptive sports programs. These structural barriers highlight the need for policies that prioritize equity and ensure that sport opportunities are accessible to all segments of the population.

Commercialization and Exploitation

The increasing commercialization of sport presents another critical ethical concern. While commercialization can bring financial investment and visibility, it can also shift the focus away from social development toward profit and entertainment. This shift may undermine the core objectives of sport as a social policy tool, particularly when commercial interests take precedence over community needs.

Athletes, especially young and aspiring individuals, may be vulnerable to exploitation in highly competitive and commercialized environments. Issues such as overtraining, pressure to perform, and lack of adequate compensation or protection can negatively impact their physical and mental well-being. In some cases, young athletes are treated as commodities, with their long-term development and welfare overlooked in pursuit of short-term success.

Moreover, commercialization can exacerbate inequalities by concentrating resources on elite sports and high-profile events, leaving grassroots and community programs underfunded. This imbalance limits opportunities for broad-based participation and undermines the inclusive potential of sport.

Governance, Accountability, and Corruption

Effective governance is essential for ensuring that sport policies and programs achieve their intended outcomes. However, weak governance structures, lack of transparency, and limited accountability mechanisms can hinder the effectiveness of sport as a social policy tool. Mismanagement of funds, corruption, and political interference are issues that have affected sports organizations in various contexts.

Poor governance can lead to the misallocation of resources, undermining the sustainability and impact of sport programs. It can also erode public trust, discouraging participation and support from communities. In some cases, sport initiatives are used for political gain rather than genuine social development, raising ethical concerns about the instrumentalization of sport.

To address these issues, there is a need for strong institutional frameworks that promote transparency, accountability, and stakeholder participation. Clear policies, monitoring systems, and ethical guidelines are essential for ensuring that sport programs are implemented effectively and responsibly.

Risk of Tokenism and Superficial Inclusion

Another challenge in sport-based social policy is the risk of tokenism, where inclusion efforts are symbolic rather than substantive. Programs may claim to promote inclusion without addressing the underlying structural inequalities that limit participation. For example, simply providing access to sport facilities does not guarantee meaningful inclusion if social, cultural, and economic barriers remain unaddressed.

Tokenistic approaches can create the illusion of progress while failing to produce tangible outcomes. They may also reinforce existing power dynamics by excluding marginalized voices from decision-making processes. To avoid this, sport programs must adopt participatory approaches that involve communities in the design, implementation, and evaluation of initiatives.

Meaningful inclusion requires more than representation; it demands equitable access, supportive environments, and sustained engagement. Policies must be designed with a deep understanding of the specific needs and contexts of target populations, ensuring that interventions are both relevant and effective.

Ethical Issues in Youth Sport

Youth sport presents unique ethical considerations, particularly in relation to the well-being and development of young participants. While sport offers numerous benefits, it can also expose youth to risks such as physical injury, psychological stress, and burnout. Excessive training, early specialization, and pressure to achieve high performance can negatively impact young athletes' health and overall development.

In educational settings, the dual demands of academics and athletics can create additional stress for student-athletes. Without adequate support systems, they may struggle to balance these responsibilities, leading to academic underperformance or mental health challenges. It is therefore essential to adopt a child-centered approach that prioritizes well-being over competition.

Safeguarding is another critical ethical concern. Ensuring the safety and protection of young athletes from abuse, harassment, and exploitation is a fundamental responsibility of sports organizations and institutions. This requires the implementation of clear policies, training for coaches and staff, and mechanisms for reporting and addressing concerns.

Cultural Sensitivity and Contextual Relevance

Sport policies and programs must also consider cultural sensitivity and contextual relevance. Interventions that are not aligned with local values, traditions, and social norms may face resistance or fail to achieve their intended outcomes. In some cases, externally designed programs may impose values that are not culturally appropriate, leading to unintended consequences.

For example, efforts to promote gender equality in sport must be approached with an understanding of local cultural dynamics. While challenging discriminatory practices is important, it must be done in a way that is respectful and inclusive of community perspectives. Similarly, the promotion of certain sports may need to be adapted to reflect local interests and traditions.

Context-sensitive approaches that involve community participation and local knowledge are essential for the success and sustainability of sport programs. By engaging stakeholders and respecting cultural diversity, policymakers can ensure that sport interventions are both effective and ethically sound.

Policy Implications and Recommendations

The growing recognition of sport as a social policy tool necessitates the development of coherent, inclusive, and evidence-based policy frameworks. While previous sections have highlighted the multifaceted benefits of sport in advancing public health, social inclusion, youth development, and community cohesion, these outcomes are not automatic. They depend on deliberate policy design, effective implementation, and sustained institutional support. This section outlines key policy implications and provides actionable recommendations to optimize the role of sport in achieving equitable and sustainable welfare outcomes.

Integrating Sport into National and Local Policy Frameworks

One of the primary policy implications is the need to formally integrate sport into broader national and local development agendas. Sport should not be treated as a peripheral sector but as a cross-cutting policy domain that intersects with health, education, social welfare, and community development.

Governments must institutionalize sport within policy frameworks by aligning it with national development priorities and international commitments, such as the Sustainable Development Goals (SDGs). This includes recognizing sport as a strategic tool for addressing issues such as non-communicable diseases, youth unemployment, and social inequality.

In the Philippine context, stronger coordination among agencies such as the Department of Education, Department of Health, and Philippine Sports Commission is essential. Collaborative governance structures can ensure that sport programs are aligned with broader policy objectives and that resources are used efficiently.

At the local level, local government units (LGUs) should incorporate sport into their development plans, particularly in areas related to youth engagement, public health, and community building. Decentralized approaches allow for context-specific interventions that respond to the unique needs of communities.

Promoting Inclusive and Equitable Access

Ensuring equitable access to sport is a fundamental policy priority. Policymakers must address structural barriers that limit participation among marginalized groups, including women, persons with disabilities, and individuals from low-income communities.

This requires investment in accessible infrastructure, such as community sports facilities, safe recreational spaces, and adaptive equipment. Policies should also provide financial support mechanisms, such as subsidies or scholarships, to reduce the cost of participation.

Inclusive programming must be intentionally designed to accommodate diverse needs. For example, gender-sensitive policies can promote the participation of women and girls by addressing safety concerns and cultural barriers. Similarly, inclusive sport initiatives should provide opportunities for persons with disabilities through adaptive sports programs and inclusive physical education.

Equity-focused policies must also consider geographic disparities, ensuring that rural and underserved communities have access to sport opportunities comparable to those in urban areas. By prioritizing inclusion, sport can serve as a genuine vehicle for social equity rather than reinforcing existing inequalities.

Strengthening Multi-Sectoral Collaboration

The complexity of social issues addressed through sport requires collaboration across multiple sectors. Effective sport policy must involve partnerships among government agencies, educational institutions, non-governmental organizations, private sector entities, and community stakeholders.

Multi-sectoral collaboration enables the pooling of resources, expertise, and networks, enhancing the reach and impact of sport programs. For instance, partnerships between schools and community organizations can expand access to sport facilities and programs. Collaboration with health agencies can integrate sport into public health campaigns, while private sector involvement can provide funding and innovation.

Engaging communities in the planning and implementation of sport programs is equally important. Participatory approaches ensure that interventions are contextually relevant and responsive to local needs. Community ownership also enhances the sustainability of programs, as stakeholders are more likely to support initiatives in which they have a vested interest.

Enhancing Governance and Accountability

Strong governance structures are critical for ensuring the effectiveness and integrity of sport policies. Policymakers must establish clear frameworks for decision-making, resource allocation, and program implementation.

Transparency and accountability mechanisms should be embedded in all levels of sport governance. This includes regular monitoring and evaluation, public reporting of outcomes, and mechanisms for stakeholder feedback. Anti-corruption measures and ethical guidelines are also essential to prevent misuse of resources and ensure that sport programs serve their intended purposes.

Capacity-building initiatives for administrators, coaches, and program managers can enhance governance by equipping stakeholders with the skills and knowledge needed to implement policies effectively. Professional development programs should emphasize ethical leadership, inclusive practices, and evidence-based decision-making.

Developing Monitoring and Evaluation Systems

To maximize the impact of sport as a social policy tool, robust monitoring and evaluation (M&E) systems must be established. These systems are essential for assessing the effectiveness of sport programs, identifying best practices, and informing policy adjustments.

M&E frameworks should include both quantitative and qualitative indicators that capture a wide range of outcomes, including health improvements, social inclusion, educational attainment, and community engagement. Data collection should be systematic and ongoing, allowing for the tracking of progress over time.

Evidence-based policymaking requires the integration of research and practice. Collaboration with academic institutions can support the development of rigorous evaluation methodologies and contribute to the generation of knowledge in the field of sport for development.

In the Philippine context, strengthening research initiatives within universities and collaborating with government agencies can enhance the evidence base for sport policy. This aligns with your role as a researcher, where empirical studies on student-athletes and community programs can inform policy and practice.

Prioritizing Youth-Centered and Holistic Approaches

Given the significant role of sport in youth development, policies must adopt a youth-centered approach that prioritizes holistic well-being. This includes balancing athletic performance with academic achievement, mental health, and personal development.

Educational institutions should implement dual-career pathways that support student-athletes in managing both academic and athletic responsibilities. Guidance and counseling services, mentorship programs, and career development initiatives are essential components of this approach.

Policies should also emphasize safe sport environments by implementing safeguarding measures to protect young participants from abuse, exploitation, and harm. Training for coaches and educators should include child protection and ethical practices to ensure the well-being of youth.

Leveraging Innovation and Technology

The evolving landscape of sport presents opportunities to leverage innovation and technology in policy implementation. Digital platforms, mobile applications, and virtual training programs can expand access to sport, particularly in contexts where physical infrastructure is limited.

The COVID-19 pandemic demonstrated the potential of technology in maintaining physical activity through online fitness programs and virtual engagement. Policymakers can build on these innovations to develop hybrid models that combine in-person and digital approaches.

Technology can also enhance monitoring and evaluation by enabling real-time data collection and analysis. This supports more responsive and adaptive policy implementation, ensuring that sport programs remain effective in changing contexts.

CONCLUSION

This chapter has examined sport as a dynamic and multifaceted social policy tool capable of addressing a wide range of contemporary societal challenges. Moving beyond its traditional role as a form of recreation or competitive activity, sport has been positioned as a strategic mechanism for advancing public health, promoting social inclusion, supporting youth development, and strengthening community cohesion. Through its accessibility, adaptability, and universal appeal, sport offers a unique platform for fostering both individual well-being and collective social progress.

The discussion highlighted that sport contributes significantly to public health by encouraging active lifestyles and preventing non-communicable diseases, while also supporting mental health and post-pandemic recovery. In the realm of social inclusion, sport has demonstrated its capacity to empower marginalized groups, challenge inequalities, and create opportunities for participation across diverse populations. Its role in youth development and education further underscores its value as a space for life skills acquisition, identity formation, and career development. At the community level, sport fosters social capital, reduces anti-social behavior, and strengthens shared identity and belonging.

However, this chapter also emphasized that the benefits of sport are not automatic. The effectiveness of sport as a social policy tool depends on the intentionality and integrity with which it is designed and implemented. Structural inequalities, unequal access, commercialization, governance issues, and ethical concerns can limit its impact and, in some cases, reproduce the very challenges it seeks to address. These complexities highlight the importance of adopting a critical and reflective approach to sport policy and practice.

The policy implications and recommendations outlined in this chapter reinforce the need for integrated, inclusive, and evidence-based strategies. Embedding sport within national and local development frameworks, promoting equitable access, strengthening multi-sectoral collaboration, and ensuring robust governance and accountability are essential for maximizing its potential. Equally important is the prioritization of youth-centered and holistic approaches that safeguard the well-being of participants and support long-term development outcomes.

Looking forward, there is a need for continued research and innovation in the field of sport as social policy. Empirical studies, particularly those grounded in local contexts such as the Philippines, can provide valuable insights into the effectiveness of sport-based interventions and inform more responsive and culturally relevant policies. The integration of technology, the expansion of inclusive programs, and the strengthening of monitoring and evaluation systems will further enhance the impact and sustainability of sport initiatives.

In conclusion, sport holds significant promise as a transformative force in advancing welfare, equity, and social development. When strategically harnessed, it can contribute to building healthier, more inclusive, and more resilient societies. However, realizing this potential requires a sustained commitment from policymakers, practitioners, and communities to ensure that sport is used not only as a tool for participation but as a vehicle for meaningful and lasting social change.

REFERENCES

Coakley, J. (2011). Youth sports: What counts as "positive development?". *Journal of Sport and Social Issues*, *35*(3), 306–324. DOI: 10.1177/0193723511417311

Coakley, J. (2021). *Sports in society: Issues and controversies* (13th ed.). McGraw-Hill Education.

Coalter, F. (2013). *Sport for development: What game are we playing?* Routledge. DOI: 10.4324/9780203861257

Department of Education. (2016). *K to 12 physical education curriculum guide*. Republic of the Philippines.

Department of Health. (2020). *Philippine physical activity guidelines*. Republic of the Philippines.

Giulianotti, R. (2011). The sport, development and peace sector: A model of four social policy domains. *Journal of Social Policy*, *40*(4), 757–776. DOI: 10.1017/S0047279410000930

Levermore, R., & Beacom, A. (2009). *Sport and international development*. Palgrave Macmillan. DOI: 10.1057/9780230584402

Schulenkorf, N., Sherry, E., & Rowe, K. (2016). Sport for development: An integrated literature review. *Journal of Sport Management*, *30*(1), 22–39. DOI: 10.1123/jsm.2014-0263

Spicker, P. (2014). *Social policy: Theory and practice* (2nd ed.). Policy Press.

United Nations. (2003). *Sport for development and peace: Towards achieving the Millennium Development Goals*. United Nations.

United Nations. (2015). *Transforming our world: The 2030 agenda for sustainable development*. United Nations.

United Nations Children's Fund (UNICEF). (2019). *Getting into the game: Understanding the evidence for child-focused sport for development*. UNICEF.

United Nations Educational, Scientific and Cultural Organization (UNESCO). (2015). *Quality physical education (QPE): Guidelines for policy-makers*. UNESCO.

Women in Sport. (2023). *Gender equality and women's participation in sport report*. Women in Sport Foundation.

World Bank. (2020). *Social inclusion overview*. World Bank. https://www.worldbank.org

World Health Organization. (2010). *Global recommendations on physical activity for health*. WHO.

World Health Organization. (2020). *WHO guidelines on physical activity and sedentary behaviour*. WHO.

World Health Organization. (2022). *Global status report on physical activity 2022*. World Health Organization. https://www.who.int

Chapter 12
Sport as a Social Policy Tool:
Enhancing the Well-Being of Individuals With Disabilities Within Welfare State Frameworks

Mehmet Emin Bekik
http://orcid.org/0000-0001-6959-1716
Inonu University, Turkey

Yener Şişman
http://orcid.org/0000-0003-4528-4521
Anadolu University, Turkey

ABSTRACT

This chapter analyzes sport as a social policy instrument and its impact on the well-being of individuals with disabilities across different welfare state regimes. Rather than treating sport as a neutral or purely recreational activity, it conceptualizes it as a structured policy field shaped by institutional arrangements, state capacity, and ideological orientations. Using a qualitative literature review and a comparative framework based on Esping-Andersen's welfare regime typology, the study examines how liberal, corporatist, and social democratic systems differ in their sport policy approaches. The findings show that participation in sport improves physical, psychological, and social well-being, while fostering self-confidence, social inclusion, and quality of life. However, these benefits are not universal and depend on inclusive infrastructure, public investment, and rights-based policies. The chapter concludes that the effectiveness of sport as a social policy tool is shaped by welfare regime characteristics and broader commitments to equality and inclusion.

DOI: 10.4018/979-8-2600-3174-2.ch012

INTRODUCTION

In contemporary welfare states, social policy has increasingly expanded its scope beyond traditional domains such as income redistribution and employment protection, incorporating broader dimensions of human development, quality of life, and participation. Within this evolving framework, sport has emerged as a significant yet still under-theorized instrument of social policy, particularly in relation to the promotion of well-being and social inclusion. Despite its growing visibility in policy discourse, the role of Sport Policies in addressing the needs and well-being of persons with disabilities remains unevenly conceptualized and fragmented within the existing literature. This chapter is situated within this gap and examines sport as a social policy instrument through a critical and comparative lens. It focuses on the relationship between sport participation and the well-being of persons with disabilities, situating this relationship within broader welfare state approaches. Rather than treating sport as a neutral or inherently inclusive practice, the study conceptualizes it as a policy field shaped by institutional arrangements, state capacities, and ideological orientations embedded in different welfare regimes. The analysis is grounded in a qualitative research design based on systematic literature review and conceptual examination. Academic studies in the fields of social policy, welfare state studies, disability studies, and sport policies, along with policy documents produced by international organizations such as the United Nations, the World Health Organization, and the European Union, constitute the primary sources of analysis. Within this framework, sport is understood not merely as a recreational or health-oriented activity but as a structured domain of social policy that reflects varying degrees of state intervention and institutional responsibility. Building on Esping-Andersen's classical typology of welfare regimes—liberal, conservative/corporatist, and social democratic—the chapter comparatively evaluates how sport policies contribute to the well-being and social inclusion of persons with disabilities. It argues that the effectiveness and accessibility of sport-based interventions vary significantly across different welfare state approaches, depending on the extent of universalism, rights-based policy orientation, and public commitment to inclusion. In this sense, sport becomes a revealing indicator of how welfare regimes conceptualize citizenship, equality, and social rights. Ultimately, this chapter problematizes the assumption that sport functions as a universally inclusive and value-neutral tool of social policy. Instead, it proposes that its impact on the well-being of persons with disabilities is structurally conditioned by welfare regime characteristics and policy design. By doing so, it aims to contribute to the theoretical discussion on social policy and sport policies while offering a critical perspective on the role of welfare states in promoting social inclusion.

1.CONCEPTUAL AND THEORETICAL FRAMEWORK

1.1.Social Policy and Sport

Conceptually, the notion of social policy originates from the combination of the Latin terms *socious* and *politeia*, which in the context of Ancient Greek city-states denoted services delivered to the public on an egalitarian basis. In academic discourse, the term "social policy" is more commonly employed in Europe, whereas in North America it is often referred to as "social welfare policy." Although these terms are sometimes used interchangeably, it has been argued that social policy constitutes a broader framework that also encompasses social welfare policy (Ersöz, 2003).

Following the Industrial Revolution, social policy increasingly came to signify the decisions and practices undertaken by the state to address the socio-economic challenges experienced by its population (Çubuk, 1979). During this period, it was largely understood as a set of principles aimed at improving the working and living conditions of the labour force and mitigating conflicts between labour and capital (Altan, 2007). More broadly, social policy may be defined as a collection of measures implemented by the state and other social institutions to protect vulnerable groups, promote social justice, and secure the minimum conditions necessary for individuals to maintain a dignified life (Talas, 1990). In this respect, it encompasses a body of ideas and practices designed to reduce social inequalities, with the ultimate goal of achieving social justice (Sunal, 2011). As noted by Koray (2012), modern social policy should be understood both as a historical and social phenomenon and as a political construct; over time, its initially limited scope has expanded in parallel with broader social, political, and economic transformations (Koray, 2012).

The emergence of social policy is closely linked to the Industrial Revolution. As industrialization intensified, the concept evolved as a response to the severe working conditions faced by workers—particularly women and children—within the context of capitalist accumulation. In subsequent periods, both the meaning and scope of social policy broadened to include other disadvantaged segments of society. Its development has therefore been shaped by the economic structures, social needs, and political orientations of different historical periods. For this reason, social policy is often conceptualized in both narrow and broad terms (Şişman, 2017).

In its narrow sense, social policy refers to measures aimed at alleviating the fundamental problems of the working class by reducing tensions between labour and capital. Traditionally, this has involved two principal mechanisms: the establishment of protective legislation and the facilitation of workers' ability to exercise their right to organize in order to defend their interests (Talas, 1990). In its broader sense, social policy constitutes an academic field concerned with analyzing public policies designed to provide comprehensive protection for dependent workers, economically disadvantaged groups, and individuals requiring special protection against social risks and adverse living conditions (Altan, 2009).

In contemporary contexts, social policy adopts a comprehensive approach to addressing societal needs. It seeks to enhance overall welfare levels across different social groups while reducing disparities in income and living standards. Accordingly, areas such as education, health, housing, environmental regulation, employment policies, and democratization are considered central components of social policy in its broadest sense (Güven, 2001).

The principal aim of social policy is to address societal challenges while simultaneously promoting social welfare and supporting economic development. In this context, social development refers to improving individuals' access to fundamental services such as education, healthcare, and housing; reducing unemployment; ensuring a more equitable distribution of income; and raising overall living standards (Bekik, 2025). These factors not only contribute to the establishment of a more secure, peaceful, and stable social order but also foster increased productivity. Consequently, investments directed toward strengthening social welfare are widely considered a key driver of economic growth.

One of the most comprehensive objectives of social policy is the enhancement and broader distribution of welfare across society. Progress in addressing core social issues constitutes a central focus in this regard. For example, decreasing unemployment and poverty levels, as well as promoting the social inclusion and participation of individuals with disabilities, are among the fundamental goals of social policy. Furthermore, the pursuit of social peace within this framework emphasizes cohesion rather than division among different segments of society. In this sense, the maintenance of social peace serves as a preventive mechanism against the emergence and escalation of social problems. The effective and sustained achievement of social peace is directly linked to the economic and political conditions in which society exists. Establishing lasting and effective social peace not only shields society from potential problems but also prevents economic losses, thereby creating a favorable environment for both economic and social development (Bedir, 2013).

The most fundamental characteristic of social policy is that it constitutes a set of policies that must be implemented by the state. The formulation of policies concerning health, education, defense, public works, and the labour market falls within the essential responsibilities of the state. As a requirement of the social state principle, these duties must be fulfilled by public authorities. State interventions carried out with consideration of public interest constitute the main sphere of activity of social policy. For this reason, social policy has the nature of public policy, and its primary implementer is the state. However, public authorities are not the sole actors influencing the formation of social policies. In countries with democratic political regimes, professional organizations, civil society organizations, universities, various social actors, and trade unions also play significant roles in the development of social policy (Altan, 2009).

Social policy consists of regulations implemented by the state within a defined national context. Accordingly, the characteristics of social policies in any given country are shaped by the specific conditions under which that country operates, resulting in distinct national patterns of policy development. Variations in economic and social structures, systems of governance, prevailing economic approaches, demographic profiles, family structures, traditions, and cultural values all contribute to the emergence of unique configurations of social policy. Core issues within social policy, particularly income distribution and unemployment, are closely linked to the underlying economic system. While the overall size of an economy—often measured by its gross national product—serves as a significant indicator, it is not sufficient on its own. More decisive factors include how income is distributed across different segments of society, the proportion allocated to wage earners, and the capacity of the economy to generate employment. These elements play a central role in shaping the relationship between economic structures and the social problems they produce (Talas, 1990; Altan, 2009).

Sport is derived from the Latin term *dis-porte*, meaning diversion from work, relaxation, recreation, and renewal, which later evolved into the modern term "sport" (Günışık, 1990). Over time, sport has developed as an interdisciplinary field supported by areas such as anatomy, physiology, kinesiology, and psychology. Beyond its scientific foundations, sport serves multiple purposes, including fostering self-confidence, creativity, competition, enjoyment, physical fitness, and overall health, while also contributing to the development of individual abilities. When practiced at a professional level, sport is structured around principles oriented toward achievement and success, requiring continuity as well as physical, mental, technical, tactical, and theoretical competencies. Accordingly, it demands both high physical capacity and psychological well-being from athletes. From the perspective of spectators, however, sport represents a recreational activity through which a range of emotions—such as joy, excitement, sadness, and entertainment—are experienced (Erkal, 1992; Aracı, 1999).

Sport is fundamentally an activity based on competition, resulting in either winning or losing outcomes. It can be broadly classified into two categories: individual sports and team sports. In particular, individual sports are considered to enhance individuals' sense of competitiveness and fighting spirit. With the economic advancement of contemporary societies, people increasingly engage in social and leisure activities, including sport. As a result, sport has gained substantial popularity over time, and this expansion has led to the growing significance of specific sport sectors, with its impacts becoming clearly observable within society. Individual sports refer to activities performed without direct competition, cooperation, or interaction with others. Through participation in individual sports, individuals develop various personal attributes such as self-confidence, autonomy, rapid decision-making, accuracy, and the ability to protect their rights in accordance with rules and regulations, while also becoming more aware of their personal capacities (Şahan, 2007). These sports are performed independently, either with or without physical contact with an opponent, and are based on technical, tactical, and skill-oriented performance. Olympic disciplines such as athletics, shooting, cycling, boxing, gymnastics, fencing, judo, weightlifting, wrestling, skiing, table tennis, tennis, and taekwondo are included within this category. In individual sports, responsibility lies entirely with the athlete; therefore, both success and failure are attributed solely to the individual. This situation may lead athletes to experience high levels of stress. Moreover, individuals engaged in individual sports often encounter feelings of isolation, as they are required to solve problems independently. Challenges faced in both sporting and everyday life contexts must be overcome without external assistance, similar to competitive situations where athletes are expected to rely entirely on their own capabilities (Yıldırım, 2011).

Team sports refer to sporting competitions organized between groups consisting of at least two or more participants, such as football, basketball, volleyball, handball, and ice hockey. Within these disciplines, tactical understanding plays a crucial role, and athletes are required to be knowledgeable about strategies and game plans. Since both success and failure are attributed to the entire team rather than to a single individual, athletes generally experience lower levels of personal responsibility and psychological stress compared to those participating in individual sports. In team sports, skills such as cooperation, understanding teammates, effective communication during competition, and anticipating teammates' actions are highly important. Because responsibilities and tasks are shared among team members, athletes are less likely to experience emotional exhaustion during competition. Furthermore, abilities such as working collaboratively, cooperating effectively, and sharing both success and failure are more prominently developed in team-based sporting contexts (Kat, 2009).

1.2. The Concept of Well-being and Its Dimensions

Bradburn's (1969) seminal work on psychological well-being. Rather than focusing on the diagnosis of psychiatric disorders, Bradburn aimed to examine how psychologically healthy individuals respond to life stressors and adversities, as well as to explore the strategies they employ in managing everyday challenges. In this framework, psychological well-being was positioned as a central construct and was linked to the Aristotelian notion of *eudaimonia*, often interpreted in contemporary scholarship as well-being and regarded by Aristotle as the ultimate aim of human life. Bradburn further advanced the field by distinguishing between positive and negative affect, proposing that subjective happiness emerges from the dynamic equilibrium between these two emotional states.

In contemporary definitions, well-being refers to an individual's capacity to recognize and utilize personal abilities, effectively manage daily stressors, engage in productive activity, and contribute meaningfully to society (World Health Organization WHO, 2014). It is also conceptualized as the coexistence of positive affective states (hedonic well-being) and optimal psychological and social functioning (eudaimonic well-being) (Keyes, 2002). Importantly, well-being should not be equated with the mere absence of mental illness, but rather understood as a distinct and multidimensional construct that may exist independently of psychopathology (Ryan & Deci, 2001).

Psychological well-being is more appropriately conceptualized as a multidimensional and dynamic structure rather than a simple combination of positive and negative affect or life satisfaction. It encompasses subjective, social, and psychological dimensions, as well as health-related behaviors and attitudes toward life (Ryff, 1989). In this framework, well-being reflects a broader system of functioning that extends beyond emotional states to include cognitive and behavioral components of how individuals engage with their lives. Moreover, psychological well-being has been associated with a range of biological processes, including cardiovascular, neuroendocrine, and immune system functioning. It is also linked to adaptive health-related outcomes such as experiencing a meaningful and purposeful life, ongoing personal growth, and the development of trusting and high-quality interpersonal relationships (Ryff & Singer, 2008). These associations suggest that psychological well-being is embedded not only in subjective experience but also in underlying physiological and social systems that support overall health and functioning.

Affective well-being is generally conceptualized as a construct that encompasses both positive and negative emotions and is widely used by researchers as an indicator for assessing overall well-being (Diener, 1984; Emmons, 1986). According to Keyes (2003), affective well-being refers to the balance between pleasant and unpleasant affective states, as well as individuals' overall evaluation of life satisfaction. In a similar vein, Kahneman and Deaton (2010) describe affective well-being as the emotional quality of individuals' everyday experiences. This includes the frequency and intensity of various feelings such as joy, admiration, stress, sadness, anger, and love, which may either enhance or diminish momentary well-being.

1.3. Disability: From the Medical Model to Social and Rights-Based Approaches

In the historical process within the field of disability, a wide range of terms have been used, such as "blind," "deaf," "mute," "crippled," "lame," and "speech-impaired." In contemporary usage, however, terms like "disabled," "handicapped," "impaired," "individuals with functional limitations," and "individuals with special needs" are more commonly encountered. Nevertheless, it can be argued that no universally accepted definitions for these terms have been established; or, more precisely, that achieving such consensus has not been possible (Şişman, 2023). Individuals with disabilities have historically constituted a marginalized and "undesired" segment of society. Across society at large, the condition of being disabled has often been characterized as unfortunate, unproductive, different, oppressed, and ill (Abberley, 1987). Definitions of disability have varied throughout the historical process within the frameworks of different approaches, as will be discussed below. Although numerous definitions of disability exist, the United Nations (UN) defines persons with disabilities as "those who have long-term physical, mental, intellectual, or sensory impairments which, in interaction with various barriers, may hinder their full and effective participation in society on an equal basis with others" (UN, 2006).

As can be inferred from the definition, the condition of disability undermines equality of opportunity with others and adversely affects the full and effective participation of individuals with disabilities in society. While disability often entails barriers to accessing opportunities available to others, these inequalities are further exacerbated in the case of women, resulting in more pronounced disparities. The rights-based model emphasizes that all individuals—regardless of whether they have disabilities, as well as irrespective of their status, national origin, or other differences—are entitled to equal rights, including social and economic rights, freedom, access to decent work and living conditions, and protection from discrimination (Okur & Erbil Erdugan, 2010). This approach underscores that individuals should be valued not merely for their economic or instrumental contributions, but for their inherent dignity as human beings. Accordingly, within this framework, the disadvantages experienced by persons with disabilities are interpreted as violations of fundamental human rights rather than as consequences of individual impairments (Şişman, 2003).

2. WELFARE STATE APPROACHES AND SPORTS POLICIES

2.1. Welfare State Regimes: Basic Typologies

The concept of the welfare state refers to a multidimensional framework encompassing transformations in social and economic structures. It is closely associated with the objective of ensuring equality of opportunity, particularly through an expanded understanding of social security and reforms aimed at improving the education sector. Furthermore, the welfare state is understood as an approach that denotes the comprehensive range of social services and supports provided by the state, including in-kind assistance, healthcare services, educational opportunities, food and housing aid, as well as monetary transfers directed toward individuals (Barr, 1992).

Esping-Andersen published his seminal work, *The Three Worlds of Welfare Capitalism*, in 1990. This study, which has become one of the most widely accepted contributions in the academic literature, classifies welfare regimes into three distinct categories: social democratic, corporatist/conservative, and Anglo-Saxon/liberal regimes. Esping-Andersen's work is primarily focused not on welfare states or individual social policy instruments, but on "welfare regimes." In this context, the concept of regime refers to the way in which welfare production and distribution are organized through the interaction of the state, the market, and households. The main analytical commonality underlying the "three worlds" typology is the mixed provision of welfare, involving both public and private actors. This classification reflects the historical development of welfare states, particularly the political and ideological drivers that became dominant during their peak in the 1970s and 1980s. It also captures the prevailing socioeconomic conditions of the period, regardless of specific political origins. These conditions include a social and economic structure characterized by mass industrial production, the predominance of the male breadwinner as the prototypical citizen-worker, and the standard household model of a single-income family (Esping-Andersen,1999).

2.1.1. Liberal Welfare Regime

The welfare state literature commonly distinguishes between three ideal-typical regime models: the liberal, conservative (or corporatist), and social democratic welfare state regimes. The liberal welfare state model—often also referred to as the Anglo-Saxon or residual welfare model—is primarily associated with countries such as the United States, Australia, and Canada Within liberal regimes, the state's role in social protection is limited and is typically activated only when support from the family and the market fails. Assistance is generally targeted, means-tested, and designed to reach only those in greatest need, often resulting in relatively modest benefits that may carry a degree of social stigma. (Esping-Andersen,1999).

In contrast, conservative welfare regimes emphasize social insurance schemes that are primarily contribution-based. In these systems, access to social protection is largely determined by prior earnings and employment status, with the aim of maintaining individuals' existing social positions through earnings-related benefits funded by payroll contributions. The central focus is on preserving status differences rather than redistributing resources broadly across society. Social democratic welfare regimes, by comparison, adopt a universalistic approach to social protection. These systems combine a guaranteed minimum income floor with comparatively generous, tax-financed benefits that are extended to the entire population regardless of occupational status. The overarching objective is to promote equality and social inclusion by ensuring comprehensive coverage and reducing dependence on market or family-based provision (Emmenegger et al., 2015).

The limited role of the state, which becomes visible primarily in situations where market mechanisms fail, has a constraining effect on the realization of social citizenship rights. In this context, the institutionalization of social citizenship remains weak within the liberal welfare state model, preventing its full and effective implementation in practice. As a result, rather than being embedded as an operational and enforceable component of everyday social life, social citizenship tends to remain largely a theoretical construct within liberal welfare regimes (Leibfried, 2014).

2.1.2.Conservative/Corporatist Welfare Regime

The corporatist welfare state model, whose influence has been most prominently observed in continental Europe, has been conceptualized under a variety of labels in the academic literature. These include the conservative welfare state model, the social insurance-based welfare regime, the Bismarckian welfare state, the continental European welfare model, and, more recently, the Christian welfare state. Despite terminological differences, these classifications generally refer to a shared institutional logic grounded in contribution-based social insurance systems and the preservation of status differentials (Özdemir, 2007).

In Gøsta Esping-Andersen's seminal analysis of welfare state regimes, conservative systems are characterized by a relative de-emphasis on market-driven priorities and a stronger commitment to maintaining or reconstructing existing hierarchies and status distinctions. Accordingly, these regimes tend to develop fragmented welfare arrangements composed of occupation- and status-based programs, which provide differentiated levels of benefits across social groups. By contrast, liberal welfare regimes are grounded in a normative commitment to the primacy of the free market and advocate minimal state intervention in the distribution of welfare. Within this framework, the persistence of inequalities generated by market mechanisms is largely accepted as an inherent feature of the system. Only when such inequalities result in sustained deprivation do states intervene, typically through means-tested and targeted assistance programs that are often associated with stigmatization (O'Connell, 1991). Within the corporatist welfare state model, individuals living below the poverty threshold are expected to seek support primarily from intermediary social institutions such as the family, religious organizations, and the broader community to which they belong. The state assumes a subsidiary role, intervening only in cases where these traditional support mechanisms prove insufficient. This reflects the principle of subsidiarity, whereby primary responsibility for welfare provision rests with non-state actors, and public authorities act as a last resort (Esping-Andersen,1999).

2.1.3. Social Democratic Welfare Regime

Social democratic welfare regimes, the expansion of democratic rights and the promotion of solidarity among the principal actors of industrial relations—namely the state, capital, and labor—are regarded as core political responsibilities. Within this framework, welfare policies are designed to foster social cohesion by aligning living standards across different segments of society. Consequently, social democratic welfare arrangements exhibit a distinctly universalistic character, seeking to integrate the population within broadly defined middle-class standards through comprehensive and inclusive social provision (O'Connell, 1991). Countries commonly associated with the social democratic welfare state model include Sweden, Denmark, Finland, and Norway. This regime type is characterized by comparatively high levels of social protection expenditure and a strong commitment to ensuring welfare on a universal basis across the population. In addition, states operating within this model actively intervene in labor markets through a diverse set of policy instruments, reflecting an emphasis on full employment, income security, and social equality (Sapir, 2006).

The designation of this model as "social democratic" is rooted in the influential role of social democracy in advancing reforms within the social sphere. Social democratic thought does not adhere to a rigid dichotomy between state and market, nor between the working class and the middle class; instead, it promotes an integrative perspective that seeks to reconcile these domains. Accordingly, the underlying principle of this model extends beyond the provision of equality at a minimal subsistence level, aiming rather at a welfare state framework in which needs are met at comparatively high standards, reflecting an emphasis on both equality and enhanced quality of life (Esping-Andersen,1999).

2.2.Positioning Sport as a Social Policy Instrument within the Context of Welfare Regimes

Sport constitutes a significant component of contemporary social life, deeply embedded in everyday practices and playing a formative role in shaping the broader sociological structure. In the modern era, sport has evolved into a domain that not only fosters intercultural cohesion but also reflects intensifying levels of competition. As such, it has become an arena through which national identity and prestige are articulated and demonstrated on a global scale (Wicker et al., 2012). Sports policy refers to the overall approach to sport, encompassing its guiding principles and objectives, as well as the strategies and methods employed to achieve these goals. It also includes considerations related to infrastructure, facilities, equipment, and educational and training frameworks. Furthermore, sports policy reflects the national and international perspectives on sport, along with the underlying philosophy governing its organization and implementation within a given system (Ekici, 2002).

Sport, within the context of welfare regimes, is not merely a recreational activity but a strategic instrument serving broader social policy objectives. Esping-Andersen's (1990) typology of welfare regimes—liberal, corporatist, and social democratic—highlights variations in social rights, state intervention, and market relations, all of which significantly shape sport policy configurations. The positioning of sport as a social policy tool is closely associated with objectives such as reducing social exclusion, strengthening social cohesion, and promoting healthy lifestyles. In social democratic welfare regimes, sport is primarily framed through universal access and public responsibility, whereas in liberal regimes, market mechanisms and individual responsibility are more prominent. In corporatist regimes, the organization of sport is typically structured through occupational groups and civil society institutions.

The relationship between sport policies and welfare regimes is also significant in terms of social capital formation. According to Coakley (2017), sport functions as a sphere that fosters trust, networking, and a sense of belonging among individuals, thereby contributing to social integration. In this regard, sport becomes not only a matter of physical health but also an integral component of social cohesion policies. In contemporary contexts, many states develop sport-based social programs that aim to integrate disadvantaged groups into society by leveraging the inclusive potential of sport. In particular, sport-oriented social policies targeting youth, migrants, and low-income populations aim to reduce risks and promote equal opportunities. However, the effectiveness of these policies varies depending on the structural characteristics of welfare regimes and the capacity of states to allocate resources. In conclusion, sport is a multidimensional instrument that supports social policy objectives within welfare regimes and is positioned differently across regime types according to varying policy priorities (Coakley, 2017).

3. SPORT AS A SOCIAL POLICY AND WELL-BEING DIMENSION FOR INDIVIDUALS WITH DISABILITIES

3.1. Sport, Social Inclusion and Equal Citizenship

Social exclusion is conceptualized as a multidimensional phenomenon that restricts individuals' full and equitable participation in social, economic, and cultural spheres. This concept extends beyond mere income deprivation or material poverty, encompassing the marginalization of individuals from social networks, decision-making processes, and access to public resources. Furthermore, structural barriers experienced in key domains such as education, healthcare, employment, and social participation constitute fundamental dimensions of social exclusion (Morris, 2001). In general terms, social exclusion can be defined as the inability of certain individuals or groups to integrate with society due to limited access to economic, political, and social rights (Walker & Walker, 1997). Individuals experiencing social exclusion are those who are marginalized from social relationships and networks. In addition to a lack of social capital and weakened ties with institutions, these individuals often encounter difficulties in exercising their legal rights and participating fully in social life (Sapancalı, 2005). The concept of social exclusion is often used in a narrow sense to denote income deprivation, referring to individuals who are unemployed or engaged in low-income occupations. However, when considered in a broader sense, it extends beyond income inequality to encompass multiple forms of deprivation that individuals may experience across various domains of social life.

Deprivation in one aspect of social life can also have spillover effects, influencing other areas of an individual's well-being (Peace, 2001). An important dimension of social exclusion is the lack of social and cultural participation. The difficulties individuals with disabilities face in engaging in social activities—such as physical accessibility barriers, prejudice, and social labeling—contribute to their isolation from society (Balcı, 2019). Historically, addressing the problem of social exclusion experienced by individuals with disabilities has required the promotion of their full integration into society. Accordingly, individuals with disabilities who are excluded from processes of social inclusion encounter challenges across multiple domains of life. Understanding societal attitudes toward specific groups necessitates an examination of the broader political and economic conditions in which these attitudes are formed. Within this context, disability is associated not only with structural barriers but also with identity-related and emotional challenges (Barton, 1993).

Social inclusion is positioned as the conceptual counterpart to social exclusion. It aims to address situations in which individuals are unable to participate in the social structure on an equal basis with others due to various factors, through institutional arrangements and policy interventions. The primary objective is to promote equal citizenship by implementing a range of institutional measures that facilitate full participation in society (Aysoy, 2008). Social inclusion encompasses the equal participation of marginalized groups, such as individuals with disabilities, in both essential public services—such as education, healthcare, and employment—and in broader public life. Within this framework, social inclusion has gained particular importance in the context of social policies developed to combat social exclusion. In addition, participation in sport constitutes a significant dimension of social inclusion, as it facilitates social interaction, enhances physical and psychological well-being, and supports the integration of individuals into community life. Through accessible and inclusive sporting opportunities, barriers to participation can be reduced, thereby contributing to greater equality and active citizenship. Promoting the integration of individuals with disabilities into society requires the organization of inclusive artistic, cultural, and sporting activities that enable interaction with other members of the community. In this regard, the effective implementation of the principles of the social state, alongside the active engagement of civil society organizations, plays a crucial role (Seyyar, 2006). One important approach in this process is the development of communication grounded in a positive and inclusive perspective. Establishing meaningful interaction with individuals with disabilities and recognizing their value systems can foster more favorable attitudes and behaviors. As social distance increases, the likelihood of negative perceptions and discriminatory behaviors also rises (Arıkan, 2001).

3.2. Causes of Disability and the Aspects of Sport's Connection to the Well-being of Individuals with Disabilities

Disability is a multifaceted condition that can arise from a wide range of determinants, and it may be experienced in different forms depending on its impact on an individual's physical, cognitive, sensory, or social functioning. In social life, there are numerous risk factors that may contribute to the development of disability. These include lack of access to education, limited availability of healthcare services, transportation barriers, inappropriate or uninformed medication use, inadequate nutrition, substance and alcohol abuse, and communication difficulties. Although the causes of impairment and functional limitations are diverse, they are generally categorized into three main groups: prenatal factors, perinatal (birth-related) factors, and postnatal factors (Doğan & Çitil, 2011).

Prenatal causes of disability encompass a wide range of biological, environmental, and behavioral factors that may negatively affect fetal development. These include consanguineous marriages, blood type and Rh incompatibility between parents, chromosomal abnormalities, and hereditary disorders. Maternal age is also a significant determinant, with both early and advanced pregnancies associated with increased risk. In addition, exposure to teratogenic substances and harmful behaviors during pregnancy—such as the use of alcohol, tobacco, and illicit drugs, as well as the unsupervised use of medications—can contribute to congenital impairments. Nutritional deficiencies, exposure to radiation, lack of regular prenatal care, frequent and closely spaced pregnancies, and deficiencies in essential vitamins and minerals further increase the risk of adverse outcomes. Moreover, infectious diseases, poisoning, psychological stress, physical trauma, accidents, and chronic maternal illnesses are also important prenatal risk factors that may lead to disability in the newborn. Perinatal (birth-related) causes of disability refer to complications occurring during the process of delivery that may adversely affect the newborn's health and development. One of the most critical factors is the absence of skilled birth attendance or delivery in an adequately equipped healthcare facility. Additional risk factors include preterm birth and obstructed or complicated labor. Perinatal asphyxia, characterized by insufficient oxygen supply to the infant during birth, is another significant cause of long-term impairment. Postnatal causes of disability refer to factors that occur after birth and may negatively influence an individual's physical, cognitive, or social development. These include the absence of routine medical examinations and essential diagnostic screenings, as well as severe neonatal jaundice or other significant illnesses during early childhood. Furthermore, failure to administer required vaccinations or irregular immunization practices can increase vulnerability to preventable conditions that may result in long-term impairments. Accidents, natural disasters, and inadequate environmental and familial conditions, particularly those related to insufficient education and care, also constitute important risk factors (WHO, 2011).

Individuals with disabilities' integration into society plays a significant role not only in their personal development but also in their relationship with broader social values. Social inclusion for persons with disabilities requires not only the removal of physical barriers but also the elimination of psychosocial obstacles. In this context, sport emerges as an important tool that enhances social cohesion by promoting both physical and social empowerment. The dynamic social interactions and positive representations provided through sport contribute to individuals with disabilities perceiving themselves as active and valued members of society (Altındağ, 2017).

From the perspective of social equity and inclusion, the participation of individuals with disabilities in sport supports theories of social justice examined within the social sciences. The capacity of sport to function as a platform that strengthens the principle of equality among individuals is grounded in fundamental human rights principles emphasized in international documents such as the Declaration on the Rights of Disabled Persons and similar frameworks (Donnelly, 2008; Lord & Stein, 2009). From a psychological viewpoint, self-esteem and self-confidence are key factors. Participation in sport has been shown to have positive effects on the psychological well-being of individuals with disabilities. It is well established in the literature that sport enables individuals to discover their abilities, develop their strengths, and enhance their self-esteem through active engagement (Smoll et al., 1993). This, in turn, contributes to an improved overall quality of life and facilitates more effective social integration into society (Sauder & DeLuca, 2023).

For individuals with disabilities, sport provides an environment that offers not only physical benefits but also a sense of increased competence and self-efficacy. In this regard, sport contributes to the strengthening of both bodily capabilities and social identity. In particular, participation in team sports enhances social interaction skills, enabling individuals to express themselves as active and socially accepted members of society. Accordingly, sport expands opportunities for social interaction for persons with disabilities, thereby contributing to their increased visibility and acceptance within the community. The effectiveness of sport in facilitating social inclusion has been supported by various studies. Sport-related activities, which have the potential to reduce discrimination and eliminate social barriers, accelerate the participation processes of individuals with disabilities in society while also fostering their self-confidence (Özdemir, 2019).

In the context of changing social perceptions, sport has the potential to enhance societal acceptance of individuals with disabilities. Through sport, individuals with disabilities are increasingly perceived not only in terms of physical limitations but also as capable individuals with significant potential, thereby contributing to the evolution of social norms (Klenk et al., 2019). Overall, participation in sport generates a range of positive physical, emotional, and social outcomes for individuals with disabilities. These benefits not only improve overall quality of life but also contribute to the transformation of societal perceptions (Jespersen et al., 2019). Innovations aimed at enhancing the sporting experience of individuals with disabilities, along with the development of adaptive sports equipment, have significantly contributed to making sport more accessible, inclusive, and enjoyable. Equipment specifically designed for athletes with disabilities provides tailored solutions that address individual needs, thereby improving both the effectiveness and safety of participation in sport.

In this context, sport-specific wheelchairs can be customized according to the requirements of different sporting disciplines. Lightweight, durable, and highly maneuverable wheelchairs play a crucial role particularly in high-intensity and agility-based sports such as wheelchair basketball (Vanderstraeten & Oomen, 2010). These technological advancements not only improve performance but also support athletes' physical and psychological well-being by enabling greater independence, confidence, and reduced perceived limitations during participation. Beyond individual health outcomes, such innovations also contribute to the development of social capital, a stronger sense of belonging, and empowerment among individuals with disabilities. Participation in adapted sports fosters meaningful social networks, reinforces inclusion within sporting communities, and strengthens feelings of collective identity. As a result, adaptive sports technologies serve not only as functional tools but also as mechanisms that enhance both physical and psychological well-being, while simultaneously promoting social integration, empowerment, and long-term participation in sport. Sport is a multifaceted tool that positively influences not only the physical health of individuals with disabilities but also their psychosocial development. In this regard, it plays a crucial role in enhancing quality of life and promoting greater independence and active participation within society. The benefits of sport are particularly significant in supporting individuals with disabilities to become more engaged and self-sufficient in their daily lives. Positive outcomes in areas such as physical health, self-confidence, and stress management demonstrate that sport can lead to meaningful improvements in the lives of individuals with disabilities. These effects collectively contribute to both personal well-being and broader social participation (Çalışkan, 2020).

The successful integration of individuals with disabilities into sports organizations represents a critical step toward ensuring that sport is accessible at all levels. In this regard, such inclusion also reflects broader principles associated with the welfare state, particularly in terms of promoting equal opportunities, social protection, and inclusive participation in public life. First and foremost, the successful integration of individuals with disabilities into sports organizations constitutes a critical step toward ensuring that sport is accessible at all levels. Sports organizations support the motivation of individuals with disabilities to participate in sport by providing appropriate facilities and opportunities tailored to their needs. Establishing environments that are easily accessible, usable, and conducive to effective training for athletes with disabilities plays a crucial role in making sport more inclusive and accessible for this population (Misener & Darcy, 2014). Sports managers and staff can better respond to the specific needs of individuals with disabilities and raise public awareness through targeted education and disability-awareness programs. Training in interacting and working effectively with persons with disabilities contributes to the development of inclusive and disability-friendly environments within sports organizations (McConkey et al., 2013). Greater inclusion of athletes with disabilities in leadership roles within sports organizations can enhance representation, serve as a model of achievement, and increase diversity within organizational structures. The active involvement of disabled athletes in managerial and decision-making positions also enables organizations to provide more responsive and effective support for individuals with disabilities. Moreover, leaders with disabilities can act as inspirational figures and role models for younger athletes with similar experiences, fostering motivation and long-term engagement in sport. In addition, sports tournaments and leagues specifically organized for individuals with disabilities provide a competitive platform that can increase participation rates. Such events facilitate the coming together of individuals with different types of impairments and varying ability levels, thereby expanding opportunities for engagement in sport and promoting inclusive participation (Winnick & Porretta, 2016). Ensuring that sports events provide appropriate accessibility for individuals with disabilities can significantly enhance participation. This involves not only the physical accessibility of facilities but also access to information and effective communication systems. In this context, it is essential to select and design venues that can be easily reached, utilized, and navigated by individuals with disabilities, while also enabling meaningful interaction within the sporting environment. Furthermore, providing social and financial support to athletes with disabilities can facilitate their engagement in sport. Assistance with access to sports equipment, travel expenses, and training costs can play a crucial role in enabling athletes with disabilities to develop their skills and sustain long-term participation (Misener & Darcy, 2014).

For individuals with disabilities, sport not only enhances physical health but also plays a significant role in the process of social inclusion. Sporting activities increase social interaction, strengthen self-confidence, and facilitate integration into society. The benefits provided by sport enable individuals to assume a more active role in social life. Moreover, the social skills acquired through participation in sport contribute to the development of important competencies such as communication, cooperation, and empathy. These outcomes support the formation of stronger social bonds and enable individuals with disabilities to participate more effectively in social environments. In addition, sport contributes to both physical and psychological well-being by improving overall health status and enhancing emotional resilience. Regular participation in sport can reduce stress, improve mood, and foster a sense of personal achievement, thereby supporting holistic well-being. From a broader perspective, sport also promotes social capital, a sense of belonging, and empowerment. Through engagement in sporting activities, individuals with disabilities develop supportive social networks, feel more connected to their communities, and experience increased agency in their daily lives. This process of empowerment strengthens their ability to participate more actively in society and reinforces their social inclusion. In the future, various studies, projects, and practical initiatives can be developed to increase participation in sport among individuals with disabilities. In particular, comprehensive efforts are needed to enhance the accessibility and sustainability of sports programs. These efforts should include recommendations for infrastructure development and the strengthening of economic support mechanisms. Increasing the number of accessible sports facilities and adapting existing infrastructures to meet the needs of individuals with disabilities are essential steps in encouraging greater participation and fostering inclusive sporting environments (Telepbergen & Ermiş, 2024).

CONCLUSION

This chapter has examined sport as a social policy instrument within the framework of different welfare state approaches, with a particular focus on its contribution to the well-being of persons with disabilities. Drawing on a comparative and conceptual analysis, it has highlighted that sport cannot be understood as an inherently inclusive or universally beneficial practice; rather, its outcomes are closely shaped by institutional structures, policy priorities, and the broader orientation of social policy within each welfare regime. The findings of the study indicate that sport policies play a potentially significant role in enhancing the physical, psychological, and social dimensions of well-being for persons with disabilities. Participation in sport contributes to improved self-confidence, social interaction, empowerment, and quality of life. Moreover, sport serves as an important mechanism for fostering social inclusion, enabling individuals with disabilities to develop social networks, strengthen their sense of belonging, and engage more actively in community life. However, these positive outcomes are not automatic; they depend on the existence of inclusive infrastructures, adequate public investment, and rights-based policy frameworks. From a comparative perspective, the analysis demonstrates that welfare state approaches significantly influence the scope and effectiveness of sport policies. In social democratic regimes, where universalism and equality-oriented social policy are more strongly institutionalized, sport is more likely to function as an inclusive public good. In contrast, liberal regimes tend to rely more heavily on market mechanisms and individual responsibility, which may limit access and reproduce inequalities. Corporatist regimes, meanwhile, often structure sport participation through occupational and intermediary institutions, which can result in fragmented access patterns. These differences reveal that the contribution of sport to social inclusion is not uniform but regime-dependent. The study also underscores that sport should be understood as part of a broader social policy architecture rather than an isolated intervention. Its effectiveness in promoting the well-being of persons with disabilities is closely linked to the extent to which states recognize disability as a rights-based issue and implement inclusive sport policies accordingly. In this regard, sport functions not only as a health-promoting activity but also as a site of citizenship, equality, and social justice. In conclusion, this chapter argues that the potential of sport to enhance the well-being of persons with disabilities is significant but conditional. Realizing this potential requires inclusive policy design, sustained public commitment, and a strong alignment between sport policies and broader social policy objectives. Future research and policy development should therefore focus on strengthening accessibility, expanding rights-based approaches, and ensuring that sport contributes more effectively to social inclusion across different welfare state approaches.

REFERENCES

Abberley, P. (1987). The concept of oppression and the development of a social theory of disability. *Disability, Handicap & Society*, *2*(1), 5–19. DOI: 10.1080/02674648766780021

Altan, Ö. Z. (2007). Sosyal Politika. Eskişehir: Anadolu Üniversitesi Yayınları Yayını No: 1744.

Altan, Ö. Z. (2009). Sosyal Politika Dersleri. Eskişehir: Anadolu Üniversitesi Yayınları Yayın No: 1987.

Altındağ, S. (2017). Engelli bireylerin toplumsal uyum süreçlerinde sporun rolü. *Toplum ve Sosyal Bilimler Dergisi*, *6*(2), 30–45.

Aracı, H. (1999). *Öğretmen ve Okullarda Beden Eğitimi*. Bağırgan Yayınevi.

Arıkan, Ç. (2001). Aile ve özürlülük: 'Görme Özürlüler Derneği' üye özürlü aileleri üzerine bir araştırma. *Ufkun Ötesi Bilim Dergisi*, *1*(1), 45–60.

Aysoy, M. (2008). *Hayatı Paylaşmak İçin "Engel Çok"*. Açı Kitaplar.

Balcı, S. (2019). Engellilerin sosyal dışlanma algılarının bazı sosyodemografik değişkenlere göre incelenmesi. *Tıbbi Sosyal Hizmet Dergisi*, *0*(14), 59–79. DOI: 10.46218/tshd.1139360

Barr, A. N. (1992). *Economic theory and the welfare state: a survey and interpretation*. LSE.

Barton, L. (1993). The Struggle for Citizenship: The Case of Disabled People. *Disability, Handicap & Society*, *8*(3), 235–248. DOI: 10.1080/02674649366780251

Bedir, E., Özaydın, M. M. ve Metin, B. (2013). Sosyal Politika 1. Eskişehir: Anadolu Üniversitesi, Açıköğretim Fakültesi Yayınları, No: 1589

Bekik, M. E. (2025). Social Policy Developments. In *The Ottoman Empire In The Context Of The Tanzimat And Islahat Edicts. Türkiye ve Dünyada Sosyal Politika* (pp. 1–17). Yaz Yayınları.

Bradburn, N. M. (1969). *The Structure of Psychological Well-Being*. Aldine Publishing Company.

Çalışkan, N. (2020). Engelli bireylerin fiziksel sağlıklarına sporun etkileri. *Toplum ve Sağlık Dergisi*, *7*(1), 27–34.

Coakley, J. (2017). Sports in society: Issues and controversies. McGraw: Hill Education.

Çubuk, A. (1979). *Sosyal Politika*. Ankara İktisadi ve Ticari İlimler Akademisi Yayını.

Diener, E. (1984). Subjective Well-Being. *Psychological Bulletin*, *95*(3), 542–575. DOI: 10.1037/0033-2909.95.3.542 PMID: 6399758

Emmenegger, P., Kvist, J., Marx, P., & Petersen, K. (2015). Three Worlds of Welfare Capitalism: The Making Of A Classic. *Journal of European Social Policy*, *25*(1), 3–13. DOI: 10.1177/0958928714556966

Emmons, R. A. (1986). Personal strivings: An approach to personality and subjective well-being. *Journal of Personality and Social Psychology*, *51*(5), 1058–1068. DOI: 10.1037/0022-3514.51.5.1058

Erkal, M. (1992). *Sosyolojik Açıdan Spor*. Kutsun Matbaa Reklam Merkezi.

Ersöz, H. Y. (2003). Doğuşundan Günümüze Sosyal Politika Anlayışı ve Sosyal Politika Kurumlarının Değişen Rolü. İstanbul Üniversitesi İktisat Fakültesi Mecmuası, 53(2), 119-144.

Esping-Andersen, G. (1990). *The Three Worlds Of Welfare Capitalism*. Policy Press.

Esping-Andersen, G. (1999). *Social Foundations of Postindustrial Economies*. Oxford University Press. DOI: 10.1093/0198742002.001.0001

Günışık, E. (1990). 'Spor Psikolojisi. *Journal of Physical Education and Sports Studies*, *1*(3), 34.

Güven, S. (2001). *Sosyal Politikanın Temelleri (3. Baskı)*. Ezgi Kitabevi Yayınları.

Jespersen, L. N., Michelsen, S. I., Tjørnhøj-Thomsen, T., Svensson, M. K., Holstein, B. E., & Due, P. (2019). Living with a disability: A qualitative study of associations between social relations, social participation and quality of life. *Disability and Rehabilitation*, *41*(11), 1275–1286. DOI: 10.1080/09638288.2018.1424949 PMID: 29357697

Kahneman, D., & Deaton, A. (2010). High income improves evaluation of life but not emotional well-being. *Proceedings of the National Academy of Sciences of the United States of America*, *107*(38), 16489–16493. DOI: 10.1073/pnas.1011492107 PMID: 20823223

Kat, H. (2009). *Bireysel sporcularla takım sporcularının stres düzeyleri ve problem çözme becerilerinin karşılaştırılması. (Yayınlanmamış Yüksek Lisans Tezi)*. Erciyes Üniversitesi Sağlık Bilimleri Ensitüsü.

Keyes, C. L. (2003). *Complete mental health: An agenda for the 21th century. C. L. Keyes, & J. Haidt (Dü) içinde, Flourishing: Positive psychology and the life well-lived.* American Psychological Association.

Klenk, C., Albrecht, J. B., & Nagel, S. (2019). Social participation of people with disabilities in organized community sport. A systematic review. *German Journal of Exercise and Sport Research, 49*(4), 365–380. DOI: 10.1007/s12662-019-00584-3

Koray, M. (2012). *Sosyal Politika (4.baskı).* İmge Kitabevi.

Leibfried, S. (2014). Towards a European welfare state?Jones. C (Eds), New perspectives on the welfare state in Europe (pp. 120-143). Routledge: London and New York.

Lord, J. E., & Stein, M. A. (2009). Social rights and the relational value of the rights to participate in sport, recreation, and play. *BU Int'l LJ, 27*, 249.

McConkey, R., Dowling, S., Hassan, D., & Menke, S. (2013). Promoting social inclusion through unified sports for youth with intellectual disabilities: A five-nation study. *Journal of Intellectual Disability Research : JIDR, 57*(10), 923–935. DOI: 10.1111/j.1365-2788.2012.01587.x PMID: 22672339

Misener, L., & Darcy, S. (2014). Managing disability sport: From athletes with disabilities to inclusive organisational perspectives. *Sport Management Review, 17*(1), 1–7. DOI: 10.1016/j.smr.2013.12.003

Morris, J. (2001). Social exclusion and young disabled people with high levels of support needs. *Critical Social Policy, 21*(2), 161–183. DOI: 10.1177/026101830102100202

O'Connell, P. J. (1991). The Three Worlds of Welfare Capitalism. by Gøsta Esping-Anderson. *Social Forces, 70*(2), 532–534.

Okur, N. ve Erbil Erdugan, F. (2010). "Sosyal Haklar ve Özürlüler: Özürlülük Modelleri Bağlamında Tarihsel Bir Değerlendirme", II. Sosyal Haklar Ulusal Sempozyumu Bildiri Kitabı (s. 245-263), Denizli: Pamukkale Üniversitesi Yayınları.

Özdemir, H. (2019). Sosyal uyum ve spor: Engelli bireyler üzerine bir inceleme. *Sosyal Bilimlerde Güncel Araştırmalar Dergisi, 10*(1), 65–72.

Özdemir, S. (2011).Refah devletinin gelişme ve bunalım dönemlerinde iş piyasaları. İktisat Fakültesi Mecmuası (Prof.Dr. Toker Dereliye Armağan Özel Sayısı), 55(1), 695-733.

Peace, R. (2001). Social Exclusion: A Concept in Need of Definition? *Social Policy Journal of New Zealand, 16*, 17–36.

Ryan, R. M., & Deci, E. L. (2001). On happiness and human potentials: A review of research on hedonic and eudaimonic well-being. *Annual Review of Psychology, 52*(1), 141–166. DOI: 10.1146/annurev.psych.52.1.141 PMID: 11148302

Ryff, C. D. (1989). Happiness is everything, or is it? Explorations on the meaning of psychological well-being. *Journal of Personality and Social Psychology, 57*(6), 1069–1081. DOI: 10.1037/0022-3514.57.6.1069

Ryff, C. D., & Singer, B. H. (2008). Know thyself and become what you are: A eudaimınic approach to psychological well-being. *Journal of Happiness Studies, 9*(1), 13–39. DOI: 10.1007/s10902-006-9019-0

Şahan, H. (2007). *Üniversite öğrencilerinin sosyalleşme sürecinde spor aktivitelerinin rolü. (Doktora Tezi).* Selçuk Üniversitesi Sosyal Bilimler Enstitüsü.

Sapancalı, F. (2005). *Sosyal Dışlanma.* Dokuz Eylül Yayınları.

Sapir, A. (2006). Globalization and the reform of european social models. *Journal of Common Market Studies, 44*(2), 369–390. DOI: 10.1111/j.1468-5965.2006.00627.x

Sauder, M. H., & DeLuca, J. R. (2023). Framing Course Content on Diversity and Inclusion: Varying Outcomes From Teaching on Disability in Sport Management. Sport Management Education Journal, 1(aop), 1-6.

Seyyar, A. (2006). Özürlülere adanmış sosyal politika yazıları. Sakarya: Adapazarı Büyükşehir Belediyesi.

Şişman, Y. (2017). Türkiye'de Sosyal Politika'nın Dünü, Bugünü: Hayırseverliğin Kurumsallaşması mı? Gelişmesi mi? *Optimum Ekonomi ve Yönetim Bilimleri Dergisi, 4*(2), 1–22.

Şişman, Y., (2023). Engellik Alanındaki Kavramsal Karmaşanın Nedenleri ve Mevcut Durum. Üçüncü Sektör Sosyal Ekonomi, vol.58, no.3, 2444-2459.

Smoll, F. L., Smith, R. E., Barnett, N. P., & Everett, J. J. (1993). Enhancement of children's self-esteem through social support training for youth sport coaches. *The Journal of Applied Psychology, 78*(4), 602–610. DOI: 10.1037/0021-9010.78.4.602 PMID: 8407704

Sunal, O. (2011). Sosyal Politika: Sosyal Adalet Açısından Kuramsal Bir Değerlendirme. *Ankara Üniversitesi SBF Dergisi, 66*(03), 283–305. DOI: 10.1501/SBFder_0000002223

Talas, C. (1990). *Sosyal Politika.* İmge Kitabevi.

Telepbergen, A., & Ermiş, A. (2024). Engelli Bireylerin Sosyal Yaşantıya Dahil Edilmesinde Sporun Önemi. *Optimal Zenith Spor Bilimleri Dergisi*, *1*(2), 49–56. DOI: 10.70736/jozss.2007

UN. (2006). Engellilerin haklarına ilişkin sözleşme. www.un.org/disabilities/documents/natl/turkey.doc

Vanderstraeten, G. G., & Oomen, A. G. (2010). Sports for disabled people: A general outlook. *International Journal of Rehabilitation Research. Internationale Zeitschrift für Rehabilitationsforschung. Revue Internationale de Recherches de Réadaptation*, *33*(4), 283–284. DOI: 10.1097/MRR.0b013e32834012b1 PMID: 22470933

Walker, A., & Walker, C. (1997). *Britain divided: The growth of social exclusion in the 1980s and 1990s*. Child Poverty Action Group.

WHO. (2011). *World report on disability*. World Health Organization.

WHO. (2014). *Strengthening Mental Health Promotion* [Fact Sheet No. 220]. World Health Organization.

Winnick, J. P., & Porretta, D. L. (2016). *Adapted physical education and sport*. Human Kinetics.

Yıldırım, S. (2011). *Lisanslı olarak takım sporu ve bireysel spor yapan ile spor yapmayan ortaöğretim öğrencilerinin sosyal beceri düzeylerinin karşılaştırılması. (Yayımlanmamış Yüksek Lisans Tezi)*. Abant İzzet Baysal Üniversitesi Sosyal Bilimler Enstitüsü.

Chapter 13

Sport as a Strategic Social Policy Tool for Strengthening Social Cohesion and Reducing Social Risk

Sohom Saha
http://orcid.org/0009-0006-9438-1554
Lakshmibai National Institute of Physical Education, India

Mahendra Kumar Singh
http://orcid.org/0000-0001-9989-9420
Lakshmibai National Institute of Physical Education, India

ABSTRACT

Sport is perceived as an aspect of physical health, yet it may be an effective social policy instrument. This chapter develops the idea of the ability of sport to enhance social cohesion and decrease social risks within the segment of the modern welfare states and community and grassroots sports programs in particular. It demonstrates the reputation of well-constructed sport programs to establish the trust between groups, decrease youth crime and school drop-out, enhance mental health, foster gender equality, and help them acquire employment skills. Based on the theoretical framework of welfare, social capital theory, and prevention policy, the chapter contends that sport has the potential to generate actual social benefits in case it is inclusive, evidence-based, and well-managed. It also suggests a mechanism to

DOI: 10.4018/979-8-2600-3174-2.ch013

quantify the impact of sport using access, social cohesion, reduction of risk and cost effectiveness. The chapter provides policy guidelines on how sport can be incorporated in the national welfare systems.

1. INTRODUCTION

The conceptualization of the welfare state has traditionally been that of a redistributive institutional structure that aims to safeguard citizens against social risk and market failures by the income transfer, provision of healthcare, unemployment insurance and other social security programs. But, beginning in the late twentieth century, much has changed as a paradigmatic shift in the direction of the preventive and participatory social policy adjusts the manner in which contemporary welfare systems are tackling issues like social exclusion, marginalization of youth, health disparities, and community disintegration (Esping-Andersen, 1990; Taylor-Gooby, 2004).

Sport has become not only a form of leisure, but also a tool of welfare governance in this changing policy environment, becoming part and parcel of national and supranational social policy agendas. Sport stands in a special nexi between the social inclusion, community development and public health. Governments across the world have started appreciating the ability of sport to be what Coalter (2007) sees as a so-called sport plus intervention- a channel through which greater social agendas are strategically being realized. Sport has been officially recognized by the European Union, the United Nations, and the International Olympic Committee as well as by many governments of countries as a tool by which social cohesion and reduction of inequality can be achieved and by which risks like youth crime, social isolation, gender marginalization, and poor mental health can be countered (United Nations, 2015; European Commission, 2022).

Although there has been an increasing policy discussion of the social utility of sport, theoretical location of sport in welfare studies is also underdeveloped. The processes by which sport brings about welfare goods, social capital formation, psychological hardiness, intergroup contact, development of employability skills are hardly considered systematically within the welfare regime models. This knowledge gap draws a discontinuity between the policy passion of sport-based interventions and the assessment of their welfare impact on a rigorous basis. This chapter attempts to fills this gap by making sport a significant part of the structure of welfare governance. It is based on three significant theoretical frameworks welfare state and social justice theory, social capital and social cohesion theory, and preventive social policy to develop a holistic case on sport as legitimate and measurable welfare policy instrument. The chapter further suggests an appraisal framework of the evaluation of the sport based social policies and ends off with some pragmatic suggestions to the policy makers in an attempt to further incorporate the sport into welfare governance paradigms.

2. AIM AND OBJECTIVES

The main goal of this chapter is to theorize and assess sport as a strategic social policy instrument that helps in social cohesion and social risks alleviation in welfare states. Precisely, the chapter has five objectives which are interrelated.

First, it discusses the theoretical premises which connect sport to the principles of welfare state and social justice and places sport in the typology of welfare regimes and normative frameworks of distributive justice developed by Esping-Andersen (1990). Second, it examines how sport fosters social cohesion by participating, being solid, and being included at an individual, community and societal level. Third, it determines the ways sport decreases social risks, specifically focusing on those least advantaged such as at-risk youth, women, impoverished people, and socially marginalized groups. Fourth, it suggests a multidimensional conceptualization of the effectiveness of sport-based welfare policies, which has been a longstanding dilemma of evaluating policies based on evidence. Fifth, it offers some policy suggestions on how sport can be systematically incorporated into the models of welfare governance with international comparative examples.

3. THEORETICAL FRAMEWORK

3.1 Welfare State Theory and Social Justice

Esping-Andersen (1990) seminal typology of welfare regimes which categorized welfare regimes into three ideal types, liberal (residual, market-oriented), conservative-corporatist (contribution-based, familialist), and social-democratic (universalist, decommodifying) has become the theoretical baseline of the analysis of welfare states. Though the sport is not directly theorized in this paradigm, there is a significant difference in its connection to the welfare governance by the type of regimes. Social-democratic societies, including Nordic countries, consider sport to be a social good, and it is provided equally to everyone via state support of community sport facilities and grassroots. In liberal regimes, the market can mediate to a large extent in the participation of sport which leads to inequitable access based on social economic status. Conservative-corporatist governments tend to leave the management of sport to civil society entities, and voluntary clubs.

Table 1. Sport Within Welfare Regime Typologies

Welfare Regime Type	Core Characteristics	Governance of Sport	Access Pattern	Social Policy Implication
Liberal	Market-oriented, residual welfare	Market & private sector dominant	Unequal, SES-based access	Risk of exclusion without subsidies
Conservative-Corporatist	Familial, contribution-based	Civil society & voluntary clubs	Moderately unequal	Community-driven but uneven reach
Social-Democratic	Universalist, decommodifying	State-funded grassroots sport	Broad universal access	Strongest cohesion & equity potential

To succeed as a social policy tool, the governance of sport should be synodal with the principles of social justice especially equality of opportunity and distributive justice (Rawls, 1971). The sport policy that privileges elite performances at the expense of the grassroots participation is not only necessary but also creates more social inequalities. On the other hand, sport can be transformed into a potent redistributive tool of the welfare state when structured around the principles of equity- targeting the underserved communities, subsidizing the participation of the low-income population, and incorporating all groups into program structure (Houlihan and White, 2002).

The so-called social investment state, which was conceptualized by Esping-Andersen et al. (2002), and Giddens (1998) offers a more than appropriate theoretical point of departure. The social investment policy emphasizes preventive expenditure as opposed to compensatory expenditure as it invests in the construction of human capital and social capabilities as opposed to compensating social failures when they happen. Sport fits well into the paradigm of social investment: organized physical activities among children, sports clubs in the poor area, and sport activities by women not only bring immediate benefits to welfare but also cut down on social costs in the long term through delinquency, illness, and social exclusion (Moustakas, 2022).

3.2 Social Capital and Social Cohesion Theory

The second highly important theoretical pillar to the analysis of the welfare role of sport is the social capital theory, coined by Bourdieu (1986), Coleman (1988), and most prominently Putnam (2000). According to Putnam, social capital is the networks, reciprocity norms and trust that make cooperation to attain mutual benefits. He makes a distinction between bonding capital which refers to the tight ties within homogeneous groups and bridging capital which refers to networks that link individuals across social boundaries. The two forms are applicable to the social policy potential of sport. The bonding capital is created through community sport clubs, recreational leagues and sport-for-development programs that establish the participant of the programs to social networks that are stable due to the sharing of common spaces and activities.

More importantly, to the benefit of welfare, sport events and mixed-team programs have the potential to create bridging capital, uniting people on the basis of ethnic, class, gender, and generational differences (Moustakas and Robrade, 2022). The groundbreaking experimental article by Mousa (2020) proved that mixed Christian-Muslim soccer teams in the post-conflict Iraq have already induced a substantial decrease in prejudice and a rise in the cross-group social connections between players, which gives strong empirical evidence of the bridging capital potential of sport.

Table 2. Mechanisms Through Which Sport Builds Social Capital

Type of Social Capital	Sport Setting	Mechanism	Expected Outcome
Bonding Capital	Community clubs	Shared identity & repeated interaction	Strong intra-group trust
Bridging Capital	Mixed-team programs	Cross-group cooperation	Reduced prejudice
Linking Capital	State-supported sport programs	Institutional engagement	Increased institutional trust

The macro-level manifestation of accumulated social capital is social cohesion which is commonly defined as a level of social integration, trust, participation and solidarity that exist in a given society. Moustakas (2024) suggests a conceptual model that connects sport program practices, mechanisms, including contact, cooperation, and identity formation, and particular social cohesion outcomes. It is a framework on which both program design and program evaluation are based, where the interactions at the micro-level within the sport setting are related to the meso-level of community integration and the macro-level of solidarity of society.

3.3 Preventive Social Policy and Social Risk Management

The third theoretical framework is the preventative paradigm of social policy which reinvents the orientation of welfare intervention that focuses on active risk management to mitigate the risks rather than to cure them (Beck, 1992; Taylor-Gooby, 2004). The contemporary welfare states have been presented with a new terrain of social risks of youth unemployment, family instability, health disparities, social isolation and community fragmentation, unlike those social risks that characterized the design of the classic welfare state in the industrial era. The younger generations, women, migrants, and poor urban groups are disproportionately exposed to these new social risks.

Sport acts as a buffer of various emerging social threats. Organized sport programs offer social support systems, positive role models, routine, and discipline, and experiential learning opportunities that, when combined, prevent risks such as delinquency, substance abuse, school dropout, and social withdrawal (Spruit et al., 2018; Zhang et al., 2023). When prompted into intersectoral welfare governmental schemes, sport and health, education, housing, and labor-market policies, sport is no longer a cumulative method of recreational service provision but a structural risk management tool, indeed, an institutionalized risk management instrument, within the welfare system.

Table 3. Theoretical Foundations Linking Sport and Welfare Governance

Theoretical Framework	Key Scholar(s)	Core Concept	Relevance to Sport Policy
Welfare State Theory	Esping-Andersen	Regime types & redistribution	Determines sport access models
Social Justice Theory	Rawls	Equity & equality of opportunity	Justifies inclusive sport policy
Social Capital Theory	Putnam	Bonding & bridging capital	Explains cohesion outcomes
Preventive Social Policy	Beck, Taylor-Gooby	Risk mitigation	Positions sport as preventive investment
Social Investment State	Giddens	Human capital building	Frames sport as long-term investment

4. SPORT AND SOCIAL COHESION

Social cohesion is one of the most controversial, but policy-relevant, concepts in the modern welfare discussion. According to Fonseca, Lukosch, and Brazier (2019), it consists of horizontal dimensions (social relations among individuals and groups), and vertical ones (relations between citizens and institutions). The contribution of sport to cohesion works on three empirically related, analytically separate levels, namely individual, community and societal.

4.1 Individual Level: Identity, Belonging, and Psychological Well-Being

On an individual level, sport participation gives a sense of belonging and identity creation which is especially important in young people and those who belong to a marginalized group. Organized sport offers structured forms of socialization where members of organizations gain self-efficacy, emotional stability, interpersonal competence, and positive sense of identity (Mahindru et al., 2023). To the socially disadvantaged youth, sport clubs tend to be one of the few consistent, prosocial establishments that offer them something to rely on in their lives. The physical venue and social community offered by the sports club or community team offers an identity anchor and counter to the anomie that is part of the marginalization of social life.

The positive effects of sport involvement on psychological well-being are properly documented. Vella et al. (2023) proved that the effect of physical activity on mental health outcomes is mediated by the context of physical activity, namely, its social aspects, perceived competence, and association with other people. Regular exercise will decrease depressive and anxiety symptoms, boost self-esteem and mood, and increase psychological resilience (Menhas et al., 2024). These individual level advantages are not personal in nature but there are definite welfare implications which lead to a decrease in demand in mental health services and enhancement in productivity and social functioning.

4.2 Community Level: Social Networks and Intergroup Relations

On the community level, sport clubs and recreational programs serve as what Putnam (2000) calls as schools of democracy the social arenas that foster interpersonal networks, develop norms of reciprocity and civic competencies. Karstensen et al. (2024) report on the role of local sports clubs in serving as a shared space that fosters a sense of community and community competence especially in a setting where other traditional civic institutions are deteriorating. The unique ability of sport to bring about a common experience despite social disparity makes it especially useful in community level cohesion. Community sport has an intercultural potential which is worthy of consideration.

Sport programs based on the principles of the contact theory, in which intergroup cooperation is formed under the conditions of equal status, shared objectives, and institutional backing, have also been reported to decrease prejudice and enhance intergroup attitudes in ethnically diverse neighborhoods and post-conflict societies (Allport, 1954; Mousa, 2020). The conceptual framework introduced by Moustakas (2024) differentiates between the so-called evangelical programs that simply expose the various groups of people to each other and structural programs that methodically try to establish the circumstances of meaningful cross-group contact.

The latter is much more successful in creating bridging social capital, and real community cohesion. Infrastructure of community sport is also relevant as the physical capital of social cohesion. Communal sporting centers, city parks, and community sports facilities are what urban sociologists refer to as what are known as a third place: social places beyond work and home, where people engage in informal social practices that form the community ties (Oldenburg, 1989). The institutional supply and fair sharing of such spaces is a social policy issue in its own right, and has a great deal to say regarding welfare outcomes.

4.3 Societal Level: National Solidarity and Collective Identity

On the macro level, national solidarity and collective identity can be seen through the policies of inclusive sport. The ability of sport to create an imagined community (Anderson, 1983) or a sense of national belonging that cuts across local and group lines has been a long-established fact by states that employ sport events and national teams as a symbol of national unity. Nevertheless, this symbolic role of sport as a cohesive element is most effective when it is reinforced by substantive policy roles in ensuring equitable access to sport participation.

The studies of a comprehensive measurement framework of social cohesion repeatedly find participation and trust as crucial dimensions of the research (Beierlein et al., 2023). When the policies of sports lead to lowering the socioeconomic barriers to participation, i.e. by making the programs free or subsidized, the facilities accessible, and culturally tailored programming, the aspect of social cohesion on the participatory level is directly enhanced. As different populations co-exist in sporting spaces and activities, they create the experiential ground of generalised social trust, which is a constituent part of sustainable social cohesion. The cohesive potential of sport is however not in itself automatic. In hopeful thinking, Coalter (2015) suggests the sport-for-change scepticism that reminds people not to blindly believe that participants in sports will automatically enjoy the cohesive benefits.

The results of cohesion of sport are mediated by program design, quality of facilitation and the larger policy environment. Institutional cultures of sport that are embedded into elite, performance oriented, or exclusionary cultures can also recreate, instead of decrease, social inequalities and class, gender, and ethnic hierarchies. It is the role of the welfare state thus not only to finance sport but also to regulate it in a manner that ensures that it is inclusive and cohesion-building.

Table 4. Sport's Contribution to Social Cohesion Across Levels

Level	Mechanism	Outcomes	Welfare Impact
Individual	Identity formation, belonging	Self-esteem, resilience	Reduced mental health burden
Community	Intergroup contact, shared spaces	Trust, civic participation	Stronger local networks
Societal	Inclusive national policy	National solidarity	Sustainable social cohesion

5. SPORT AND THE REDUCTION OF SOCIAL RISK

Social risk which is defined as the likelihood of encountering negative social outcomes as a factor of structural placement, life course transformations, or external shocks is among the main issues of modern-day welfare governance (Taylor-Gooby, 2004). The interventions based on sport focus on social risks in a range of how it can be considered a protective factor, which prevents the intensification of the risks, and promotive factor, which develops capabilities and resilience.

5.1 Youth at Risk: Delinquency, School Dropout, and Substance Abuse

The best-known literature on the use of sport as a social risk-reduction mechanism perhaps involves the case of at-risk youth. It has been established that structured sport programs can decrease delinquency, substance abuse, and school dropout rates through mentorship, structured time use, positive peer associations, and experiential moral learning (Spruit et al., 2018). The comprehensive review of life skills development in the sport programs in the areas where the youth are socially at risk was carried out by Hermens et al. (2017), who found the consistent evidence of the behavioral improvements in case of the explicitly designed sport programs aimed at promoting the development of the life skills rather than at the merely providing the sport activity.

In Spruit et al. (2018), a quasi-experimental assessment was done on a Dutch sport-based crime prevention program (AJB) with 368 at-risk youth. They found that police registrations in the intervention group were significantly lower compared to the comparison group, which proved that sport-based crime prevention can be implemented in large-scale applications. The quality of coaching relationship and the prosocial sport club climate mediated the effect of the program, which highlighted the role of implementation fidelity and trained practitioners.

Harrison et al. (2024) conducted a systematic review to analyze life skills acquired in response to physical activity and sport programs in youth at risk of or involved in delinquency. The results of their study, which include primary, secondary, and tertiary levels of intervention, prove that purposely developed life skills programs in the sport settings can produce protective delinquency factors. More importantly, the review notes that sport activity cannot take its own; it is the purposeful, systematic development of competencies, including self-regulation and conflict resolution, and prosocial norms, that determine the outcomes of welfare. The main theoretical process that connects sport and delinquency prevention is the theory of social bonding (Hirschi, 1969).

The involvement in sport enhances affiliation to prosocial institutions and role models, conventional behavior through observable investment in sport success, involvement in structured time use, which restricts delinquent opportunity, and the belief in the authenticity of the social rule which is upheld by the culture of fair play. Sport programs when incorporated in the community institutions and presented by professional caring practitioners are successful operationalization of all four aspects of social bonding.

5.2 Health Inequalities: Physical and Mental Welfare

The second significant sphere of social risk where sport is a preventive welfare tool is health inequalities. The connection between socioeconomic disadvantage and the lack of physical and mental health is well established and documented, and sport participation is already a population-scale intervention to curb such disparity at a low cost. Guidelines of physical activity adopted by the world health agency highlight its protection against non-communicable diseases such as cardiovascular disease, type 2 diabetes, cancer and obesity, which have a lot of social welfare implications. The welfare policy is especially concerned with mental health outcomes.

Mental illnesses pose a very high burden to the world and they are also increasing despite the fact that mental health services are still inadequate in most welfare regimes. Sport participation provides a preventive intervention that has been shown to have a scale effect on depression, anxiety, self-esteem, and psychological resiliency. The article by Vella et al. (2023) conducted a review of evidence in contextual factors in physical activity interventions on mental health, as proved by the fact that social context, i.e., peer relationships, coach support, and sense of belonging created through sport, plays a significant mediating role. These results put sport as a true mental health promotion device as opposed to just a supplement to clinical intervention.

In the view of welfare economics, preventive investment to engage in sport provides considerable savings in healthcare spending in the long run. Lower rates of obesity, cardiovascular disease, type 2 diabetes and mental conditions of regular sport participants will be converted into quantifiable health care use. In the United

Kingdom and Australia, cost benefit analyses have always demonstrated that an investment in community sport and physical activity programs will result in positive returns on investment in terms of reduced healthcare expenditure, enhanced workforce productivity and educational outcomes among children and youth.

5.3 Gender and Social Marginalization: Empowerment Through Sport

Social marginalization, especially gender inequality, is one of the dimensions of social marginalization that sport policy deals with. Traditionally, sport has been a male-dominated field, and women and girls have been systematically excluded with the help of cultural norms, institutionalization, and resource inequalities (Indelicato, 2025). The international sport policy statement of equality between men and women and the further international frameworks that followed, such as the Brighton Declaration (1994), have adopted gender equality in sport as a policy requirement because it has been realised that sport exclusion is a perpetuation of increased gender inequity.

Policies that are aimed specifically at women as participants in sport and bring about inclusive sport induce various benefits in the form of welfare. Sport leads to agency building, self-confidence, leadership skills and social networks that go far beyond the sporting environment. Evans and Knepper (2023) discuss the topic of women sports through the prism of social equity by clarifying that sport is a social place where women may acquire skills and presence that is central to social and economic empowerment in the larger sense. The authors concluded that gender equity in sport organizations could be promoted through structured community of practice initiatives, which yielded quantifiable positive changes in the proportion and representation of women in leadership and overall participation in the organizations (Sotigui et al., 2021).

Sport programs that are culturally sensitive and exclusively women-oriented have proven especially promising to women in especially marginalized roles, such as those in low-income communities, women with disabilities, and women with strong cultural norms against full participation in the community. Alhumaid et al. (2024) report about how physically disabled women in Saudi Arabia started to build identity, social relationships, and disrupt cultural scripts of disability and femininity through the Para sport programs, which led to discovering the empowering potential of sport even in the most limiting social settings. Intergenerational benefits of women participating in sport strengthen the welfare argument of the gendered sport policy. The mothers involved in sport will find it easier to bring up physically active children, and the health-generating multi-generation effect is created. The women who have a history of sport participation exhibit a higher level of education, the level of participation in the labor market, and civic participation -all of which lead to a lower level of welfare dependency and social capital.

5.4 Economic Vulnerability and Labor Market Integration

A fourth dimension of social risk reduction has to do with economic vulnerability and marginalization in labor market. Sport-based interventions help in improving employability by instilling soft skills, which employers are always after, such as teamwork, leadership, communication, time management, goal-setting, resilience in the wake of failure, and ability to work under pressure (Spaaij, Magee, and Jeanes, 2013). These are competences that are acquired in the competitive and participatory sport environment that has been organized in a goal-focused way, and they reflect in improved performances at the labor market.

In young people facing a combination of two or more disadvantages, such as poverty, poor educational performance, and social marginalization, sport programs which involve physical activity, purposeful training in life skills and employment opportunities are an integrated form of welfare intervention whose benefits are high-order returns. This combined model has been demonstrated by some of the programs like the Street League in the United Kingdom and Midnight Basketball in the United States, which have combined sport participation with formal qualifications, mentorship, and job placement. Systematic reviews of these programs show better engagement in education, less NEET (not in education, employment, or training), and better life skills of participants.

Table 5. Sport as a Social Risk Reduction Mechanism

Social Risk Domain	Target Group	Sport-Based Intervention	Measured Outcome
Youth Delinquency	At-risk youth	Structured mentoring sport programs	Reduced crime rates
School Dropout	Vulnerable adolescents	Life-skills sport curriculum	Higher retention
Mental Health	Low-income populations	Community sport participation	Lower depression & anxiety
Gender Inequality	Women & girls	Women-only sport programs	Empowerment & leadership
Economic Marginalization	NEET youth	Sport-employment integration	Increased employability

6. MEASURING POLICY EFFECTIVENESS: AN EVALUATION FRAMEWORK

A proposed framework of the evaluation of sport-based social policies is one of the major contributions of this chapter. Sport policies unless measured systematically run a risk of being symbolic instead of transformational in that they will produce rhetorical commitment but not real welfare benefits. The framework is based on the Coaters' (2008) sport- in-development evaluation manual, Cohesion outcomes model by Moustakas (2024) and the basic welfare indicators, and it provides a combined method to evaluate the effectiveness of sport social policy in four interrelated areas.

Table 6. Multidimensional Evaluation Framework for Sport-Based Social Policy

Evaluation Dimension	Key Indicators	Measurement Approach	Time Frame
Access	SES participation rates, facility distribution	Administrative & survey data	Short-term
Social Cohesion	Trust, cross-group interaction	Longitudinal surveys	Medium-term
Risk Reduction	Crime rates, health outcomes	Quasi-experimental designs	Medium–Long term
Cost-Benefit	ROI, healthcare savings	Economic modelling	Long-term

6.1 Access Indicators

Access indicators are used to determine how sports programs are accessed by the desired welfare beneficiaries. Some key measures are participation rates by socioeconomic status, gender, ethnicity, disability state, and physical location; facility provision by the 5-income quintiles; use of subsidies and fee waivers by the eligible groups; and the representation of marginalized groups in sport leadership and governance. The indicators of access are also primary: without fair access, sport cannot be used to fulfil its social policy promise. Cross-regional comparison of welfare regimes demonstrates that there are regular variations in access patterns, with universal provision systems in social-democratic regimes always doing better in terms of broad-based participation in comparison to means-tested systems.

Table 7. Access and Inclusion Indicators in Sport Policy

Indicator Category	Specific Measure	Target Benchmark
Socioeconomic Access	Participation by income quintile	Equalized participation rates
Gender Equity	Female participation ratio	50% parity
Disability Inclusion	Facility accessibility rate	100% compliance
Geographic Equity	Rural vs Urban facility density	Proportional distribution
Leadership Representation	Marginalized group representation	Reflect population share

6.2 Social Cohesion Indicators

Indicators of social cohesion measure the role of sport in social integration, trust and solidarity. Based on Fonseca et al. (2019) and the conceptual framework proposed by Moustakas (2022), the following metrics can be considered relevant changes in social trust generalization among the participants of the program; the rates of cross-group social interaction and formation of friendships in the mixed-group sport programs; civic engagement and rates of volunteering among the members of the sport clubs; attachment to the community and the sense of belonging among the members of the program; and intergroup attitude change measured with the help of the valid instruments. Cohesion indicators require longitudinal designs, because the effects of social capital and the effect of cohesion are normally realized in the long term.

6.3 Social Risk Reduction Indicators

Risk reduction indicators are used to quantify how successful sport is in preventing or alleviating unfavourable outcomes in target populations in relation to welfare. Youth crime rates, school retention, and educational attainment among those who attend youth sport programs, mental health outcomes such as scores on depression, anxiety, and psychological resilience, physical health outcomes such as BMI, cardiovascular fitness, and prevalence of chronic diseases, substance abuse rates, and gender-specific outcomes such as women empowerment scores, labor market participation rates, and political engagement are all examples of domain-specific measures. These signs have to be gathered via strict quasi-experimental or randomized designs to allow causal inference of the role of sport in reducing risk that separates the impact of programs and selection effects.

6.4 Cost-Benefit Analysis

The fourth dimension of the assessment model is the cost benefit analysis of preventive sport investment versus downstream welfare spending. This method is a health-economic principle, which has been extensively used to quantify returns to investment by estimating the healthcare utilization, criminal justice system use, social service dependency, and lost productivity caused by sport participation. In the United Kingdom, studies have estimated returns of £4 to £8 per £1 invested in community sport programs aimed at at-risk populations when downstream health, justice and employment benefits are factored into the calculation.

These analyses are also necessary in making the economic argument of sport as a welfare tool so as to fund ministries and treasury departments, rather than social policy activists. These four dimensions of integration, access, cohesion, risk reduction, and cost-benefit, can assist welfare policy makers and sport administrators to transcend anecdotal assertions regarding the social value of sport into evidence-based programming and accountability. Cross-national comparative analysis and finding policy best practices would also be facilitated through standardized indicators, which are shared through national sport systems, and this would contribute to the accumulation of generalizable evidence on the effectiveness of sport in terms of welfare.

7. POLICY IMPLICATIONS

The synthesis of theory and empirical findings in this chapter lead to the development of a set of substantive policy implications to governments wishing to utilize sport as a policy tool of the welfare state. All these recommendations are structured around five thematic priorities.

7.1 Integrating Sport into National Social Policy Frameworks

The most basic policy suggestion is the clear integration of sport into national social policy frameworks which places it as a welfare tool as opposed to an optional cultural facility. It demands that national sport policies formulate particular social policy goals: to reduce youth offending, to enhance better mental health outcomes, to enhance social cohesion, to empower women, to find targets which are identified with other welfare performance indicators. Other nations like the United Kingdom and Australia have been heading this way with structure to bridge sport and physical activity with health, education and social inclusion objectives, but the approach is still incomplete and sport ministries often do not have the intersectoral mandate to enforce wholesome policy alignment.

7.2 Prioritizing Grassroots and Community Sport

Priorities in investment should be shifted off elite performance sport to community and grassroots sport infrastructure. Whereas elite sport provides cultural visibility and benefits of national identity, it is community sport (recreational leagues, school sport programs, local sport clubs and inclusive physical activity programs) that provides the welfare outcomes that have been described in this chapter. Community sport programs that focus on the disadvantaged populations have a social payoff that is far greater than the investment in elite sport. Fair distribution of facilities, special subsidies to low-income participants and community sport development grants are fundamental tools of achieving welfare potential of the grassroots sport.

7.3 Intersectoral Collaboration

The effectiveness of sport social policy requires an intersectoral governance environment to link sport to health, education, labor market as well as social welfare systems. The sport policies of single ministries that have no coordinated relationship with the wider welfare governance rarely make any significant social contributions. Active intersectoral frameworks comprise school sport collaborations connecting physical education with social inclusion objectives; sport-based diversion initiatives that are co-developed by sport, criminal justice and social work agencies; sport-health integration initiatives that incorporate physical activity into the mental health and primary care pathways; and sport-employment initiatives that connect community sport organizations to labor market support services. The effective intersectoral governance requires the creation of cross departmental sport and welfare task forces, with administrative authority as well as specific budgetary allocation.

7.4 Evidence-Based Monitoring and Evaluation

The assessment model proposed in the Section 6 gives a basis to the systematic evidence-based practice of sport social policy. Governments must make compulsory all publicly funded sport programs with welfare aims to gather standardized data on access, cohesion, and risk reduction outcomes and to provide them to rigorous impact assessments with suitable research designs. Similar monitoring systems of national sport policy, such as those designed in the Netherlands and Australia, as well as England, offer an infrastructure to aggregate evidence to support adaptive management. Evaluation system design should be accompanied with investment in evaluation capacity (aspects such as sport practitioner training in basic monitoring and data collection).

7.5 Targeting Disadvantaged Communities

Lastly, sport social policy should embrace models of needs-based allocation that should guide resource allocation to communities and population with highest welfare deficit as well as those with highest sport-based social returns. This entails effective social deprivation mapping, community needs appraisals, participatory program development processes that actually involve target communities in the process of determining sport interventions. Programming that is adapted to the culture, female-only sports, access to facilities by people with disabilities, outreach by multiple languages, transport subsidies are effective tools in lowering the barriers to access that keep the welfare benefits of sport inaccessible to the most marginalized segments of the population. Universal provision would have to accompany targeting in order to prevent stigmatization of only residual sport programs.

Table 8. Policy Recommendations for Integrating Sport into Welfare Governance

Policy Priority	Strategic Action	Expected Welfare Outcome
National Integration	Embed sport in welfare frameworks	Institutional legitimacy
Grassroots Investment	Shift funding to community sport	Greater equity impact
Intersectoral Governance	Cross-ministerial task forces	Policy coherence
Evidence-Based Evaluation	Mandatory monitoring systems	Accountability
Targeted Inclusion	Needs-based allocation	Reduced structural inequality

8. CONCLUSION

This chapter has believed that sport is no longer to be seen simply as a type of leisure or a means of enhancing physical health, but rather as a policy instrument of social policy in modern welfare states. The chapter has combined the welfare state theory, social capital theory and preventive social policy frameworks to show that sport has both theoretical viability and practical possibilities as a quantifiable welfare mechanism. Sport can make positive contributions in building social cohesion and mitigating structural social risks provided it is well-designed and managed. It was revealed that sport exists on several levels of social life. On an individual level, being involved in organized sport leads to identity, belonging, self-efficacy, and psychological strength. These advantages are especially important with regards to marginalized groups of people such as disadvantaged young people, women, and economically disadvantaged people. At community level, sport serves as collective social space which creates networks, trust, reciprocity and intergroup understanding. By means of systematic opportunities at communication and inclusive program construction, sport may create bridging social capital and diminish prejudice along ethnic, class, and gender lines. Inclusive sport policies at the societal level can enhance national unity and civic engagement, especially where access is fairly spread out and enablers to participation are reduced in an organized manner. Another of the aspects noted in the chapter was the preventive nature of sport in the tackling of modern social risks. The purpose-oriented and structured sport programs have reported positive results in terms of reducing youth delinquency, preventing school dropout, empowering women, and improving employability skills. But the facts are always that sport does not always have these results. Sport-based interventions require purposeful program planning, qualified facilitation, positive institutional settings, and inability to achieve the interventions with wider welfare goals. Sport should then not be looked at as a separated kind of activity, but as a portion of a combined social investment approach. One of the most important contributions of this chapter is the suggested multidimensional evaluation framework. The framework provides practical assessments of the welfare impact of sport to policymakers by structuring it into four interrelated areas namely access, social cohesion, social risk reduction, and cost-benefit analysis. The strategy takes the debate past the rhetorical statements about whether sport has social value and into evidence based accountability. Valid data gathering, longitudinal studies and economic analysis are necessary to prove that preventive sporting investments could have quantifiable social and financial benefits. The implications of the policy are evident. The governments are expected to formally incorporate sport in the national social policy frameworks and make sure that the social aims are incorporated in the sport strategies. The priorities of investors must be revolutionized towards grassroots and community sport instead of making major emphasis on elite performance. Sport, health, education, labor and social welfare ministries need intersectoral cooperation in order to have maximum effect. Moreover, systematic monitoring and evaluation systems should be accompanied with the public funding. Lastly, the sport policy should ride on a needs-based allocation model which should focus on the disadvantaged communities but still be universal to avoid stigmatization. With the age of demographic transition, social fragmentation, economic insecurity, and escalating mental health problems, the welfare states are putting a strong emphasis on preventive approaches that are both cost-efficient and effective. One of such strategies is sport. It is internalized in culture, is very accessible and can result in both individual and collective gains. Placed in inclusive governance frameworks and with stringent assessment in place, sport can make the societies more balanced, stronger and integrated. Finally, the acceptance of sport as a welfare state governance extends the scope of social policy. It challenges policymakers to start perceiving community sport as a desirable and quantifiable tool of social investment, rather than an optional cultural activity. The task still at hand is not to demonstrate the social worth of sport, but to make sure that this worth is achieved in a systematic way, equitably and in a demonstrable way.

REFERENCES

Allport, G. W. (1954). *The nature of prejudice*. Addison-Wesley.

Anderson, B. (1983). *Imagined communities: Reflections on the origin and spread of nationalism*. Verso.

Beck, U. (1992). *Risk society: Towards a new modernity*. SAGE Publications.

Beierlein, C., Werner, C. S., Brähler, E., & Zick, A. (2023). An integrated approach to the conceptualisation and measurement of social cohesion. *Social Indicators Research, 167*(1–3), 147–172. DOI: 10.1007/s11205-023-03110-z

Bourdieu, P. (1986). The forms of capital. In Richardson, J. G. (Ed.), *Handbook of theory and research for the sociology of education* (pp. 241–258). Greenwood Press.

Coalter, F. (2007). *A wider social role for sport: Who's keeping the score?* Routledge. DOI: 10.4324/9780203014615

Coalter, F. (2015). Sport-for-change: Some thoughts from a sceptic. *Social Inclusion (Lisboa), 3*(3), 19–23. DOI: 10.17645/si.v3i3.222

Coleman, J. S. (1988). Social capital in the creation of human capital. *AJS; American Journal of Sociology, 94*(Supplement), S95–S120. DOI: 10.1086/228943

Esping-Andersen, G. (1990). *The three worlds of welfare capitalism*. Polity Press.

Esping-Andersen, G., Gallie, D., Hemerijck, A., & Myles, J. (2002). *Why we need a new welfare state*. Oxford University Press., DOI: 10.1093/0199256438.001.0001

Evans, M. D., & Knepper, H. J. (2023). Women's sports and public administration: Intertwined paths to social equity. *Administrative Theory & Praxis, 46*(2), 107–124. DOI: 10.1080/10841806.2023.2282920

Fonseca, X., Lukosch, S., & Brazier, F. (2019). Social cohesion revisited: A new definition and how to characterize it. *Innovation (Abingdon), 32*(2), 231–253. DOI: 10.1080/13511610.2018.1497480

Giddens, A. (1998). *The third way: The renewal of social democracy*. Polity Press.

Harrison, D.. (2024). Using sport and physical activity interventions to develop life skills and reduce delinquency in youth: A systematic review. *International Review of Sport and Exercise Psychology*. Advance online publication. DOI: 10.1080/1750984X.2024.2349994

Hermens, N., Super, S., Verkooijen, K. T., & Koelen, M. A. (2017). A systematic review of life skill development through sports programs serving socially vulnerable youth. *Research Quarterly for Exercise and Sport*, *88*(4), 408–424. DOI: 10.1080/02701367.2017.1355527 PMID: 28796575

Hirschi, T. (1969). *Causes of delinquency*. University of California Press.

Houlihan, B., & White, A. (2002). *The politics of sports development: Development of sport or development through sport?* Routledge.

Indelicato, A. (2025). Does gender equality in sports matter? Examining the socio-economic impact on public perceptions. *Frontiers in Sports and Active Living*, *7*, 1537064. DOI: 10.3389/fspor.2025.1537064 PMID: 40093422

Karstensen, J. M., Sandvik, M., & Itkonen, H. (2024). Unlocking the power of sports: An exploration of the nexus between shared place, community competence, and sense of community. International Journal of Sport Policy and Politics. Advance online publication. DOI: 10.1080/19406940.2024.2396836

Mahindru, A., Patil, P., & Agrawal, V. (2023). Role of physical activity on mental health and well-being: A review. *Cureus*, *15*(1), e33475. DOI: 10.7759/cureus.33475 PMID: 36756008

Menhas, R., & Saqib, Z. A.. (2024). Does physical activity influence health behavior, mental health, and psychological resilience under the moderating role of quality of life? *Frontiers in Psychology*, *15*, 1349880. DOI: 10.3389/fpsyg.2024.1349880 PMID: 38529092

Mousa, S. (2020). Building social cohesion between Christians and Muslims through soccer in post-ISIS Iraq. *Science*, *369*(6505), 866–870. DOI: 10.1126/science.abb3153 PMID: 32792403

Moustakas, L. (2022). Sport for social cohesion: Transferring from the pitch to the community? *Social Sciences (Basel, Switzerland)*, *11*(11), 513. DOI: 10.3390/socsci11110513

Moustakas, L. (2024). Sport for social cohesion: A conceptual framework linking common practices and theory. *Sport in Society*, *27*(10), 1549–1567. DOI: 10.1080/17430437.2024.2304231

Moustakas, L., & Robrade, D. (2022). Sport for social cohesion: From scoping review to new research directions. *Sport in Society*. Advance online publication. DOI: 10.1080/17430437.2022.2100304

Oldenburg, R. (1989). *The great good place: Cafes, coffee shops, bookstores, bars, hair salons and other hangouts at the heart of a community*. Paragon House.

Putnam, R. D. (2000). *Bowling alone: The collapse and revival of American community*. Simon & Schuster.

Rawls, J. (1971). *A theory of justice*. Harvard University Press. DOI: 10.4159/9780674042605

Spaaij, R., Magee, J., & Jeanes, R. (2013). Urban youth, worklessness and sport: A comparison of sports-based employability programmes in Rotterdam and Stoke-on-Trent. *Urban Studies (Edinburgh, Scotland)*, *50*(8), 1608–1624. DOI: 10.1177/0042098012465132

Spruit, A., van der Put, C. E., van Vugt, E. S., & Stams, G. J. J. M. (2018). The effect of a sport-based intervention to prevent juvenile delinquency in at-risk adolescents. *Child Abuse & Neglect*, *83*, 84–93. DOI: 10.1016/j.chiabu.2018.09.009

Taylor-Gooby, P. (Ed.). (2004). *New risks, new welfare: The transformation of the European welfare state*. Oxford University Press., DOI: 10.1093/019926726X.001.0001

United Nations. (2015). Transforming our world: The 2030 agenda for sustainable development. United Nations General Assembly Resolution A/RES/70/1.

Vella, S. A., Sutcliffe, J. T., Fernandez, D., Liddelow, C., Aidman, E., Teychenne, M., Smith, J. J., Swann, C., Rosenbaum, S., White, R. L., & Lubans, D. R. (2023). Context matters: A review of reviews examining the effects of contextual factors in physical activity interventions on mental health and wellbeing. *Mental Health and Physical Activity*, *25*, 100520. DOI: 10.1016/j.mhpa.2023.100520

Zhang, T., Liu, H., Lu, Y., & Wang, Q. (2023). The nexus of sports-based development and education of mental health and physical fitness. *International Journal of Environmental Research and Public Health*, *20*(4), 3737. DOI: 10.3390/ijerph20043737 PMID: 36834432

Chapter 14

Sport Social Justice and Welfare Regimes in the Promotion of Equitable Public Policy

Sohom Saha
http://orcid.org/0009-0006-9438-1554
Lakshmibai National Institute of Physical Education, India

Mahendra Kumar Singh
http://orcid.org/0000-0001-9989-9420
Lakshmibai National Institute of Physical Education, India

ABSTRACT

Sport is no longer regarded as means of leisure or entertainment. Today it is seen as a significant aspect of the state policy which can enhance health, decrease disparities, and facilitate social inclusion. There is, however, no equal access to sport. Barriers to participation are experienced by people in low-income families, rural regions, women, ethnic minorities, and individuals with disabilities. The chapter outlines the different welfare systems, namely, liberal, corporatist and social democratic, that determine policies on sport and impact the beneficiaries. It bases its argument on the notions of social justice and the capability approach by asserting that sport ought to be a public good, such as health and education. The chapter suggests policy measures to achieve equitable access and minimize inequalities and to utilize sport as the means to foster health and inclusion as well as equal opportunities among all citizens.

DOI: 10.4018/979-8-2600-3174-2.ch014

1. INTRODUCTION

The relationship between sport and the public policy has significantly changed within the last forty years. What was traditionally viewed as, at best, leisure time or an elite activity has been increasingly re-conceptualised as the field of strategic policy interest, with consequences of civic engagement, social cohesion, distributive and public health implications. The governments of various political traditions have invested in sport infrastructures, school physical education programmes and community sport initiatives as they believe that mass participation in sport produces quantifiable social goods.

The World Health Organization (2020) has characterized physical inactivity as being among the most prevalent global risks of non-communicable diseases which adds additional emergency to policy frameworks within which sport and physical activity is a preventive health intervention. However, sport and social justice are not always related in a straightforward manner. The field of sport continues to be very deeply stratified in terms of socioeconomic status, geography, gender, ethnicity, and disability. Studies by Richard et al. (2023) have shown that there were continued socioeconomic inequalities in mainstream sport participation among the European populations, where people in lower-income brackets were always underrepresented in organised sport. In the same vein, Eime et al. (2013) discovered that there were high correlations between socioeconomic disadvantage and low engagement in community sport in Australia. These trends point to the fact that sport, when allowed to the play of markets, is more likely to reproduce, than to threaten the status quo of inequalities. The way states react to these inequalities is largely informed by the welfare architecture that exists therein.

The typology of welfare regimes that is known as liberal, corporatist, and social democratic by Esping-Andersen (1990) has embodied a robust concept among scholars to provide answers on cross-national differences in social policy provision. When applied to sport, this typology sheds light on why in some countries being able to access sport is regarded as a virtual universal social right and in others sport participation is largely left to the market and the individual. It is important to realize that without knowledge of these institutional differences, any systematic attempt to utilize sport as a tool of just welfare governance would be futile. There are three contributions made in this chapter. First, it constructs a theoretically based explanation of sport as a welfare good that combines the theory of welfare regime as well as philosophy of social justice, specifically, capability approach to social justice set forth by Amartya Sen and Martha Nussbaum. Second, it engages in a comparative study of how various welfare regimes are organizing the policy of sport and derive dissimilar equity results. Third, it develops an integrated policy model that places sport in a justice-based framework of welfare governance, suggests criteria of evaluation that go beyond the rates of participation to include distributional equity, health impacts, and social cohesion.

The next step in the chapter is as follows. Section 2 introduces the conceptual framework, which combines the welfare regime theory with the social justice theories. Section 3 concentrates on the issue of sport as a tool of social justice in various interrelated avenues. Section 4 examines the varying ways welfare regimes organize the sport policy and have varying equity implications. Section 5 touches on structural inequalities that have remained constant regarding sport participation. Section 6 formulates a combined policy framework and governance model. The thought-provoking normative and practical inferences of integrating sport into fair communal policy are put into consideration in section 7.

2. CONCEPTUAL FRAMEWORK: WELFARE REGIMES, SOCIAL JUSTICE, AND SPORT

2.1 Welfare Regime Theory

The theoretical base of the chapter is based mainly on the comparative understanding of the regimes of the welfare states that Esping-Andersen (1990) puts forward in The Three Worlds of Welfare Capitalism. Esping-Andersen restricted the linear explanations of the development of welfare states by focusing on the diverse differences in the quantity of social expenditure among advanced capitalist democracies but on the qualitative nature of their institutional organization- the manner in which they allocate allocations of responsibilities between the state, the market, and the civil society and the decomposition of a given character of social stratification they generate. The three ideal-typical regimes that Esping-Andersen had identified have different implications to the design of social policy.

The liberal regimes such as the United States, Canada and Australia focus on means-tested welfare benefits, modest universalism and market-driven service delivery. The state intervention is residual as it only intervenes in cases where the market fails, and social rights are not guaranteed without work effort and contributory history. Segmented into corporatist or conservative, as typified by Germany, France and Austria, social provision is based on occupational hierarchy and family and the employer association, trade union and, in most, the Church all play strong roles. The Nordic countries are linked to the so-called universalist or social democratic regimes that focus on equal citizenship, the universal access to high-quality state-provided services, and the decommodification of labour, i.e. citizens being able to sustain decent standard of living regardless of having to engage in the market (Esping-Andersen, 1990). Later researchers have developed and criticized this typology.

As Ferrera (1996) found, there existed a unique Southern European welfare model with primitive universalism and high levels of familialism. As it was observed by Ferragina and Seeleib-Kaiser (2011), although regime typology is analytically strong, it is not to be considered as a fixed categorization but rather as a heuristic that reflects the major institutional tendencies in the face of diversity. Gumus (2020) conducted the literature review of the welfare regime research over 30 years and found the constant usefulness of the framework offered by Esping-Andersen, however, the author should not ignore the arguments concerning the gender-blindness of the framework, the lack of attention to healthcare, and its inapplicability to other regions of the world. The following critiques apply to the current analysis: similarly to other fields (e.g. healthcare and childcare), sport policy comprises both gendered and disability aspects that need intersectionally sensitive frameworks.

The welfare regime theory is used in this chapter as a comparative prism through which to comprehend why governments vary in their definition of sport as a social good or a commodity and by which they can use sport as a tool of social justice.

2.2 Social Justice Theories: Distributive and Capability-Based Approaches

The chapter has a normative basis which relies on two sets of social justice theory. The tradition of distributive justice is the first, and best developed by John Rawls in A Theory of Justice (1971). According to Rawls, social and economic disparities can only be just in a sense that they produce the maximum gain to the least-privileged members of society- the difference principle. This would translate into sport policy which would end up prioritizing the allocation of sport resources, facilities, and programmes based on the benefit of the most deprived groups rather than on aggregate participation figures. The policy regime that drastically enhances sport participation without prioritizing disadvantaged communities may be effective but not just according to the Rawlsian principles.

The second approach is the capability approach that was created by Amartya Sen (1999) and Martha Nussbaum (2011). Sen claimed that justice was not to be evaluated as to the distribution of primary goods but as to what people can really do and be, their actual freedoms to live lives that they have reasons to appreciate. Nussbaum (2003) developed this point of view, presenting a list of most important human capabilities, i.e., bodily health, bodily integrity, affiliation and play, which are the minimal requirements of a dignified life. The capability approach re-places the frame of evaluation between resources contributions and the outcome freedoms, which is why it will be especially effective when analyzing sport policy as an sphere that intersects physical health and social connection with civic participation. The capability approach has been gaining more and more ground in public health as Till et al. (2021) showed in a systematic review of measurement tools, where combining individual, social, and structural factors and returning attention to the actual options open to people is critical. Bringing it to sport, a capability framework does not just enquire about the existence of facilities, but focused on the ability of individuals to utilize them in fact, and particularly disadvantaged individuals, due to time, cost, transportation, cultural norms and disability. Combining the welfare regime theory and the capability approach makes welfare regimes a potent instrument of sport policy: welfare regimes influence the institutional context where capabilities are open up or closed down, and sport policy is either promoting or weakening the capabilities in relation to its design and funding.

2.3 Sport as a Public Good

The major theoretical shift in this chapter is the redefinition of sport as a type of personal leisure as a public good. The theory of public goods in economics is used to differentiate between non-excludible and non-rival goods in terms of consumption, implying that their provision in the market will be underprovided. The sport infrastructure, such as parks, public pools, recreation grounds, school gymnasiums, and others, have numerous traits of the form of the public or quasi-public good. When sport is regarded as a public good which is to be enshrined in the rights of citizens, the law of the sport must be a matter of welfare policy. When it is privatized as a commodity, the access is decided by the purchasing power and the equity consequences are expected to be retrogressive.

In his argument, Coalter (2007) posited that the social advantages of sport namely, health promotion, community building and youth development can be realized not by the dynamic market forces, but by policy intervention. This finding is in line with welfare regime theory: whether the potential social goods of sport can be realised or not, this depends on the institutional context. It is also related to an expanding range of literature assessed by Hasson et al. (2024) that sport and physical activity, when designed in an equitable manner, can be effective interdisciplinary interventions to tackle health inequities and help bear greater social transformation.

3. SPORT AS AN INSTRUMENT OF SOCIAL JUSTICE

3.1 Equality of Opportunity and Access

The equalisation of the opportunity is the first tool by which sport can promote social justice. In cases where sport facilities, physical education programmes, and community sport organisations are financed, apportioned and managed in such a distribution that cuts across all socioeconomic levels and geographical locations, sport is a shared ground that overcuts instead of upholds class differences. In an attempt to show that sport and physical activity participation is socially stratified, Collins (2004) revealed that the stratification is in a manner that reflects broader trends of socioeconomic exclusion. The deprived communities are usually situated in low sport infrastructure, lesser qualified coaching, greater costs of participation in proportion to disposable income, and higher time constraints among working parents- all of which act to create systematic disparities of access.

The findings of the Mudd et al. (2024) investigation in the Netherlands showed that educational disparities in sport participation are mediated by both structurally based resources such as economic, social and cultural capital and individual agency, which agrees with the Bourdieu conceptualisation of capability and with the Bourdieu (1986) theory of capital. This observation highlights the need to have policies that can correct structural bottlenecks as opposed to individual motivation or awareness promotion. Similar data were reported by Richard et al. (2023), who found that free access policy in Geneva minimized financial barriers to sport participation but was constrained by socio-cultural factors such as self-segregation, implying that access policy needs to be integrated into a wider strategy of cultural and social aspects of exclusion.

The implication on the sport governance is evident: in order to equalise opportunity not only should facilities be built but they should be geographically distributed in accordance with need, subsidies and waiver of fees should be offered to those who need them most and culturally appropriate programmes should be created in collaboration with those who are underserved. In a discourse analysis on Norwegian policy on sport over 20 years, Dowling (2024) has identified that the social democratic vision of sport as a means of universal access has been increasingly strained by neoliberalism requirements of accountability and efficiency, pitting the objectives of universal access to sport with the logics of performance-based funding.

3.2 Health Equity

The second channel is that of health equity. There is a broad literature on the preventative health advantages of exercise. Physical inactivity has been linked to high risks of cardiovascular disease, type 2 diabetes, obesity, and depression and its health burden is unequally distributed across lower socioeconomic groups (World Health Organization, 2020). Ball et al. (2015) conducted an evidence review of what can be done to tackle social determinants of inequities in physical activity and discovered promising interventions include community-wide interventions, neighbourhood design that is amenable to active living, school programmes, and group-specific interventions targeting the disadvantaged populations. These results directly address the welfare policy argument, investment in sport infrastructure that is accessible and community-based acts as a preventive health spending that may decrease downstream expenditures of healthcare systems and decrease health inequalities.

In an editorial titled Physical activity, health equity, and health-related outcomes, Barengo and Alkhatib (2022) presented the role of socioeconomic status, race, ethnicity, gender, and geographic location in influencing the availability of healthy environments and physical activity opportunities. By viewing sport as a health equity intervention, the fiscal argument can be redefined: rather than discussing the possibility of justifying investment in sport as discretionary spending, it becomes a matter of whether investment in sport is part and parcel of an intervention strategy of health promotion with calculable outcomes in the form of lower morbidity and mortality among disadvantaged groups.

Heinemann (2005) observed that European welfare states vary widely in the extent to which they incorporate sport in health policy, Nordic countries being most developed in the promotion of physical activity as a population health instrument incorporated into welfare governance. This finding confirms the regime-based approach formulated in Section 4: the institutional position of sport as a part of the welfare state apparatus, or as something external, defines its potential to act as a health equity tool.

3.3 Social Cohesion and Civic Participation

The contribution of sport to social cohesion works in several ways. Involvement in organised sport fosters interpersonal trust, common norms and collective identity the social capital ingredients as discussed by Putnam (2000). Putting emphasis on social well-being, Coalter (2007) claimed that sport participation created social capital, social cohesion as well as social participation. Such effects have been reported among various groups of people, such as immigrant populations (Blachnicka-Ciacek and Trabka, 2024) and disadvantaged youth (Anderson-Butcher et al., 2021).

Sport as a civic aspect is also important. The sports clubs, especially those in European context, have long been the centre of the life of the community, voluntary association and civic involvement. The Gaelic Athletic Association (GAA) in Ireland is one example where sporting organisation can serve as both athletic organisation, cultural organisation, and community development organisation. Morgan and colleagues (2025) were able to observe that where sport is integrated into the everyday life of a region and can be used outside of the competitive sports, it provides an opportunity to have an inclusive development of communities and civic participation. The ability of sport to create social cohesion is, however, dependent on the structure of sport programmes and the motives of governing bodies.

In a critical review of sport based social inclusion programmes in England and Wales, Coalter (2010) established that although these programmes were successful in different measures in encouraging social cohesion and pathway to work outcomes, they had a naturally constrained effect on the structural processes through which exclusion was generated where structural causes were not addressed.

3.4 Empowerment of Marginalised Groups

Sport may act as a venue of empowerment to groups that suffer structural disadvantage in the broader society such as women, youth at risk, persons with disabilities, refugees and ethnic minority. In their review of social work and youth sport, Anderson-Butcher et al. (2021) suggested that involvement in sport among young people living in socially vulnerable conditions also forecasts an array of positive outcomes, such as improved mental health, lessened explanation behaviours, and social integration. These impacts are magnified as the sport programmes are strategically structured in creating social-emotional skills, leadership abilities and civic participation than concentrating on simple sport performance.

Sport participation offers certain opportunities and certain challenges to persons with disabilities. Reducing the definition of social inclusion in disability sport, Klenk et al. (2019) established that personal motivation, physical and social competence, coach attitudes, and accessibility of facilities can be considered determinants of participation, and insufficient funding is a systemic barrier.

Sandford et al. (2022) have reviewed the literature on disability and inclusive education in sport settings, and highlight that institutional cultures that feature ableism in sport organisations may serve to compromise official pledges of inclusion even where policy frameworks are formally inclusive. The continued access of women to sport has been limited by long held gender norms, infrastructure inadequacy, imbalanced media coverage and structural leadership barriers. Gender equality in sport research (Ince-Yenilmez et al., 2025) indicates that structural and socio-cultural influences are closely interconnected and that policy should consider both: more funding on gender-equitable programmes, economic motivators like scholarships and lowered training costs, investment in infrastructure of women sport, and governance reforms so that women have a more prominent role in sport leadership.

4. WELFARE REGIMES AND SPORT POLICY: A COMPARATIVE ANALYSIS

4.1 Liberal Welfare Regimes

The sport policy in liberal welfare regimes is usually defined by a residual role of the state, extreme dependence on the operations of the market and personal philanthropy, and a policy discourse that more or less stresses the responsibility and choice of individuals. This has resulted in a mix of private club outlay fees, commercial sponsorship and charitable-based community programmes and focused government grants to elite sport and particular social interventions in countries like the United States, Australia and, to some extent, the United Kingdom (especially after the neoliberal era of welfare reforms since the 1980s).

The equity implications of the underlying of this model are documented. In their study of youth sport access in the United States, Whitaker et al. (2021) determined that children in low-income households were less likely to participate in as many days per week of physical activities, fewer types of sports sampled and more likely to have never played sports, with financial cost, transportation, and not wanting to be on a team being the most frequently reported barriers. The students for the high-income high schoolers were three times more likely to have ever been involved in sports than their low-income counterparts.

Liberal regimes in terms of funding elite sport also add to inequity. When state money is redirected towards elite sport development and flagship sport events to the disadvantage of community sport, the distributive effects are retrogressive: spectators can get subsidies on elite performance, and the lack of participation in grassroots sport continues. Liang et al. (2024) evidence review on the question of legacies of major sporting events on disadvantaged communities found that positive community legacies are not at all natural, but rather require careful policy decisions regarding the manner in which event-related investment is directed.

4.2 Corporatist Welfare Regimes

Corporatist welfare regimes usually have sport organised by federations, clubs and voluntary associations that receive partial state subsidy and institutional recognition. A good example is the German sport system which is organized in an expansive network of Vereine (voluntary clubs) under a single umbrella of the Deutscher Olympischer Sportbund, which is publicly subsidized at federal, Lander and municipal tiers. The model has enjoyed significant levels of participation and substantial institutional stability but at the same time, has tendencies of recreating the preferences and priorities of the member groupings that are already present given that they may not be a complete representation of the national population.

According to Ferragina and Seeleib-Kaiser (2011), corporatist welfare institutions are capable of creating internal rigidity that would disadvantage outsiders-those who are not already part of occupational or associational network. In sport, this implies that immigrant communities, low-income communities who cannot pay the membership fee and those who do not have established social networks may not be well served by club-based systems. Corporatist regimes have tried to overcome these shortcomings with policy innovations in the form of integration programmes, diversity requirements, and special funding to sport by disadvantaged populations with mixed outcomes.

4.3 Social Democratic Welfare Regimes

Social democratic welfare regimes are the most conducive institutional environment to use sport as a tool of social justice. The universalist morality of Nordic welfare states (with its focus on equal citizenship rights and decommodification of social goods) is converted into a policy agenda, which views access to sport and physical activity as part of social contract. Sport infrastructure is comparatively well-invested by the state, school physical education is richly endowed, and sport programmes in the community are usually subsidised to lower the barriers of participating financially. The Norwegian example is educative.

Dowling (2024) reported the influence of a social democratic vision of welfare that has been a dominant factor in the formulation of sport policy in Norway in relation to sport as part of welfare political goals such as health, social inclusion, and integration of immigrant groups. Government White Papers on sport are clearly connecting any government investment in sport to even wider welfare targets and the National Olympic Committee and Confederation of Sports (NIF) have official equations to equality and non-discrimination. However, in this favourable institutional environment, Dowling discovered that neoliberal accountability and value for money discourses have gradually infiltrated the sport governance sphere producing pressures that can undermined the aim of universal access.

The results of comparative research on sport policy outcomes in European welfare regimes by Hoekman and Scheerder (2021) affirmed the general findings of previous lower-income welfare regime studies on this topic that a social democratic system tends to lead to the creation of more equitable sport participation patterns, yet the authors observed that the association between the type of welfare regime and equitable sport participation patterns is mediated by certain policy instruments, mechanisms of funding, and arrangements of governance. Universal availability of sport facilities, government subsidisation of club membership by low-income households, and combined strategies between sport and both the health and social welfare units were also found to be especially efficient policy levers.

4.4 Implications of the Comparative Analysis

The comparative welfare regime analysis and sport policy analysis provides a number of substantive conclusions. To begin with, institutional form of welfare governance is one of the main factors that determine whether sport is a social leveller or a social stratifier. Sport systems that dominate the market are consistent in generating inequity in participation that reflects the underlying inequality in socioeconomic status. Second, in the context of welfare regimes that officially adhere to the principles of universality, the decline of state investment and the infiltration of market values into the sport administration may compromise the equity objectives. Third, there is fairness in the institutionalization of sport policy in more comprehensive welfare governance- when sport policy is not a discretionary or ambitious add-on, but an element of the social infrastructure that is required as a matter of whole social engagement.

5. ADDRESSING STRUCTURAL INEQUALITIES IN SPORT PARTICIPATION

5.1 Socioeconomic Barriers

There are numerous dimensions of socioeconomic factors that inhibit sports participation. The most obvious impediment is the direct financial expenses of club membership, equipment, coaching and traveling, however, less obvious indirect expenses such as opportunity costs when a parent has several jobs, expenses of the proper sportswear and footwear and transport costs to reach the facilities may be as cost-prohibitive to low-income families also. According to Jayanthi et al. (2018), young people in less affluent social groups are at higher risks of non-participation and early dropout; as well as injury as a result of specialisation due to financial reasons but not based on developmental rationale. Another structural dimension is the built environment.

In most national settings, the distribution of sport facilities is skewed in a systematic biased way whereby the richer communities are located at the center (Powell et al., 2006). Social groups with high levels of poverty, disinvestment in cities, or remote locations tend to have limited parks, recreational facilities and club facilities. A review of evidence on equity in physical activity promotion policies in European countries by Farrer et al. (2015) revealed that in countries where national policies were devoted to the equity consideration, the policy documents often lacked clarity on the equity goals and strategies of allocating additional funds to disadvantaged groups.

5.2 Geographic Inequalities

Urban rural disparity in sport infrastructure is another important but less discussed aspect of sport inequity. The rural communities generally have a lower capacity of sport facilities, fewer variety of sport provision, fewer club memberships and lacked transport links with regional facilities. Such policy frameworks which allocate sport investment in a population density based systematically undermine the rural populations. Intersectorally, facility deficits are compounded by the lack of public transport in rural areas, which increases the physical inaccessibility of the provision where it exists, as well as to the provision itself. Liquid sport policy demands formulae of investment that place more emphasis on need as opposed to population density.

5.3 Gender and Disability

The issue of gender norms still influences the sport participation in a manner that does not favor women and girls. The socio economic and gender limitations in sport (Ince-Yenilmez et al., 2025) were found through research that found interdependent structural and socio-cultural factors such as pay gaps between elite male and female athletes, unequal media attention, lack of women in sport governing bodies and coaching, and cultural beliefs about women not valuing their involvement in some sports.

These institutional characteristics interplay with the socioeconomic limitations to create compound disadvantage among lower income women. Among the disabled, the obstacles are physical, in the form of facilities that are inaccessible, no adapted equipment, inadequate specialist coaching, and institutional. Ramsden et al. (2023) looked at the sport participation of individuals with disabilities observing that inclusive models exist such as wheelchair basketball but that policy is required to fund adapted sport programmes, facility design, and coach disability inclusion training on a long-term basis. In the absence of these systemic investments even the formal commitments to disability sport inclusion are not operational but only ideal.

5.4 Cultural and Intersectional Dimensions

The ethnic minorities and immigrant groups are especially sensitive to cultural barriers that prevent them in sport participation. The literature on how sport can be used to aid social integration of the disadvantaged populations (reviewed by Ley et al., 2025) determined the existence of an array of determinants such as language barriers, cultural lack of familiarity with dominant forms of sport, sport-related discrimination, and conflicting needs of cultural and religious practices. These populations can be reached through the design of culturally appropriate sport programmes, which is carried out through collaborating with community organisations.

An intersectional approach to sport equity acknowledges that disadvantages add up, such that those with concurrent disadvantages of class, gender, disability, ethnicity and geography are disadvantaged. The qualitatively different and compounded barriers a young disabled woman of an immigrant background in a deprived rural area will encounter is not comparable to any one dimension of disadvantage by itself. Fair sport policy should no longer be built on targeting strategies along a single axis but develop strategies to recognize and focus on the particular forms of disadvantage that limit sport performance to the largest degree.

6. POLICY IMPLICATIONS AND AN INTEGRATED FRAMEWORK FOR EQUITABLE SPORT GOVERNANCE

6.1 Principles of the Framework

The formulated analysis in the foregoing sections leads to a kind of normative principles, which ought to determine the incorporation of sport into equitable welfare governance. These values are based on theoretical models of the welfare regime theory, the capability approach as well as distributive justice, and are informed by the comparative and empirical evidence that is examined in the chapter. The first one is universalism: the facilities and programmes of community sport must be identified as a social right to which access is granted to all citizens and not a privilege subject to the buying power.

This suggests a long-term state investment in community sport infrastructure that is allocated based on its need, and also prioritizing geographically under-served geographical locations and underserved population groups. In markets where market supply is inadequate to guarantee universal services, where it does not seem to do so systematically, the rationale of public investment is both on the equity side and on the efficiency side. The second principle is the principle of capability development: sport policy should be evaluated in terms of whether or not participation actually widens individual capacities not the aggregate participation rates that can conceal distributional inequalities.

A system of sport that has high overall participation and leaves the most disadvantaged even further behind does not pass the test of capability even though it might show success by traditional measures. The third principle is intersectoral integration: sport policy can no longer exist in institutional isolation but must be organizationally connected to health, education, social welfare, urban planning and transport policy.

The evidence has continually demonstrated that the welfare benefits of sport are realised in the fullest when sport programmes are integrated into wider strategies that deal with multiplicity of factors of social disadvantage. The fourth principle is accountability and evidence: sport policy must be accountable and evidence-based just as any other welfare service. This involves expenditure on research infrastructure, longitudinal tracking of participation and health outcomes stratified by socioeconomic status, gender, disability, ethnicity, as well as geography and authentic public reporting of distributional outcomes.

6.2 Policy Instruments

The framework presented here points to a number of specific policy tools with the help of which these principles can be realised. In the context of infrastructure investment, governments must consider need-weighted funding formulae of community sport facilities which would lead to the disproportional distribution of investment to community areas of maximum socioeconomic deprivation, rural remoteness and infrastructure deficit. Physical activity policy reviews have evidence of showing that structural interventions such as facility provision and neighbourhood design are some of the most effective levers of increasing physical activity at the population level provided, they are explicitly geographically and demographically focused (Kokko et al., 2016).

In the area of financial access, direct impact by means of lowering the financial barriers of participation in sports among low-income households should be employed through means-tested subsidies, free club membership schemes, and voucher schemes. The evidence analyzed by Higgerson et al. (2018) of the effectiveness of free access to leisure facilities in the United Kingdom showed that their results positively impact on physical activity, which is especially important to lower socioeconomic groups, but financial subsidies do not ensure that socio-cultural barriers will be eliminated.

In terms of programme design, community sport programmes ought to be established through authentic collaboration with the target communities and they ought to include culturally-compensated forms of sport, flexible-timing to suit working parents, transport, and reach to non-participating communities. The above-mentioned evidence on the sport-based social integration of disadvantaged populations (Ley et al., 2025) allows underlining that the reach and relevance to target populations are as significant as the quality of the programmes.

In the areas of governance and leadership, sport governing bodies on all levels must be obliged to incorporate equity goals in their governance systems, to show advancement with regard to distributional goals, and to promote diversity, as well as women, ethnic minorities, and persons with disabilities, in their leadership. Sotiriadou and De Haan (2019) presented the evidence that gender quotas in the formal reforms of governance potentially can facilitate gender equity in sport leadership, but their impact depends on organisational culture and the level of investment in the principles of equity.

6.3 Evaluation Framework

The proposed integrated model of policy needs to be evaluated through the framework that goes beyond the traditional measures of participation rate. There are three types of outcome indicators suggested. The indicators of distributional equity need to reflect the participation rates by the socioeconomic quintile, gender, disability status, ethnicity, and urban-rural location, which will allow detecting the gaps in participation and monitoring the improvement in the same. It is necessary to keep the levels of physical activity in populations, the prevalence of chronic diseases, and mental health outcomes of the target populations and to evaluate the sport investment aspects in relation to the welfare system objectives in promoting health and preventing disease.

The indicators of social cohesion must involve self-reported trust, sense of belonging, intergroup contact and civic engagement among participants in sport in relation to non-participants as evidence to the role of sport in social capital and community wellbeing. It should be an intersectoral design of evaluation systems, based on administrative data of health, education, and welfare systems and specific sport participation surveys. The depth of evidence required to comprehend the interactions between sport participation patterns and social background and institutional context throughout the life course can be found in longitudinal panel studies such as the Norwegian Inequality in Youth study reviewed by Eriksen et al. (2025). The policy issue in itself should be the investment into this evidence infrastructure: good intentions are not sufficient towards equitable sport governance: there should be the empirical means of checking whether the intentions really lead to equitable performance.

6.4 Institutional Conditions for Reform

Sport governance can be implemented fairly based on institutional conditions which differ based upon the welfare regime contexts. The main institutional problem in liberal welfare regimes is to construct the political coalition and evidence base required to legitimize increasing public investment in community sport as a welfare good, in a dominant policy culture that social provision is viewed as a residual good, and market efficiency as the ultimate measure of policy success. The issue with corporatist regimes is accessing established structures of sport federations to those previously underserved by the organisations, and developing funding systems that can channel resources to those outside of existing organisational structures.

The biggest dilemma is how to protect the universalist sport provision against the neoliberal welfare reform pressures and accountability logics of the fiscal environment, which is most conducive to social democratic regimes. Intersectoral coordination is one of the core issues in any type of regime. Sport-health, education, social welfare and urban planning integration demand institutional architectures to jointly plan, have common data systems and have coordinated fund flows. In the absence of such architectures, the sport policy will continue to be siloed, its possible synergies with other welfare objectives will not be realised, and it will not be held accountable to equity standards.

7. CONCLUSION

This chapter has stated that sport plays an important and undervalued role in the nexus of welfare governance and social justice. Sport has the capacity to facilitate equitable policy in the society, but it is not something inherent in sport as an activity, but is conclusively determined by the institutional structures through which it is organised, funded and governed. Welfare regime theory provides a necessary tool of analysis concerning these institutional settings and their distributional implications. The capability approach gives the normative standard against which the sport policy is supposed to be judged: not aggregate participation but the actual growth of freedoms and social opportunities of people who are the most limited on the basis of their structural disadvantage. Comparative analysis of liberal, corporatist and social democratic welfare regimes shows that sport is best used as a tool of social justice when it is institutionally anchored within a universalist welfare framework that views sport access as a social right, invests in community infrastructure based on need, and one which also holds governance of sport to the distributional equity standard. Where sport is entrusted mainly to market forces or elite sporting interests, it strengthens systematically instead of causing changes in the existing inequalities. Socioeconomic, geographic, gender gender-based, disability-based and cultural structural barriers to equitable sport participation are all real and enduring. They cannot even be resolved by mere aspiration. They demand systematic policy responses: needs-weighted infrastructure investment, financial subsidy programmes, the design of culturally-appropriate programmes, intersectoral coordination of governance, and strict evaluation based on distributional equity indicators. Such are not marginal to welfare governance but core to it at the proper data when sport is well conceptualized as a preventive and promotive welfare instrument. The final statement in the chapter is normative but analytical: just sport policy is not just a recreational dream but an imperative of modern welfare states that do not mock their promises of equal citizenship, distributive fairness, and the broadening of human dysfunctions. Whether sport can play a role in social justice or not is not the question posed by policymakers or scholars, but whether the institutional context and policy commitments that are required to make this contribution a reality will be put in place and maintained. This chapter has attempted to furnish the theoretical frame and comparative data that are required to further that undertaking.

REFERENCES

Anderson-Butcher, D., Iachini, A., & Riley, A. (2021). Social work and youth sport. *Child & Adolescent Social Work Journal, 38*(4), 359–365. DOI: 10.1007/s10560-021-00777-6 PMID: 34075276

Ball, K., Carver, A., Downing, K., Jackson, M., & O'Rourke, K. (2015). Addressing the social determinants of inequities in physical activity and sedentary behaviours. *Health Promotion International, 30*(Suppl 2), ii18–ii19. DOI: 10.1093/heapro/dav022 PMID: 25855784

Barengo, N. C., & Alkhatib, A. (2022). Editorial: Physical activity, health equity and health related outcomes. *Frontiers in Public Health, 10*, 828108. DOI: 10.3389/fpubh.2022.828108 PMID: 35284398

Blachnicka-Ciacek, D., & Trąbka, A. (2024). 'Football was the key': The role of sports in facilitating migrants' belonging and inclusion in Poland. *Leisure Studies, 43*(6), 932–945. DOI: 10.1080/02614367.2022.2088834

Bourdieu, P. (1986). The forms of capital. In Richardson, J. G. (Ed.), *Handbook of theory and research for the sociology of education* (pp. 241–258). Greenwood.

Coalter, F. (2007). *A wider social role for sport: Who's keeping the score?* Routledge. DOI: 10.4324/9780203014615

Coalter, F. (2010). 'Social inclusion' through sports-based interventions? *Critical Social Policy, 30*(3), 440–458. DOI: 10.1177/0261018310385442

Collins, M. (2004). Sport, physical activity and social exclusion. *Journal of Sports Sciences, 22*(8), 727–740. DOI: 10.1080/02640410410001712430 PMID: 15370484

Dowling, F. (2024). Is sport's 'gateway for inclusion' on the latch for ethnic minorities? A discourse analysis of sport policy for inclusion and integration. *International Review for the Sociology of Sport, 59*(2), 239–257. Advance online publication. DOI: 10.1177/10126902231198864

Eime, R. M., Young, J. A., Harvey, J. T., Charity, M. J., & Payne, W. R. (2013). A systematic review of the psychological and social benefits of participation in sport for children and adolescents: Informing development of a conceptual model of health through sport. *The International Journal of Behavioral Nutrition and Physical Activity, 10*(98), 98. Advance online publication. DOI: 10.1186/1479-5868-10-98 PMID: 23945179

Eriksen, I. M., Stefansen, K., & Smette, I. (2025). Sports participation as a reflection of social inclusion in youth: A holistic exploration of sport within young people's lives. *Sport Education and Society*, 1–12. Advance online publication. DOI: 10.1080/13573322.2025.2451354

Esping-Andersen, G. (1990). *The three worlds of welfare capitalism*. Polity Press.

Esping-Andersen, G. (1999). *Social foundations of postindustrial economies*. Oxford University Press. DOI: 10.1093/0198742002.001.0001

Esping-Andersen, G. (2015). Welfare regimes and social stratification. *Journal of European Social Policy*, *25*(1), 124–134. DOI: 10.1177/0958928714556976

Farrer, L., Marinetti, C., Cavaco, Y. K., & Costongs, C. (2015). Advocacy for health equity: A synthesis review. *The Milbank Quarterly*, *93*(2), 392–437. DOI: 10.1111/1468-0009.12112 PMID: 26044634

Ferragina, E., & Seeleib-Kaiser, M. (2011). Welfare regime debate: Past, present, futures? *Policy and Politics*, *39*(4), 583–611. DOI: 10.1332/030557311X603592

Ferrera, M. (1996). The 'southern model' of welfare in social Europe. *Journal of European Social Policy*, *6*(1), 17–37. DOI: 10.1177/095892879600600102

Gumuş, İ. (2020). Esping-Andersen and welfare regime discussions: A theoretical assessment. *Ekonomi Maliye Isletme Dergisi*, *3*(1), 101–117. DOI: 10.46737/emid.753591

Hasson, R. E.. (2024). Harnessing the power of sport and physical activity for social change: An interdisciplinary approach to address health equity. *Kinesiology Review (Champaign, Ill.)*, *14*(1), 23–35. DOI: 10.1123/krj.2023-0048

Heinemann, K. (2005). Sport and the welfare state in Europe. *European Journal of Sport Science*, *5*(4), 181–188. DOI: 10.1080/17461390500344347

Higgerson, J., Halliday, E., Ortiz-Nunez, A., Brown, R., & Barr, B. (2018). Impact of free access to leisure facilities and community outreach on inequalities in physical activity: A quasi-experimental study. *Journal of Epidemiology and Community Health*, *72*(3), 252–258. DOI: 10.1136/jech-2017-209882 PMID: 29330166

Hoekman, R., & Scheerder, J. (2021). Sport policy practice and outcome: Theoretical and empirical approaches. *EJSS European Journal for Sport and Society*, *18*(2), 103–113. DOI: 10.1080/16138171.2021.1926772

Ince-Yenilmez, M.. (2025). Does gender equality in sports matter? Examining the socio-economic impact on public perceptions. *Frontiers in Public Health*. Advance online publication. DOI: 10.3389/fpubh.2025.1489000

Jayanthi, N. A., Holt, D. B.Jr, LaBella, C. R., & Dugas, L. R. (2018). Socioeconomic factors for sports specialization and injury in youth athletes. *Sports Health, 10*(4), 303–310. DOI: 10.1177/1941738118778510 PMID: 29851549

Klenk, C., Albrecht, J., & Nagel, S. (2019). Social participation of people with disabilities in organised community sport: A systematic review. *German Journal of Exercise and Sport Research, 49*, 365–380. DOI: 10.1007/s12662-019-00584-3

Kokko, S., Ng, K., Mehtälä, A., Villberg, J., Aira, T., Jussila, A., & Vasankari, T. (2016). An evaluation of equity and equality in physical activity policies in four European countries. *Health Promotion International, 31*(3), 567–577. DOI: 10.1093/heapro/dav001

Ley, C.. (2025). The use of sport for social integration amongst disadvantaged populations: A systematic review. *Managing Sport and Leisure*. Advance online publication. DOI: 10.1080/14413523.2025.2603799

Ley, C., Karus, F., Wiesbauer, L., Rato Barrio, M., & Spaaij, R. (2021). Health, integration and agency: Sport participation experiences of asylum seekers. *Journal of Refugee Studies, 34*(4), 4140–4160. DOI: 10.1093/jrs/feaa081

Liang, X., Quinton, M., Veldhuijzen van Zanten, J., Duan, Z., Zoob Carter, B., Heyes, A., Lee, M., Alharbi, A., & Chen, S. (2024). Legacies and impacts of major sporting events for communities and individuals from disadvantaged backgrounds: A systematic review. *Equality, Diversity and Inclusion*. Advance online publication. DOI: 10.1108/EDI-02-2024-0058

Morgan, H.. (2025). Sport as a catalyst for social justice and inclusion: A case study of the Gaelic Athletic Association's role in community and youth development. *Youth, 5*(3), 70. DOI: 10.3390/youth5030070

Mudd, A. L., Bal, M., van Lenthe, F. J., & Kamphuis, C. B. M. (2024). Understanding educational inequalities in sports participation through structurally based resources and individual agency: A sequential mediation analysis. *International Journal for Equity in Health, 23*(1), 218. DOI: 10.1186/s12939-024-02303-3 PMID: 39434092

Nussbaum, M. C. (2003). Capabilities as fundamental entitlements: Sen and social justice. *Feminist Economics, 9*(2–3), 33–59. DOI: 10.1080/1354570022000077926

Nussbaum, M. C. (2011). *Creating capabilities: The human development approach*. Harvard University Press. DOI: 10.4159/harvard.9780674061200

Putnam, R. D. (2000). *Bowling alone: The collapse and revival of American community*. Simon & Schuster.

Ramsden, R., Hayman, R., Potrac, P., & Hettinga, F. J. (2023). Sport participation for people with disabilities: Exploring the potential of reverse integration and inclusion through wheelchair basketball. *International Journal of Environmental Research and Public Health*, *20*(3), 2491. DOI: 10.3390/ijerph20032491 PMID: 36767857

Rawls, J. (1971). *A theory of justice*. Harvard University Press. DOI: 10.4159/9780674042605

Richard, V., Piumatti, G., Pullen, N., Lorthe, E., Guessous, I., Cantoreggi, N., & Stringhini, S. (2023). Socioeconomic inequalities in sport participation: Pattern per sport and time trends – a repeated cross-sectional study. *BMC Public Health*, *23*(1), 785. DOI: 10.1186/s12889-023-15650-7 PMID: 37118691

Sandford, R., Beckett, A., & Giulianotti, R. (2022). Sport, disability and (inclusive) education: Critical insights and understandings from the Playdagogy programme. *Sport Education and Society*, *27*(2), 150–166. DOI: 10.1080/13573322.2021.1902299

Sen, A. (1999). *Development as freedom*. Oxford University Press.

Sotiriadou, P., & De Haan, D. (2019). Women and leadership: Advancing gender equity policies in sport leadership through sport governance. *International Journal of Sport Policy*, *11*(3), 365–383. DOI: 10.1080/19406940.2019.1577902

Till, M., Abu-Omar, K., Ferschl, S., Reimers, A. K., & Gelius, P. (2021). Measuring capabilities in health and physical activity promotion: A systematic review. *BMC Public Health*, *21*(1), 353. DOI: 10.1186/s12889-020-10151-3 PMID: 33588799

Whitaker, A. A., Baker, G., Matthews, L. J., McCombs, J. S., & Barrett, M. (2021). Socioeconomic inequities in youth participation in physical activity and sports. *International Journal of Environmental Research and Public Health*, *18*(13), 7124. DOI: 10.3390/ijerph18137124 PMID: 34281061

World Health Organization. (2020). WHO guidelines on physical activity and sedentary behaviour. World Health Organization. https://www.who.int/publications/i/item/9789240015128

Chapter 15

Sports-Centric Welfare: Evaluating the Efficiency and Efficacy of the "Samanta Model" in Indigenous Social Inclusion

Pinaki Nandan Pattnaik
http://orcid.org/0000-0002-6632-6156
School of Leadership, KIIT (Deemed to be) University, India

Bignya Patnaik
http://orcid.org/0000-0003-3941-3323
School of Liberal Studies, KIIT (Deemed to be) University, India

ABSTRACT

This chapter reconceptualizes sport beyond the dominant paradigms of competitive excellence and recreational health by positioning it as a transformative instrument of social development. It engages with an emerging "third paradigm" in which sport facilitates social integration, identity formation, and institutional access, particularly in contexts marked by structural inequality. Building on this perspective, the study introduces the concept of sports-centric welfare, where sport becomes a central mechanism for delivering education, health, and social mobility through an integrated institutional framework anchored in KISS, KIIT, and KIMS. The model addresses multidimensional deprivation through free residential education, healthcare, and structured sports engagement. Using an ethnographic approach and drawing on theories of social inclusion and social capital, the study demonstrates how sport fosters identity reconstruction and social integration. It concludes by assessing the model's effectiveness and its potential for replication in similar socio-cultural contexts.

DOI: 10.4018/979-8-2600-3174-2.ch015

INTRODUCTION

Historically, scholarly engagement with sport has been primarily limited to the two dominant paradigms of the pursuit of competitive excellence (Orlick, 2015) and the promotion of recreational health (Elsborg et al., 2019). The pursuit of competitive excellence emphasizes elite performance, national prestige, and professional achievement, while promotion of recreational health emphasizes physical well-being, lifestyle management, and preventive healthcare (Skille, 2010). Both paradigms present critical aspects of sports and remain significant, but they inadequately capture the broader socio-political potential of sport as a transformative institutional mechanism. In recent times, a growing body of literature has begun to reconceptualize sport as an instrument of development (Shilling & Mellor, 2014), particularly within the Global South, where structural inequalities, social exclusion, and economic marginalization persist across multiple dimensions (Coalter, 2013).

This reconceptualization has given rise to what may be termed a "third paradigm" of sport that positions engagement in sports not merely as the pursuit of competitive excellence or the promotion of recreational health rather as a means of achieving broader developmental objectives (Moran, Matthews & Kirby, 2011). Within this emerging paradigm, sport is conceptualized as a vehicle for social integration (Ekholm, 2019), identity formation (Kleiber & Kirshnit, 2019), and institutional access (Borgers et al., 2018). It operates as a culturally neutral platform capable of transcending entrenched hierarchies of caste, class, ethnicity, and geography. As Miragaia, Ferreira, and Ribeiro (2025) argue, sport-based interventions increasingly intersect with public policy frameworks, thereby enabling governments and institutions to address complex socio-economic challenges through innovative delivery mechanisms.

In this context, the concept of sports-centric welfare is proposed as a critical advancement in development thinking. Unlike conventional welfare models that rely on direct transfers, subsidies, or service provisioning, sports-centric welfare integrates participation into the societal fabric and positions sport as a central organizing principle through which education, health, and social mobility are delivered (Bradbury, Coates, & Humphreys, 2023). This approach is particularly relevant in contexts characterized by what Amartya Sen (2000) describes as "poverty of opportunity," where individuals are systematically excluded from the capabilities necessary to lead meaningful lives.

India presents a compelling case for examining this paradigm, given its vast socio-cultural diversity and persistent inequalities. Among the most marginalized populations are the Scheduled Tribes (STs), who constitute almost 8.6% of the national population and remain disproportionately excluded from mainstream development processes (Tribes IOS, 2023). In states such as Odisha, tribal communities inhabit geographically isolated regions with limited access to quality education, healthcare, and economic opportunities (Bhoi & Acharya, 2024). Their marginalization is not solely economic but deeply embedded in cultural, institutional, and historical processes that restrict their participation in the broader socio-political landscape (Subramanyam & Rao, 2022).

Within this context, the "Samanta Model," pioneered by Prof. Achyuta Samanta, represents a pioneering institutional response to multi-dimensional deprivation. Anchored in the integrated ecosystem of the Kalinga Institute of Social Sciences (KISS), Kalinga Institute of Industrial Technology (KIIT), and Kalinga Institute of Medical Sciences (KIMS), the model seeks to address structural exclusion through a holistic framework that combines residential education, healthcare, and sports development. At its core, the model operationalizes sports as a unifying and empowering force capable of bridging the gap between marginalized tribal communities and mainstream society.

The uniqueness of the Samanta Model lies in its emphasis on access over privilege. By providing tribal children with free education, nutrition, healthcare, and exposure to world-class sports infrastructure, the model dismantles the structural barriers that typically limit participation in both education and sport (Datta, 2022). It creates a level playing field where talent, rather than socio-economic background, becomes the primary determinant of opportunity. In doing so, it challenges conventional assumptions about meritocracy and demonstrates the transformative potential of inclusive institutional design.

Moreover, sport within the Samanta Model serves as more than a physical activity and becomes a medium for identity reconstruction and social belonging. For tribal youth, who often experience alienation when transitioning into urban or mainstream environments, participation in team sports fosters a sense of collective identity and shared purpose (Tripathi, 2026). Further, it also provides a culturally neutral space where differences are subsumed within teamwork and performance. This process not only enhances individual self-esteem but also facilitates integration into broader social networks. The relevance of this model extends beyond its immediate context. As global development discourse increasingly emphasizes sustainability, inclusion, and resilience, there is a growing need for scalable and adaptable frameworks that can address complex social challenges. The Samanta Model offers a potential blueprint for such interventions, particularly in regions characterized by indigenous populations and systemic marginalization (Indiatimes, November 5, 2020)

By grounding the analysis in theoretical perspectives on social inclusion and social capital, and employing an ethnographic methodology to capture lived experiences, the study contributes to both academic discourse and policy practice. It advances the argument that sport, when embedded within a well-designed institutional framework, can serve as a powerful instrument of social transformation (Kihl, 2023). This chapter seeks to critically evaluate the efficiency and efficacy of the Samanta Model within the framework of sports-centric welfare. It aims to answer two central questions: (1) How does the integration of sport within a holistic institutional ecosystem contribute to social inclusion and human development? (2) To what extent can this model be replicated in other socio-cultural contexts?

THEORETICAL AND CONCEPTUAL FRAMEWORK

The evaluation of the Samanta Model requires a theoretically robust and conceptually integrated framework to capture the subjective experience of social inclusion as well as the structural mechanisms through which such inclusion is produced, sustained, and scaled. Sports-centric welfare is not merely an intervention, but a multi-layered socio-institutional process which operates at the levels of identity, community, institution, and policy. Accordingly, this study draws upon four complementary theoretical foundations that include the phenomenology of social inclusion, theory of social capital, stakeholder theory, and diffusion of innovation theory. These perspectives are further synthesized into a unifying conceptual lens referred to as the cumulative identity transformation, which provides a dynamic and longitudinal understanding of how sports-centric welfare generates enduring social change.

Phenomenology of social inclusion

At its core, social inclusion is not merely an objective condition but a lived and felt experience. Phenomenology, rooted in the works of Edmund Husserl and later expanded by Alfred Schutz and Maurice Merleau-Ponty, emphasizes the importance of understanding how individuals perceive, interpret, and internalize their social realities (Dorfman, 2009). Within the context of sport-for-development, Riffi Acharki, Spaaij, and Nieuwelink (2023) argue that inclusion must be conceptualized as an embodied experience of belonging, rather than as a set of externally measurable indicators such as participation rates or access metrics. Building on this perspective, inclusion is understood as something lived and felt through everyday interactions, relationships, and social recognition within sporting spaces. It shifts the analytical focus from quantitative proxies of involvement to the qualitative dimensions of dignity, acceptance, and identity affirmation. Such a framing foregrounds how individuals interpret their own participation (whether they feel valued, heard, and socially connected) thereby emphasizing the affective and relational aspects of inclusion. This approach also exposes the limitations of policy frameworks that equate access with equity, often overlooking subtle forms of exclusion embedded in norms, power relations, and institutional practices. This distinction is particularly significant in the context of marginalized indigenous communities. For Scheduled Tribes in India, exclusion is not solely a function of economic deprivation but also manifests as symbolic marginalization, cultural invisibility, and a persistent sense of "otherness" in mainstream institutions (Chakraborty, 2024). Conventional welfare interventions often address material deficits but fail to engage with these deeper experiential dimensions of exclusion.

The Samanta Model directly engages with this phenomenological dimension by constructing an environment where inclusion is experienced in everyday life. The residential ecosystem of KISS creates a shared social space in which tribal students engage in collective routines—living, learning, eating, and training together. Within this space, sport functions as a universalizing medium of interaction, dissolving markers of difference and enabling participants to engage on equal footing (Edexlive, 2020). Team sports, in particular, play a crucial role in this process. The act of training, competing, and striving toward common goals fosters situational equality, where hierarchical distinctions based on caste, tribe, or socio-economic status are temporarily suspended. Over time, these repeated interactions contribute to the internalization of a new social identity that is anchored in competence, contribution, and collective belonging rather than inherited disadvantage.

Furthermore, phenomenology allows us to understand the temporal dimension of inclusion. Inclusion is not a derived outcome, but an evolving process shaped by cumulative experiences. In the Samanta Model, this process unfolds through multiple stages that include initial entry into the institution, adaptation to the residential environment, participation in sports, and eventual engagement with external competitive platforms. Each stage contributes to the gradual transformation of self-perception and social positioning. Importantly, this framework also highlights the role of affect and emotion in social inclusion. Feelings of pride, recognition, and achievement while representing one's institution or country in sports serve as powerful catalysts for identity reconstruction and reinforce the individual's sense of worth and belonging, thereby deepening the process of inclusion.

Social Capital Theory

While phenomenology explains the experiential dimension of inclusion, it does not fully explore the structural resources and opportunities that such inclusion generates. For this, Pierre Bourdieu's (1986) theory of social capital offers a critical analytical framework. Bourdieu defines social capital as the "aggregate of the actual or potential resources linked to possession of a durable network of institutionalized relationships of mutual acquaintance and recognition." This definition underscores two key elements of networks and resources. Social capital is not merely about who one knows, but about the value embedded within those relationships.

In the context of marginalized communities, the absence of social capital constitutes a major barrier to upward mobility. Tribal populations often remain excluded from networks that provide access to education, employment, and institutional support (Xaxa, 2018). This exclusion is self-reinforcing, as limited access to networks restricts opportunities for building further connections. The Samanta Model can be understood as a systematic mechanism for generating and redistributing social capital. Through its integrated institutional ecosystem, the model facilitates the accumulation of bonding, bridging and linking forms of social capital.

Bonding social capital refers to strong ties within a homogenous group. Within KISS, students from similar tribal backgrounds develop deep interpersonal connections based on shared experiences, cultural practices, and collective aspirations. These bonds foster trust, solidarity, and emotional support, which are essential for navigating the challenges of institutional life. Sports further strengthen bonding capital by creating team-based identities. The shared pursuit of athletic excellence reinforces group cohesion and mutual reliance, contributing to a robust support system.

Bridging social capital connects individuals across diverse social groups. The integration of KISS with KIIT exposes tribal students to peers from urban and more privileged backgrounds. This interaction facilitates the exchange of knowledge, norms, and aspirations, enabling students to navigate multiple social worlds. Participation in national and international sports competitions further expands these networks, providing exposure to global cultures and practices. Such interactions enhance inter-cultural competence, a critical skill for social mobility in an increasingly interconnected world (India Education Diary Bureau, 2025).

Linking social capital refers to connections with institutions and individuals in positions of power. Through partnerships with organizations such as FIFA, FIVB, and FIDE, the Samanta Model provides students with access to elite institutional networks. These connections open pathways to scholarships, professional opportunities, and international recognition. Importantly, linking capital also manifests in the form of institutional legitimacy (Himanshu, 2025). The reputation of KISS and its associated institutions enhance the credibility of its students, thereby facilitating their acceptance in external environments.

Stakeholder Theory

While social capital explains the distribution of resources, it does not fully capture the organizational dynamics that enable such distribution. Stakeholder theory provides a framework for understanding how multiple actors collaborate to create and sustain value. Originally developed by Freeman (1984), stakeholder theory posits that organizations must consider the interests of all stakeholders rather than focusing solely on shareholders to achieve long-term success. In the context of sports-centric welfare, stakeholders include students & their families, educational institutions (KISS, KIIT), healthcare providers (KIMS), government agencies, international sports organizations and local communities.

The Samanta Model is distinguished by its ability to create institutional synergy among these stakeholders. Rather than operating in isolation, KISS, KIIT, and KIMS function as an integrated ecosystem where education, sport, and healthcare are delivered in a coordinated manner. Sport serves as a convergence point for stakeholder interests. For students, it offers opportunity and recognition; for institutions, it enhances reputation; for international organizations, it provides a platform for grassroots development; and for governments, it aligns with policy goals of inclusion and youth development (India Education Diary Bureau, 2023). This alignment facilitates value co-creation, where each stakeholder contributes to and benefits from the system. For instance, international partnerships bring technical expertise and global exposure, while the institution provides a large and motivated talent pool. This reciprocal relationship enhances the overall effectiveness of the model.

Diffusion of Innovation

A key indicator of success is the replicability of the Samanta Model. For this purpose, Rogers' (2004) diffusion of innovation theory provides a valuable framework. According to Rogers, the adoption of an innovation is influenced by five key attributes:

Relative Advantage

The Samanta Model demonstrates clear advantages over conventional welfare approaches by integrating multiple dimensions of development including education, health, and sport into a single framework. Its success in producing international athletes from marginalized backgrounds provides tangible evidence of its effectiveness.

Compatibility

The model aligns with cultural values of community, collective identity, and resilience prevalent in tribal societies. Sport, as a culturally adaptable activity, facilitates this alignment.

Complexity

While the model involves multiple institutional components, its core principles of access, integration, and empowerment are conceptually straightforward. However, replication may require significant organizational capacity.

Trialability

Elements of the model, such as sports-based interventions within educational institutions, can be piloted on a smaller scale. This enhances its adaptability across different contexts.

Observability

The visible success of athletes and the institutional reputation of KISS make the outcomes of the model highly observable, thereby encouraging adoption.

Diffusion is not automatic, rather influenced by contextual factors such as political will, resource availability, and cultural acceptance. Therefore, while the Samanta Model offers a compelling template, its replication requires careful adaptation to local conditions.

Conceptual Integration

Building on the preceding theoretical perspectives, this study proposes the concept of cumulative identity transformation as an integrative framework for understanding sports-centric welfare. The concept, presented in Figure 1 posits that social inclusion is achieved through the progressive accumulation of three interrelated variables.

Figure 1.

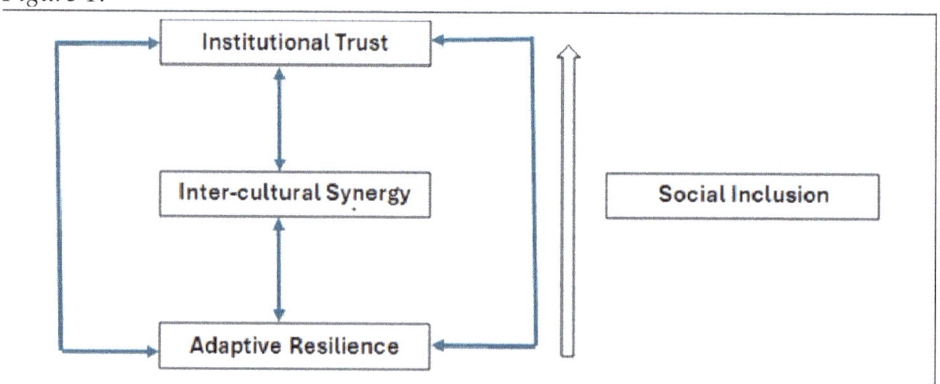

In the figure, adaptive resilience refers to the psychological capacity to cope with adversity and navigate socio-economic challenges by fostering discipline, perseverance, and goal orientation, inter-cultural synergy refers to the ability to engage with diverse social contexts without losing one's cultural identity and institutional trust refers to confidence in institutions as supportive and reliable structures. These variables interact dynamically over time, leading to a transformation in both self-identity and social positioning. Importantly, this transformation is not linear but iterative and is shaped by continuous engagement with the institutional ecosystem.

RESEARCH METHODOLOGY

Research Design and Philosophical Orientation

This study adopts a qualitative ethnographic research design to evaluate the efficiency and efficacy of the Samanta Model within the broader framework of sports-centric welfare. The choice of ethnography is both methodological and epistemological, rooted in the recognition that the core constructs of this study are experiential, relational, and socially constructed. The study is situated within an interpretivist paradigm, which assumes that social reality is co-created through meanings, interactions, and lived experiences. Ethnography, as articulated by Geertz (1973), enables the production of "thick description," allowing the authors to move beyond observations and uncover the layered meanings embedded in everyday practices. In the context of the Samanta Model, this approach is particularly relevant as it facilitates an in-depth understanding of how sports-centric welfare is experienced and internalized by participants over time within a holistic institutional ecosystem.

Research Setting

The research setting for this study is the Kalinga Institute of Social Sciences (KISS), located in Bhubaneswar, Odisha, India, which serves as the foundational institution of the Samanta Model. KISS is one of the largest fully residential educational institutions for indigenous tribal students globally, providing free education, accommodation, nutrition, and specialized sports training. The research setting is further extended to include the institutional linkages with the Kalinga Institute of Industrial Technology (KIIT) and the Kalinga Institute of Medical Sciences (KIMS), which together form an integrated ecosystem delivering education, sports infrastructure, and healthcare services. This interconnected institutional environment enables the examination of how sports-centric welfare operates not as a standalone intervention but as part of a coordinated system of support. The residential nature of

KISS is particularly significant, as it allows for continuous observation of participants across academic, athletic, and social domains, thereby offering a comprehensive understanding of their lived experiences within the model.

Sampling Strategy and Participant Selection

The study employs a purposive sampling strategy to select participants who have direct and meaningful engagement with the Samanta Model. A total of 45 participants are included, comprising 30 current student athletes and 15 alumni who have transitioned into external educational, professional, or athletic pathways. This dual-sample design enables the study to capture both immediate experiences and longer-term outcomes, aligning with the conceptual focus on cumulative identity transformation. Within these categories, maximum variation sampling is employed to ensure diversity in terms of gender, type of sport, geographic origin within tribal regions, and levels of athletic achievement. This approach enhances the analytical depth of the study by capturing a wide range of perspectives and experiences, thereby enabling a more nuanced understanding of how inclusion and mobility are negotiated across different contexts and trajectories.

Data Collection Methods

Data collection is conducted through a combination of participant observation, in-depth semi-structured interviews, and document analysis, allowing for methodological triangulation and enhanced robustness of findings. Participant observation constitutes the core method, with the researcher engaging in immersive observation within the KISS campus over an extended period. This includes attending sports training sessions, academic classes, competitions, and community activities. Such immersion facilitates the observation of informal interactions, embodied practices, and institutional norms that are often inaccessible through other methods. Detailed field notes are maintained to document observations, interactions, and reflections, forming a rich empirical basis for analysis.

In-depth semi-structured interviews are conducted with all 45 participants to elicit detailed personal narratives. The interviews explore participants' life histories, experiences of inclusion and exclusion, the role of sport in shaping identity and aspirations, and their perceptions of institutional support and trust. For alumni, additional emphasis is placed on post-institutional experiences and the extent to which the model has influenced their life trajectories. The semi-structured format allows flexibility, enabling participants to articulate their experiences in their own terms while ensuring coverage of key thematic areas. All interviews are conducted with informed consent, audio-recorded, and transcribed verbatim to ensure accuracy and reliability.

Document analysis is employed as a supplementary method to provide insights into the formal articulation of the Samanta Model. Institutional reports, policy documents, training manuals, and media coverage are analyzed to understand how the model is represented and communicated. This method enables a comparison between official narratives and lived experiences, thereby identifying potential alignments or discrepancies between policy intentions and practical implementation.

Data Analysis and Coding

Data analysis follows a thematic approach that combines both inductive and deductive strategies. The process begins with familiarization, involving repeated reading of interview transcripts and field notes to identify initial patterns and insights. This is followed by open coding, where segments of data are labeled based on emerging concepts. These codes are then organized into broader categories through axial coding and subsequently integrated into core themes through selective coding. The analysis is guided by the study's theoretical framework, particularly the constructs of adaptive resilience, inter-cultural synergy, and institutional trust. At the same time, the inductive component allows for the emergence of context-specific themes that may extend or challenge existing theoretical assumptions. The use of constant comparison ensures that patterns are systematically validated across different data sources and participant groups, thereby enhancing the rigor of the analysis.

To ensure methodological rigor, the study adheres to established qualitative research criteria, including credibility, transferability, dependability, and confirmability (Anney, 2014). Credibility is achieved through prolonged engagement in the field, triangulation of data sources, and member checking, wherein participants are invited to validate the researcher's interpretations. Transferability is supported by providing rich and detailed contextual descriptions that enable readers to assess the applicability of findings to other settings. Dependability is maintained through systematic documentation of research procedures and decision-making processes, while confirmability is ensured through reflexive practices and the maintenance of an audit trail to minimize researcher bias. Together, these measures enhance the trustworthiness and integrity of the research.

Ethical considerations are central to the research design, particularly given the study's focus on indigenous tribal populations. The research adheres to the guidelines of the Indian Anthropological Association (IAA), ensuring informed consent, confidentiality, and cultural sensitivity. Participants are fully informed about the purpose, methods, and potential implications of the study, and their participation is entirely voluntary. Measures are taken to anonymize identities and protect participant privacy. Additionally, the research is conducted with sensitivity to local cultural norms and practices, ensuring respectful and non-intrusive engagement. Particular attention is given to the power dynamics between researchers and participants, with efforts made to avoid exploitation and ensure that participants' voices are represented authentically.

THE SAMANTA MODEL

Conceptual Foundations

The Samanta Model represents a distinctive and innovative approach to social welfare that reconfigures the relationship between education, sport, and human development within marginalized communities. Conceptually, the model may be understood as an integrated, sports-centric welfare ecosystem that leverages institutional synergy to address multi-dimensional deprivation among indigenous populations. Unlike conventional welfare interventions that operate through fragmented service delivery or short-term subsidies, the Samanta Model is anchored in a longitudinal, capability-enhancing framework that seeks to transform both individual trajectories and collective social outcomes. At its core, the model is premised on the recognition that poverty, particularly in tribal contexts, is not merely a condition of economic scarcity but a manifestation of what Amartya Sen (2000, 2006) describes as "capability deprivation" or "poverty of opportunity." This form of deprivation restricts access to education, healthcare, social networks, and platforms for self-expression. The Samanta Model responds to this challenge by constructing an institutional environment that simultaneously expands capabilities across multiple domains, with sport functioning as a central integrative mechanism.

The defining feature of the model is its emphasis on access over privilege. By eliminating financial barriers and providing comprehensive support, including education, nutrition, healthcare, and sports infrastructure, the model creates a level playing field where participation is determined by potential rather than socio-economic background. This reorientation challenges dominant meritocratic narratives that often obscure structural inequalities and instead foregrounds the role of institutions in enabling equitable opportunities.

Institutional Architecture

The operational strength of the Samanta Model lies in its unique institutional architecture, which integrates the Kalinga Institute of Social Sciences (KISS), the Kalinga Institute of Industrial Technology (KIIT), and the Kalinga Institute of Medical

Sciences (KIMS). Together, these institutions form a cohesive and interdependent ecosystem that delivers a holistic model of welfare.

KISS functions as the foundation and entry point of the model. As a fully residential institution catering to over 30,000 tribal students, it provides free education, accommodation, nutrition, and access to sports training. The residential structure is critical, as it removes students from environments characterized by deprivation and situates them within a supportive and resource-rich setting. Within KISS, sport is not treated as an extracurricular activity but as an integral component of daily life, embedded within the broader educational framework (Samanta, 2024). KIIT serves as the aspirational and developmental extension of the model. With its advanced infrastructure, including world-class sports facilities and academic programs, KIIT provides students with exposure to environments of excellence that are typically inaccessible to marginalized populations (Prasad, 2022). This transition from KISS to KIIT represents a critical phase in the model, where students move from foundational support to aspirational engagement. The presence of international-standard stadiums and training facilities ensures that tribal students are not merely participants but are positioned as competitors at the highest levels. KIMS, in turn, operates as the healthcare and support pillar of the ecosystem. Recognizing that athletic performance and overall well-being are intrinsically linked, KIMS provides comprehensive medical care, including sports medicine, physiotherapy, and nutritional guidance. This ensures that students' physical health is systematically managed, reducing the risk of injury and enhancing performance outcomes. Importantly, healthcare services are provided free of cost, reinforcing the model's commitment to equitable access.

The integration of these institutions creates what may be conceptualized as a "composite developmental ecosystem," where education, sport, and health are delivered in a coordinated and mutually reinforcing manner. This synergy reduces institutional fragmentation, enhances efficiency, and ensures that students receive continuous support across different stages of their development (Team Sportstar, 2023).

Sport as a Central Organizing Principle

A defining characteristic of the Samanta Model is the positioning of sport as a central organizing principle rather than a peripheral activity. Sport functions as a unifying medium that connects various components of the institutional ecosystem and facilitates multiple dimensions of development. At the individual level, sport contributes to the development of discipline, resilience, and goal orientation. The structured nature of training, combined with the demands of competition, fosters a strong work ethic and the ability to cope with adversity. These attributes are transferable beyond the sporting context, influencing academic performance and life choices.

At the social level, sport serves as a platform for inclusion and interaction. Team-based activities create opportunities for collaboration, mutual support, and the formation of social bonds. For tribal students who may have experienced isolation or marginalization, participation in sports fosters a sense of belonging and collective identity. The shared pursuit of common goals reduces social distance and enables the construction of inclusive social networks. Finally, at the institutional level, sport enhances visibility and legitimacy. Success in national and international competitions not only elevates the profile of individual athletes but also enhances the reputation of the institution (Edugraph, 2025). This, in turn, attracts partnerships, resources, and recognition, creating a virtuous cycle of development.

Rugby as a Transformation

One of the most compelling illustrations of the Samanta Model's efficacy is its success in promoting rugby among tribal students (World Rugby, 2025). Rugby, a sport with minimal historical presence in rural India, was introduced at KISS as part of a broader strategy to foster teamwork and resilience. The adoption of rugby represents a strategic departure from conventional sports programs that often focus on established disciplines such as cricket or athletics (Nayak, 2025). By introducing a relatively unfamiliar sport, the model created a level playing field where prior exposure and socio-economic advantages were less significant. This allowed tribal students to compete on equal terms and rapidly develop proficiency. The team-based nature of rugby further reinforced the model's emphasis on collective identity and mutual support. Players developed strong interpersonal bonds, which contributed to both athletic performance and social cohesion. Over time, KISS rugby teams achieved significant success at national and international levels, with players representing India in global competitions (Odisha Diary Bureau, 2025). This transformation from marginality to global recognition exemplifies the concept of symbolic capital accumulation, where sporting success translates into social prestige and institutional legitimacy. It also demonstrates the potential of sports-centric welfare to produce outcomes that extend beyond individual achievement, contributing to broader narratives of inclusion and empowerment.

Global Partnerships and Transnational Integration

The model's effectiveness is further enhanced by its engagement with global organizations and transnational networks. Partnerships with institutions such as FIFA, the International Volleyball Federation (FIVB), and the International Chess

Federation (FIDE) provide access to technical expertise, training resources, and international exposure (FIVB, 2025). These collaborations serve multiple functions. First, they ensure that the quality of sports training meets international standards, thereby enhancing the competitiveness of athletes. Second, they provide opportunities for cross-cultural exchange, enabling students to engage with diverse perspectives and practices. Third, they enhance the credibility of the model, positioning it as a globally recognized initiative in sports for development (Odisha Diary Bureau, 2026). From a theoretical perspective, these partnerships contribute to the accumulation of linking social capital, connecting students and institutions to global networks of power and influence. They also facilitate the diffusion of the model, as international organizations act as conduits for knowledge transfer and replication.

Identity Transformation and Social Mobility

The ultimate objective of the Samanta Model is not merely to produce athletes but to facilitate holistic identity transformation and sustainable social mobility. This transformation occurs through the interplay of multiple factors, including access to resources, exposure to new environments, and participation in sports. For many tribal students, entry into KISS represents a transition from a context of deprivation to opportunity. This shift initiates a process of identity reconstruction, where individuals begin to reimagine their capabilities and aspirations. Sport plays a central role in this process by providing tangible experiences of success and recognition. As students' progress through the institutional ecosystem, they accumulate various forms of capital including educational credentials, social networks, and symbolic recognition which enable them to navigate broader social fields. Alumni who transition into professional careers, higher education, or international sports serve as evidence of the model's efficacy in facilitating upward mobility. Importantly, this mobility is not merely individual but has intergenerational implications. Successful graduates often serve as role models within their communities, inspiring others to pursue similar pathways. This creates a multiplier effect, where the benefits of the model extend beyond direct participants to influence broader social dynamics (United Nations India, 2024).

Institutional Ethos of "Art of Giving" and Morality

An often-overlooked dimension of the Samanta Model is its underlying ethos, encapsulated in the philosophy of the "Art of Giving." This philosophy emphasizes altruism, service, and collective well-being, shaping the moral and cultural environment of the institution (Edexlive, 2018; Samanta, 2021). From a sociological perspective, this ethos contributes to the creation of a moral economy, where relationships are governed not solely by market logic but by principles of reciprocity and care. This contrasts with neoliberal welfare models that prioritize efficiency and cost-effectiveness, often at the expense of relational and ethical considerations. The emphasis on giving fosters a culture of mutual support and responsibility, reinforcing the social bonds that underpin the model. It also enhances institutional trust, as participants perceive the system as genuinely committed to their well-being.

Efficiency Through Integration and Cultural Alignment

The efficiency of the Samanta Model can be understood not in conventional economic terms but as the minimization of cultural and institutional friction. By aligning educational, athletic, and healthcare interventions within a single ecosystem, the model reduces redundancies and enhances coordination. Moreover, the model is culturally aligned with the values and practices of tribal communities. The emphasis on collective identity, respect for tradition, and community engagement ensures that interventions are not perceived as externally imposed but are integrated into existing social frameworks. This alignment enhances both participation and effectiveness.

In synthesis, the Samanta Model represents a paradigmatic shift in the conceptualization and practice of welfare. By integrating sport into the core of its institutional design, the model transcends traditional boundaries between education, health, and social development. It demonstrates that sport, when embedded within a supportive and coordinated ecosystem, can serve as a powerful catalyst for inclusion, identity transformation, and social mobility. The model's strength lies not only in its outcomes but in its underlying logical commitment to access, integration, and empowerment. As such, it offers valuable insights for policymakers, practitioners, and scholars seeking to develop innovative approaches to inclusive development in the Global South.

FINDINGS AND DISCUSSION

In this study, results were assessed through the dual lens of efficiency and efficacy, in alignment with the ethnographic and theoretical foundations of the research. Efficiency is conceptualized not merely as cost minimization but as the reduction of cultural and institutional friction, while efficacy is understood as the durability and depth of social transformation, particularly in terms of agency, identity, and mobility. Such framing allowed for a more holistic evaluation that captured the multi-dimensional nature of inclusion and attempted to move beyond economic indicators to include psychosocial, cultural, and institutional outcomes. It also aligned with the theoretical framework developed earlier, particularly the concepts of phenomenological inclusion, social capital accumulation, stakeholder synergy, and cumulative identity transformation (CIT).

The Samanta Model demonstrated a high degree of efficiency by systematically minimizing cultural frictions through its institutional design. Researchers have indicated that cultural friction, which refer to the tensions and dissonances that arise when individuals from marginalized backgrounds engage with mainstream institutions and manifested as language barriers, unfamiliar social norms, discrimination, or a lack of cultural representation as vital in situations where cultural assimilation is attempted. It was observed that the residential nature of KISS created a culturally sensitive environment where tribal identities were recognized and respected, rather than being suppressed. Simultaneously, exposure to broader institutional settings such as KIIT facilitated gradual acclimatization to mainstream norms. From a phenomenological perspective, it was observed that the reduction of cultural friction enhanced the lived experience of belonging. Students were not merely present within the institution but actively experienced inclusion through daily interactions, shared practices, and recognition. The absence of overt hierarchical markers within sporting contexts further reinforced their sense of equality. This alignment suggested that efficiency in the model was achieved through the creation of an affectively inclusive environment, where individuals could engage without the psychological burden of marginalization. Efficiency was also evident in the integration of services within the institutional ecosystem. By co-locating education, sports training, and healthcare, the model reduced transaction costs associated with accessing multiple services. Students did not need to navigate fragmented systems, which was particularly important given the logistical and informational barriers faced by tribal populations. From a stakeholder theory perspective, this integration reflected effective coordination among institutional actors and resulted in streamlined service delivery and enhanced outcomes.

The model demonstrated efficacy through its ability to produce enduring changes in identity, capability, and social positioning. Efficacy in sports-centric welfare was assessed in terms of long-term and sustainable outcomes, rather than short-term outputs. These changes were not limited to individual achievements but extended to broader processes of social mobility and community transformation. Alumni who transitioned into higher education, professional careers, or international sports served as indicators of the model's long-term impact. The concept of cumulative identity transformation provided a framework for understanding how efficacy was produced within the Samanta Model. The model facilitated the iterative accumulation of the three identified variables like adaptive resilience which was developed through rigorous sports training and exposure to challenges, inter-cultural synergy was enabled by interaction with diverse social groups and global networks and institutional trust built through consistent and supportive institutional engagement.

These variables had interacted over time and had led to a transformation in both self-perception and social status. The durability of this transformation was a key indicator of efficacy. From a phenomenological standpoint, efficacy was reflected in the internalization of new identities wherein students began to perceive themselves not as marginalized individuals but as capable actors with agency and potential. This shift had been reinforced through experiences of success, recognition, and belonging. The emotional and affective dimensions of this transformation have also played a critical role in sustaining change over time.

Findings suggest that the model also facilitated the accumulation of multiple forms of capital, consistent with Bourdieu's theoretical framework, by creating an integrated environment where education and sport operated as complementary mechanisms of development. Participants acquired cultural capital in the form of skills, discipline, and knowledge through structured academic engagement and rigorous sports training. Simultaneously, they developed social capital by forming networks within the institutional ecosystem as well as through interactions beyond it, including exposure to diverse peer groups and external stakeholders. Sporting achievements further translated into symbolic capital, as recognition and prestige were conferred upon successful athletes, enhancing both individual and institutional visibility. Over time, these accumulated forms of capital were converted into economic capital, as participants accessed opportunities for higher education, employment, and financial stability. Sporting success, initially manifested as cultural capital, often led to symbolic recognition, which subsequently opened pathways to economic advancement. In addition, the model significantly contributed to the development of bridging and linking social capital. Through sustained engagement with students from varied socio-cultural backgrounds and participation in networks facilitated by international organizations, participants gained access to relationships and opportunities that extended beyond their immediate communities. From a structural perspective, findings indicated that the accumulation and conversion of capital reduced the reproduction of inequality. By systematically expanding access to networks and institutional resources, the model successfully disrupted entrenched cycles of exclusion and enabled participants to navigate broader social fields with greater agency, thereby facilitating upward social mobility.

Further, the model showed effective stakeholder engagement through the alignment of interests among diverse actors including students, institutions, global organizations, and communities who contribute to and benefit from the system. This alignment facilitated value co-creation, where outcomes were not produced by a single entity but emerged from the collective efforts of multiple stakeholders. Institutional trust seemed to play a critical role in mediating the relationship between stakeholders and consistency in delivery of high-quality services enhanced trust. It reduced resistance to institutional interventions and encouraged sustained participation and engagement. From a governance perspective, the model demonstrated the importance of coordinated leadership and institutional integration wherein the presence of a unified vision and centralized coordination ensured that different components of the model function cohesively.

Findings also suggested that the Samanta model exhibited several attributes that facilitated its diffusion, aligning closely with the principles of diffusion of innovation theory. It demonstrated relative advantage through its proven success in fostering social inclusion and producing internationally recognized athletes, while its compatibility with community-oriented values enhanced its acceptability. The visibility of its outcomes further strengthened its observability, making its impact tangible to external stakeholders. However, the model also faced notable constraints in terms of replication and scalability. Its dependence on substantial financial resources, strong institutional integration, and visionary leadership limited its direct applicability in resource-constrained contexts. Consequently, the model was better understood not as a universally replicable template but as a framework for adaptive replication. Its core principles such as institutional integration, equitable access, and sustained long-term engagement could be selectively adapted and implemented in diverse socio-cultural contexts, allowing for contextual flexibility while preserving the model's foundational logic of inclusive development.

The Social Return on Investment (SROI) framework provided a useful tool for evaluating the broader impact of the model by extending beyond traditional cost-benefit analysis to capture social, cultural, and environmental values (Gosselin, Boccanfuso & Laberge, 2020; Yates & Marra, 2017). Findings suggest that the model generated long-term value across multiple domains, including improved educational outcomes, enhanced physical and mental health, and increased opportunities for social mobility. These outcomes contributed not only to individual well-being but also to broader societal development by strengthening human capital and community resilience. Importantly, the SROI approach also captured intangible returns that were central to the model's overall impact. These included enhanced self-esteem among participants, a growing sense of community pride, and the development of institutional trust. Together, these tangible and intangible outcomes demonstrated the model's comprehensive value and its capacity to produce sustained and meaningful social transformation.

Finally, the model generated significant intergenerational and community-level impact through a strong role model effect. The success of individual participants created a powerful demonstration effect, inspiring others within their communities to pursue similar educational and athletic pathways. This, in turn, contributed to the emergence of a broader culture of aspiration and achievement among tribal populations. Over time, these individual successes accumulated to produce measurable community-level transformation, reducing social stigma and enhancing the collective status and visibility of marginalized groups. Furthermore, the model fostered positive feedback loops, wherein successful alumni remained connected to the institution and their communities, contributing through mentorship, advocacy, and support. These recursive dynamics reinforced the sustainability of the model by continuously generating new cycles of participation and success, thereby ensuring that the benefits of the intervention extended beyond individual outcomes to influence broader social structures.

CONCLUSION AND CONTRIBUTION

This chapter set out to evaluate the efficiency and efficacy of the Samanta Model as a distinctive institutional articulation of sports-centric welfare, with a particular emphasis on its capacity to advance indigenous social inclusion in the tribal regions of Odisha. In doing so, it deliberately moved beyond conventional welfare analyses that privilege narrow economic indicators such as income generation, cost efficiency, or output maximization. Instead, it adopted a multidimensional analytical lens that integrates questions of identity, culture, institutional design, and long-term processes of social transformation. Such an approach is particularly relevant in contexts of deep historical marginalization, where the barriers to inclusion are not merely material but also symbolic, psychological, and institutional. The findings of this study demonstrate that the Samanta Model represents far more than an innovative welfare intervention; it embodies a paradigmatic shift in how welfare itself is conceptualized, organized, and delivered in complex socio-cultural settings.

At its core, the model challenges the dominant binary that positions sport either as a domain of elite competition or as a supplementary tool for physical recreation and health promotion. By contrast, the Samanta Model advances a third paradigm in which sport functions as a central organizing principle of welfare. In this formulation, sport is not peripheral but foundational serving as a unifying axis around which education, healthcare, and social development are systematically integrated. This repositioning is not merely rhetorical but is operationalized through the institutional synergy between (KISS), (KIIT), and (KIMS). Together, these institutions form a cohesive ecosystem that transforms otherwise fragmented welfare services into a continuous and structured developmental pathway. This integrated architecture enables the model to address the interdependent dimensions of marginalization including educational exclusion, health vulnerabilities, and socio-cultural isolation in a coordinated and mutually reinforcing manner.

One of the most significant contributions of this study lies in its reconceptualization of efficiency. In classical welfare economics and public administration, efficiency is typically understood in terms of minimizing costs while maximizing outputs. However, such a definition proves inadequate in contexts where the primary constraints are not merely financial but are rooted in cultural dissonance and institutional alienation. In the context of sports-centric welfare, efficiency is more meaningfully understood as the minimization of cultural and institutional friction. The Samanta Model achieves this by creating an environment that is simultaneously culturally sensitive and structurally enabling. Tribal students are situated within a residential ecosystem that affirms their identities, respects their cultural practices, and provides a sense of belonging, while also exposing them to broader institutional norms and opportunities. This dual orientation reduces the psychological barriers that often deter marginalized populations from engaging with mainstream systems. As a result, participation is not only increased but also deepened, leading to higher levels of engagement, retention, and performance. Efficiency, in this sense, becomes a function of alignment between institutional design and lived experience rather than a mere calculation of inputs and outputs.

In parallel, the chapter advances a redefinition of efficacy, shifting the focus from short-term, quantifiable outcomes to the durability and depth of social transformation. Efficacy is thus conceptualized to the extent to which an intervention can generate sustained changes in identity, agency, and social positioning over time. The concept of cumulative identity transformation (CIT), developed within the theoretical framework of this study, provides a powerful lens through which to understand this process. CIT captures the gradual and iterative nature of transformation, wherein individuals accumulate layers of adaptive resilience, intercultural competence, and institutional trust through sustained engagement with the model. These changes are not instantaneous but unfold over time, as participants navigate and internalize new social roles and expectations. Importantly, this transformation extends beyond individual achievements to encompass broader trajectories of social mobility and community change. Alumni of the model, who have successfully transitioned into higher education, professional careers, and competitive sports, serve as tangible evidence of this long-term impact.

The analytical depth of the study is further enhanced by the integration of multiple theoretical perspectives, including phenomenology, Bourdieu's theory of capital, Stakeholder theory, and Diffusion of innovation. Phenomenology enables a nuanced understanding of inclusion as a lived and embodied experience, emphasizing the importance of belonging, recognition, and affective engagement in shaping individual trajectories. This perspective foregrounds the subjective dimensions of participation, which are often overlooked in quantitative evaluations. Bourdieu's framework, particularly when extended to incorporate multiple forms of capital like cultural, social, symbolic, and economic provides a robust analytical tool for examining how resources are accumulated, converted, and mobilized within the institutional context. Stakeholder theory highlights the importance of coordination among diverse actors, including educational institutions, healthcare providers, policymakers, and community stakeholders, in co-creating value and sustaining the model. Meanwhile, diffusion of innovation offers insights into the mechanisms through which the model can be adapted, replicated, and scaled across different contexts, while also identifying potential barriers to such diffusion.

The findings of the study reveal a strong alignment between these theoretical constructs and the operational dynamics of the Samanta Model. The model actively facilitates the accumulation of various forms of capital through structured participation in sport and education. Sporting engagement, for instance, contributes not only to physical development but also to the acquisition of discipline, teamwork, and self-confidence which as forms of embodied cultural capital are transferable to other domains. Educational opportunities enhance cognitive and institutional capital, while consistent and supportive service delivery fosters trust in formal institutions. The integration of global partnerships further strengthens linking social capital, connecting participants to transnational networks and expanding their horizons of opportunity. Crucially, these processes are embedded within a framework that values collective identity and community engagement, ensuring that individual advancement does not come at the cost of cultural erosion. Instead, the model promotes a form of inclusive modernization that harmonizes tradition and transformation, enabling participants to navigate multiple social worlds without losing their cultural grounding.

Another critical dimension of the model's impact lies in its intergenerational and community-level effects. The success of individual participants generates a powerful demonstration effect, inspiring others within their communities to pursue similar pathways. This, in turn, contributes to the emergence of a broader culture of aspiration, where education, sport, and professional achievement are increasingly seen as attainable goals. Over time, these individual transformations accumulate to produce shifts in community perceptions, reducing stigma and enhancing the social status of tribal populations. Families that were once hesitant to engage with formal institutions begin to see them as viable avenues for advancement. This multiplier effect underscores the importance of viewing welfare not as a series of isolated interventions but as a systemic process with cascading impacts across multiple levels of society. It also highlights the role of role models and social proof in driving behavioral and attitudinal changes within marginalized communities.

Furthermore, the model's institutional design ensures continuity across different stages of the life cycle, from early education to higher studies and professional integration. This continuity is critical in preventing the drop-offs that often characterize fragmented welfare systems, where beneficiaries are left to navigate transitions without adequate support. By providing a seamless pathway, the Samanta Model enhances both retention and progression, thereby maximizing the long-term returns on investment in human development. This life-cycle approach also reinforces the model's emphasis on sustainability, as it builds capacities that endure beyond the duration of formal participation.

In conclusion, the Samanta Model represents a compelling and empirically grounded example of how innovative institutional design can fundamentally reimagine the role of sport in social development. By embedding sport within a holistic ecosystem that integrates education, healthcare, and community engagement, the model demonstrates the transformative potential of sports-centric welfare. It challenges entrenched assumptions about both sport and welfare, offering an alternative vision of development that is integrated, inclusive, and deeply human-centered. The model's emphasis on access, dignity, and empowerment aligns with broader normative frameworks of social justice, while its operational effectiveness provides a practical blueprint for policy and practice. Ultimately, the significance of the Samanta Model lies not only in its measurable outcomes but also in its underlying philosophy: that human potential is universal, but opportunity is not. By systematically creating conditions in which this potential can be realized, the model serves as a powerful reminder that inclusive development is not merely a technical or policy objective, but a moral imperative that demands sustained institutional commitment and innovation.

Limitations and directions for future research

Despite its many strengths, this study also acknowledges the inherent limitations and contextual dependencies of the Samanta Model, particularly when viewed through the lens of scalability and replicability. The model's success is embedded in the integrated institutional architecture that combines education, healthcare, and sport within a unified ecosystem. Such integration, while central to its effectiveness, is also resource-intensive and dependent on sustained financial investment, organizational coherence, and visionary leadership. These conditions are not easily reproduced across diverse institutional or regional contexts. Consequently, while the model demonstrates significant promise, it cannot be uncritically transplanted into other settings without careful adaptation. Its reliance on long-term commitment, infrastructural capacity, and institutional alignment raises important questions about feasibility, especially in regions where governance structures are fragmented or resources are constrained.

From the perspective of Diffusion of Innovation, certain attributes of the Samanta Model such as its relative advantage, visibility of outcomes, and demonstrable social impact enhance its attractiveness to policymakers and practitioners. However, other attributes, including its operational complexity, high initial investment, and need for coordinated stakeholder engagement, may hinder widespread adoption. This duality suggests that the model is best understood not as a fixed template but as a modular framework. Its core principles including holistic integration, cultural sensitivity, and sport as a vehicle for inclusion can be adapted and reconfigured to suit local conditions, even if the full institutional structure cannot be replicated in its entirety. Such an approach allows for contextual innovation while preserving the underlying philosophy of sports-centric welfare.

The study also reflects critically on its methodological approach, particularly the use of ethnography as the primary mode of inquiry. Ethnographic research offers rich, contextually grounded insights into lived experiences, institutional processes, and cultural dynamics. However, it is not without limitations. The findings generated through this approach are inherently context-specific and do not lend themselves to statistical generalization. Instead, their strength lies in analytical generalization offering theoretical insights that may inform understanding in similar contexts. The immersive nature of ethnography also introduces the possibility of researcher subjectivity, as prolonged engagement with participants and institutions can shape interpretation. This risk is mitigated through reflexivity, systematic documentation, and triangulation of data sources, including interviews, observations, and institutional records.

Another potential limitation arises from the responses of participants themselves. Within institutional settings, individuals may consciously or unconsciously align their narratives with perceived expectations, leading to social desirability bias. This is particularly relevant in environments where participants benefit directly from institutional support and may feel a sense of loyalty or obligation. Additionally, access to certain internal processes, decision-making structures, or sensitive data may be restricted, limiting the scope of inquiry. These constraints are acknowledged transparently within the study and addressed through methodological rigor, ensuring that the findings remain credible, nuanced, and analytically robust despite these challenges.

At the same time, the study makes a significant methodological contribution by demonstrating the value of ethnographic inquiry in evaluating complex and integrated welfare models. Traditional evaluation frameworks, which often rely on quantitative indicators and short-term metrics, are ill-equipped to capture the layered and longitudinal nature of social transformation. By contrast, the ethnographic approach employed in this study combines immersive observation with narrative inquiry and document analysis, enabling a comprehensive understanding of both experiential and structural dimensions. This methodological design aligns closely with the concept of cumulative identity transformation (CIT), allowing the study to trace gradual shifts in identity, agency, and social positioning over time. In doing so, it highlights the importance of process-oriented evaluation in contexts where change is incremental, relational, and deeply embedded in lived experience.

For policymakers and practitioners, the findings of this study offer several important implications. First, they underscore the limitations of siloed approaches to welfare that address education, health, or social inclusion in isolation. The Samanta Model demonstrates the effectiveness of integrated, ecosystem-based approaches that simultaneously engage multiple dimensions of deprivation. Such models recognize the interdependence of social challenges and the need for coordinated interventions that reinforce one another. Second, the study highlights the potential of sport as a powerful policy instrument. Far from being a peripheral or recreational activity, sport can serve as a conduit for discipline, identity formation, social cohesion, and institutional engagement. When embedded within a broader developmental framework, it becomes a catalyst for both individual empowerment and collective transformation.

Third, the findings emphasize the importance of long-term, sustained interventions. Social inclusion, particularly in historically marginalized communities, cannot be achieved through short-term or episodic programs. It requires consistent engagement, trust-building, and the creation of enabling environments over extended periods. The Samanta Model's success is rooted in its continuity and its ability to support individuals across different stages of their life trajectories. This highlights the need for policy frameworks that prioritize durability and depth over immediacy and scale.

The study's theoretical framework—integrating phenomenology, social capital theory,, and —offers a multi-level analytical lens that advances the study of sport-for-development in several important ways. It bridges the gap between subjective experience and structural analysis by linking lived realities of inclusion with broader institutional and societal mechanisms. Phenomenology foregrounds the affective and experiential dimensions of participation, emphasizing belonging and recognition. Social capital theory elucidates the networks and relationships that enable access to resources and opportunities. Stakeholder theory highlights the role of coordinated institutional action in creating and sustaining value, while diffusion of innovation provides a framework for understanding how such models can spread and adapt across contexts.

Importantly, this integrated framework also foregrounds the role of institutions as mediators of inclusion. It demonstrates how well-designed and coordinated systems can reduce barriers, enhance participation, and facilitate long-term transformation. At the same time, it provides a robust basis for evaluating questions of scalability and replicability, particularly in relation to complex and resource-intensive models. The introduction of cumulative identity transformation as a conceptual contribution further strengthens this framework by capturing the longitudinal and iterative nature of inclusion. Rather than viewing inclusion as a static outcome, CIT conceptualizes it as a dynamic process that unfolds over time through repeated interactions, experiences, and institutional engagements.

From a theoretical standpoint, the study contributes to broader literature by advancing sports-centric welfare as a distinct paradigm within social policy. It challenges conventional dichotomies that separate sport from development and instead positions it as an integral component of welfare architecture. By integrating multiple theoretical perspectives, the study also demonstrates the value of interdisciplinary approaches in capturing the complexity of social phenomena. It bridges micro-level experiences—such as individual perceptions of belonging—with macro-level structures, including institutional design and policy environments, thereby offering a more holistic understanding of inclusion.

Looking ahead, future research can build on these contributions in several ways. Comparative studies across different regions, institutional models, or cultural contexts would provide valuable insights into the conditions under which similar approaches can succeed or fail. Such analyses would help refine the modular aspects of the Samanta Model and identify context-specific adaptations. The integration of quantitative methods, including longitudinal surveys and impact assessments, could complement ethnographic insights by providing measurable indicators of outcomes. Long-term tracking of participants would further enhance understanding of sustainability, particularly in relation to educational attainment, employment trajectories, and social mobility.

Future research can build on these contributions by incorporating comparative analyses across different regions and models, as well as by integrating quantitative measures to complement ethnographic insights. Longitudinal studies tracking participants over extended periods would further enhance understanding of the sustainability of outcomes. Additionally, research exploring the role of policy environments and governance structures in facilitating or constraining the adoption of similar models would provide valuable insights for scaling and adaptation. Additionally, there is a need for more focused research on the role of policy environments and governance structures in enabling or constraining the adoption of integrated welfare models. Factors such as political will, institutional capacity, funding mechanisms, and regulatory frameworks play a critical role in shaping the feasibility of replication. Understanding these dynamics would provide actionable insights for policymakers seeking to scale or adapt similar interventions.

REFERENCES

Anney, V. N. (2014). Ensuring the quality of the findings of qualitative research: Looking at trustworthiness criteria. [jeteraps]. *Journal of Emerging Trends in Educational Research and Policy Studies*, *5*(2), 272–281.

Bhoi, N., & Acharya, S. K. (2024). Health status of particularly vulnerable tribal groups (PVTGs) of Odisha: A narrative review. *Journal of Health, Population and Nutrition*, *43*(1), 176. DOI: 10.1186/s41043-024-00671-8 PMID: 39478584

Borgers, J., Pilgaard, M., Vanreusel, B., & Scheerder, J. (2018). Can we consider changes in sports participation as institutional change? A conceptual framework. *International Review for the Sociology of Sport*, *53*(1), 84–100. DOI: 10.1177/1012690216639598

Bourdieu, P. (1986). The forms of capital. In J. Richardson (Ed.), *Handbook of Theory and Research for the Sociology of Education*. Greenwood Press.

Bradbury, J. C., Coates, D., & Humphreys, B. R. (2023). The impact of professional sports franchises and venues on local economies: A comprehensive survey. *Journal of Economic Surveys*, *37*(4), 1389–1431. DOI: 10.1111/joes.12533

Chakraborty, S. (2024). Rethinking tribes in India through context of tribe-caste Continuum: Negotiation of identity and exploration of Hypervisibility among Siddi Tribe. *International Journal of Developmental Research*, *14*(12), 67270–67280.

Coalter, F. (2013). *Sport-for-development: What game are we playing?* Routledge. DOI: 10.4324/9780203861257

Datta, R. (2022, April 18). How Odisha's Kalinga Institutes provide free education to tribal children in remote areas. *India today*. https://www.indiatoday.in/magazine/happiness-quest/story/20220418-how-odisha-s-kalinga-institutes-provide-free-education-to-tribal-children-in-remote-areas-1934626-2022-04-08

Dorfman, E. (2009). History of the lifeworld: From husserl to merleau-ponty. *Philosophy Today*, *53*(3), 294–303. DOI: 10.5840/philtoday200953317

Edexlive (2018, May 17). Learn the Art of Giving from one of it's most successful practitioners, Dr Achyuta Samanta, *The New Indian Express*. https://www.edexlive.com/campus/learn-the-art-of-giving-from-one-of-its-most-successful-practitioners-dr-achyuta-samanta-2875.html

Edexlive. (2020, November, 27). How Kalinga Institute of Social Sciences is providing Odisha's youth access to quality education. *The New Indian Express.* https://www.edexlive.com/news/how-kalinga-institute-of-social-sciences-is-providing-odishas-youth-access-to-quality-education-15351.html

Edugraph, (2025, April 11). KIIT recognised as Best University for Promotion of Sports at 2025 Sportstar Aces Awards. *Telegraph India.* https://www.telegraphindia.com/edugraph/campus/kiit-recognised-as-best-university-for-promotion-of-sports-at-2025-sportstar-aces-awards/cid/2093598#goog_rewarded

Ekholm, D. (2019). Sport as a means of governing social integration: Discourses on bridging and bonding social relations. *Sociology of Sport Journal, 36*(2), 152–161. DOI: 10.1123/ssj.2018-0099

Elsborg, P., Nielsen, G., Klinker, C. D., Melby, P. S., Christensen, J. H., & Bentsen, P. (2019). Sports-based recreation as a means to address social inequity in health: Why, when, where, who, what, and how. *BMC Public Health, 19*(1), 1084. DOI: 10.1186/s12889-019-7428-3 PMID: 31399029

FIVB. (2025, December 14). Athletes take centre stage as kiit kiss centre of excellence is formalized in india. *FIVB.com.* https://www.fivb.com/athletes-take-centre-stage-as-kiit-kiss-centre-of-excellence-is-formalised-in-india/

Freeman, R. E. (1984). *Strategic Management: A stakeholder Approach.* Pitman.

Geertz, C. (1973). *The Interpretation of Cultures.* Basic Books.

Gosselin, V., Boccanfuso, D., & Laberge, S. (2020). Social return on investment (SROI) method to evaluate physical activity and sport interventions: A systematic review. *The International Journal of Behavioral Nutrition and Physical Activity, 17*(1), 26. DOI: 10.1186/s12966-020-00931-w PMID: 32106872

Himanshu (2025, December 27). KISS student Jyoshna Shabar conferred with Pradhan Mantri Rashtriya Bal Puraskar; a rising star of Indian weightlifting. *Kalinga TV.* https://kalingatv.com/odisha/kiss-universitys-sports-talent-jyotsna-shabar-receives-pradhan-mantri-rashtriya-bal-puraskar/ https://indiananthro.in/codeofethics.html

India education Diary Bureau. (2025, November 20). KIIT & KISS Set for a Grand Participation at Khelo India University Games 2025. *India Education Diary.* https://indiaeducationdiary.in/kiit-kiss-set-for-a-grand-participation-at-khelo-india-university-games-2025/

India Education diary Bureau (2023, December 13). KISS Model of Holistic Education for Tribal Children Earns Praise in Lok Sabha. *India education diary*. https://indiaeducationdiary.in/kiss-model-of-holistic-education-for-tribal-children-earns-praise-in-lok-sabha/

Kalinga Institute of Social Sciences (KISS). (2025). *Annual Report: Scaling the SDGs*. KISS Publications.

Kalinga Institute of Social Sciences (KISS) – Empowering Underprivileged Tribal Children to Aim for the Sky (2020, November 5). *News Indiatimes*. https://newsindiatimes.com/kalinga-institute-of-social-sciences-kiss-empowering-underprivileged-tribal-children-to-aim-for-the-sky/

Kihl, L. A. (2023). Development of a national sport integrity system. *Sport Management Review*, *26*(1), 24–47. DOI: 10.1080/14413523.2022.2048548

Kleiber, D. A., & Kirshnit, C. E. (2019). Sport involvement and identity formation. In *Mind-body maturity* (pp. 193–212). Taylor & Francis. DOI: 10.4324/9781315792194-14

Miragaia, D. A., Ferreira, J. J., & Ribeiro, I. J. (2025). Can sports events contribute to public policy development strategies? *Managing Sport and Leisure*, *30*(1), 1–20. DOI: 10.1080/23750472.2022.2098172

Moran, A. P., Matthews, J. J., & Kirby, K. (2011). Whatever happened to the third paradigm? Exploring mixed methods research designs in sport and exercise psychology. *Qualitative Research in Sport, Exercise and Health*, *3*(3), 362–369. DOI: 10.1080/2159676X.2011.607843

Nayak, S. (2025, October 23). Asia Rugby Emirates Sevens Trophy 2025: Indian men's team announced, 3 from KISS included. *Kalinga TV*. https://kalingatv.com/odisha/asia-rugby-emirates-sevens-trophy-2025-indian-mens-team-announced-3-from-kiss-included/

Odisha Diary Bureau. (2025, December 16), KISS Higher Secondary School Clinches Double Title at CHSE Inter Higher Secondary Schools Rugby Championship 2025. *Odisha Diary*. https://orissadiary.com/four-kiss-tribal-girls-selected-for-u-14-india-team-for-fide-iscf-world-school-chess-championship-2026/

Odisha Diary Bureau. (2026, April 4), Four kiss tribal girls selected for u-14 india team for fide iscf world school chess championship 2026. *Odisha Diary*. https://orissadiary.com/four-kiss-tribal-girls-selected-for-u-14-india-team-for-fide-iscf-world-school-chess-championship-2026/

Orlick, T. (2015). *In pursuit of excellence*. Human Kinetics.

Prasad, A. (2022, July 8). KIIT & KISS: A sports hub with world-class infrastructure. *The Hindu*. https://sportstar.thehindu.com/other-sports/kalinga-kiit-kiss-odisha-sports-infrastructure-feature-alumni-stadiums/article65598333.ece

Riffi Acharki, E., Spaaij, R., & Nieuwelink, H. (2023). Social inclusion through sport? Pedagogical perspectives of Dutch youth sport coaches. *Sport Education and Society*, *28*(2), 144–158. DOI: 10.1080/13573322.2021.2006174

Rogers, E. M. (2004). A prospective and retrospective look at the diffusion model. *Journal of Health Communication*, *9*(sup1, S1), 13–19. DOI: 10.1080/10810730490271449 PMID: 14960401

Samanta, A. (2021). *Art of Giving: A Way of Life*. KIIT University Press.

Samanta, A. (2024). The KISS Model of Holistic Education. In *Global Perspectives on Social Inclusion*. IGI Global.

Sen, A. (2000). Social exclusion: Concept, application, and scrutiny.

Sen, A. (2006). Conceptualizing and measuring poverty. *Poverty and inequality, 30*, 46.

Shilling, C., & Mellor, P. A. (2014). Re-conceptualizing sport as a sacred phenomenon. *Sociology of Sport Journal*, *31*(3), 349–376. DOI: 10.1123/ssj.2013-0034

Skille, E. Å. (2010). Competitiveness and health: The work of sport clubs as seen by sport clubs representatives-a Norwegian case study. *International Review for the Sociology of Sport*, *45*(1), 73–85. DOI: 10.1177/1012690209352395

Subramanyam, V., & Rao, S. N. (2022). Cultural identity, exclusion and inclusion of tribes in India: An empirical research study in Visakha Agency of Andhra Pradesh. *Skylines of the Anthropology*, *2*(2), 141–155.

Team Sportstar. (2023, December 5). KIIT University bags Best Sports Facility award in CII Sports Business Awards 2023. *The Hindu*. https://sportstar.thehindu.com/other-sports/kiit-university-bags-best-sports-facility-award-in-cii-sports-business-awards-2023/article67606871.ece

TRIBES, I. O. S. (2023). LIVES ON THE EDGES: SCHEDULED TRIBES.

Tripathi, R. C. (2026). Revitalising indigenous sports in India: An examination of their impact on fostering social and character development of children. *Curriculum Studies in Health and Physical Education*, *17*(1), 82–93. DOI: 10.1080/25742981.2024.2400259

United Nations India. (2024). *KISS: A Global Hub for Sustainable Development Goals*. UN Resident Coordinator's Office.

World Rugby. (2025). *The Evolution of Rugby in Odisha*. World Rugby Development Series.

Xaxa, V. (2018). Isolation, inclusion and exclusion: The case of Adivasis in India. In *Adivasi rights and exclusion in India* (pp. 27–40). Routledge India.

Yates, B. T., & Marra, M. (2017). Introduction: Social return on investment (SROI). *Evaluation and Program Planning*, *64*, 95–97. DOI: 10.1016/j.evalprogplan.2016.10.013 PMID: 27866664

Chapter 16
Football Between Decommodification and Financialization:
A Discussion Within the Context of Social Policy

Mehmet Atilla Güler
http://orcid.org/0009-0005-4527-8430
Aydın Adnan Menderes University, Turkey

ABSTRACT

This chapter examines contemporary football as a contradictory social field shaped simultaneously by financialisation and decommodifying countertendencies. It argues that football can no longer be understood merely as a cultural game or entertainment industry, because clubs, supporters, media rights, stadiums, and governance structures are increasingly reorganised through debt, investment, brand value, and revenue extraction. Yet football is not reducible to an ordinary commodity. Clubs remain historically embedded institutions shaped by locality, memory, and community attachment. From a social-policy perspective, the key issue is to identify the conditions under which football can sustain access, participation, representation, and collective ownership rather than deepen inequality.

INTRODUCTION

Football can no longer be understood merely as a cultural game, a sphere of local belonging, or a sub-sector of the sports industry. Over the past four decades, it has undergone a broader transformation through media rights, debt regimes, ownership

DOI: 10.4018/979-8-2600-3174-2.ch016

structures, stadium investment, digital platforms, and governance techniques. This has expanded not only football's economic environment but also its social meaning. Football must therefore be analysed not only through commodification, but also through the more advanced lens of financialisaton. While commodification refers to the process through which an object or social practice acquires exchange value and market-centred meaning, the literature shows that in contemporary football this process has intensified into hyper-commodification; in parallel, clubs have come to operate within a financial logic marked by chronic losses, debt, and expectations of rescue (Franck, 2013; Giulianotti, 2002; Storm & Nielsen, 2012).

Yet football cannot be read solely as a story of financialisaton. Professional clubs are not ordinary businesses. They are, on the one hand, economic organisations operating under pressures of investment, revenue, debt, brand value, and competitive performance; on the other, institutions shaped by local memory, historical attachment, symbolic ownership, and communal belonging. A football club therefore occupies an uneasy space between business and community. The core claim of this chapter follows from that tension: contemporary football is a social field in which decommodifying tendencies and financialising tendencies operate simultaneously. The word "between" in the title signals precisely this contradiction.

Here, decommodification is not taken directly from its classical use in welfare-state literature but adapted to the specific field of football. It does not mean that football becomes a non-market sphere. Rather, it means that the social value of the game and of the club is not reduced entirely to purchasing power, return on investment, and financial performance. Seeing the supporter not as a customer but as a stakeholder, grounding the relationship with the club not solely in consumption but in membership, representation, and reciprocity, ensuring that access is not governed exclusively by pricing, and recognising clubs' community embeddedness are central to this framework. Classical football sociology has shown that supporters' relations with clubs have historically been structured through membership, obligation, and representation, creating a form of informal participatory democracy (Giulianotti, 2002). More recent debates likewise suggest that clubs' claim to community status has not disappeared; rather, commodification continues to derive legitimacy from these residual elements (Kennedy & Kennedy, 2013).

Financialisaton, for its part, is not simply a matter of more money flowing into the game. It refers to the reorganisation of clubs' risk-taking, borrowing, fiscal discipline, and managerial priorities in line with financial-market logic. In European football, extraordinarily high survival rates despite persistent deficits and growing debt, the tolerance of losses by states, creditors, or private benefactors, and clubs' continued competition even near insolvency are all indicators of this logic. It transforms not only club finance but also reporting and accountability regimes. Debates over Financial Fair Play show that clubs are too socially embedded to be measured as ordinary firms, yet prevailing forms of financial reporting remain inadequate to capture this layered value. Financialisaton thus signifies a transformation both in economic behaviour and in the institutional imagination of what a club is.

This is where the discussion becomes important for social policy. Football is not merely an entertainment market. It is tied to questions of access, participation, representation, community, public space, youth, health, social inclusion, and the allocation of urban resources. Yet the role of sport and football in these areas is often presented in exaggerated and instrumental terms. The *sport for good* approach has portrayed sport as a low-cost solution to a wide range of social problems, although the evidential basis for such claims is often weak. Research repeatedly shows that participation alone is insufficient, that positive effects emerge only under specific institutional and social conditions, and that the same practices may also generate exclusionary and stigmatising outcomes (see Coalter, 2007). Football's significance for social policy therefore lies not in romantically declaring it "good", but in distinguishing the conditions under which it supports collective welfare from those under which it becomes a marketised substitute mechanism.

The chapter's argument is therefore straightforward. The dominant tendency in contemporary football is financialisaton. Yet football's historical and social character prevents it from being reduced entirely to an ordinary commodity. Supporters' symbolic and moral ownership claims, clubs' insistence on their community character, debates over redistribution in media rights, the place-making quality of the stadium, the partial but real potential of social-inclusion programmes, and democratic supporter intervention all carry traces of decommodifying countertendencies. None of these tendencies, however, is pure or free of contradiction; each may be intertwined with, compromised by, or reabsorbed into market logic. The issue, then, is not to code football either as commodified or as the people's game, but to analyse the struggle between financialisaton and decommodification in its historical and institutional forms.

The chapter proceeds in six sections. The first examines how the neoliberal transformation has restructured supportership, scale, and consumption. The second analyses financialisaton through chronic deficits, soft budget constraints, ownership forms, and fiscal discipline regimes. The third addresses media rights and media capitalism through the contradiction between football's public circulation and paid access. The fourth explores the spatial face of financialisaton through stadiums and mega-events. The fifth critically evaluates football's capacity to generate social inclusion and welfare while also showing its limits. The sixth discusses supporter exclusion, loss of representation, and democratic alternatives, thereby showing why football must be understood as a matter of social policy.

1. THE NEOLIBERAL TRANSFORMATION OF FOOTBALL: THE RESTRUCTURING OF SUPPORTERSHIP, SCALAR SHIFT, AND THE REGIME OF CONSUMPTION

In the neoliberal era, it is analytically insufficient to treat football merely as a cultural game or a sphere of local belonging. Since the 1980s, its institutional structure, revenue mechanisms, media circulation, and club-supporter relations have been reshaped within a broader restructuring in which market logic has become increasingly central. This process has gone beyond ordinary commercialisation and produced a phase of hyper-commodification, more tightly articulating football with media corporations, telecommunications networks, sponsorship systems, brand economies, and financial markets (Giulianotti, 2002; Giulianotti & Robertson, 2012).

One of the clearest consequences of this transformation has been the shift of supportership from a community-based relation of membership towards one increasingly constituted through consumption. The issue, however, is not simply that the supporter has been reduced to a customer, but that the nature of the bond with the club has changed. A relationship once grounded in locality, class attachment, repeated rituals, and mutual loyalty has been reconfigured through broadcasting packages, licensed merchandise, digital content, star-player culture, and brand circulation. Neoliberal football thus transforms not only spectating, but the wider regime of social membership through which football is lived (Giulianotti, 2002).

In this respect, the typology mapping supportership along the axes of hot/cool and traditional/consumerist remains illuminating. The local supporter, grounded in intense and historically sedimented attachment, has not disappeared, but its structural weight has weakened. By contrast, mediatized, mobile, and experience-oriented forms of supportership have become more visible. Supporters who relate to clubs not through spatial and community ties, but through image, style, brand, and temporary experience, make visible the new cultural logic of neoliberal football. Yet the process is not linear. Large clubs simultaneously seek to preserve local loyalty, sell products to fans, attract followers through star players, and incorporate supporters located in transnational circuits into the brand economy. Older forms of supportership therefore do not vanish, but are re-hierarchised within the new revenue regime (Giulianotti, 2002).

For this reason, the neoliberal transformation is not only cultural but also spatial and scalar. Football is no longer a field defined solely by national leagues and federations. It has become a multilayered global field shaped by elite clubs, media corporations, sponsors, international institutions, and transnational supporter networks. Within this configuration, clubs operate as transnational brand organisations, and decision-making, visibility, and revenue generation are increasingly tied to networks extending beyond the national context (Giulianotti & Robertson, 2012).

This rescaling does not mean that the local has disappeared. On the contrary, local belonging is being re-signified under new conditions of transnational competition. Studies of European football show that supportership has not simply moved from the national to the global; rather, local identities are being reconstructed within new relations of capital, media, and competition. Urban, regional, and club-based attachments are not dissolving, but being recoded within broader circuits of circulation (King, 2016).

Likewise, contemporary supportership can no longer be defined solely by physical presence in the stadium. Television, digital platforms, forums, blogs, e-zines, podcasts, and social media have created new channels through which relations with clubs are sustained. This does not mean that traditional supportership has disappeared, but that new layers have been added to it. The supporter still goes to the stadium, but also follows the club online, discusses it, produces identity, and sustains attachment in the digital sphere. Moreover, intense attachment to clubs outside one's own country is no longer exceptional, but one of the ordinary outcomes of football's global media economy (Millward, 2011; Niemann et al., 2024).

This transformation is not merely abstract. The restructuring of the Premier League since the 1990s around broadcasting, sponsorship, and global visibility has not only turned English football into a more profitable media product but has also reconstituted the relationship between clubs and supporters within a transnational regime of consumption and belonging extending beyond local loyalty. In this process, the club has ceased to function primarily as the representative of a particular city or community and has instead become a brand and identity object consumed within transboundary media circulation. Studies on Manchester United provide a particularly revealing example. Its supporter base can no longer be understood solely through physical proximity or stadium attendance but must be grasped as a multilayered attachment shaped by media consumption, symbolic identification, and transnational circuits of circulation. Neoliberal football thus does not eliminate local belonging so much as recode it within the global brand economy and mediatized forms of supportership (King, 2016; Hill & Vincent, 2006; Cleland, 2017; Giulianotti & Robertson, 2004).

Taken together, these developments show that neoliberal football has not simply surrendered supportership to the market; it has fundamentally reconfigured the relations among belonging, consumption, locality, media, and governance. The local supporter has not disappeared, but has been pushed into a more limited place within clubs' revenue strategies. Mediatized and mobile forms of supportership have, by contrast, become increasingly central. Local identities have not dissolved, but have been reframed by transnational competition and the brand economy.

From the standpoint of the book's overall argument, this transformation makes the first major tension visible: football's historically decommodified dimensions, which have produced community, belonging, and collective participation, have not disappeared, yet they have become increasingly subordinated to the logics of the market, media, and consumption. Put differently, the central problem of contemporary football lies in the marginalisation of decommodifying forms of belonging within a financialised restructuring. The neoliberal transformation of football is therefore the starting point of the structural tension between decommodification and financialisaton explored in the rest of the chapter.

2. THE FINANCIALIZATION OF FOOTBALL: DEBT, OWNERSHIP, AND THE REGIME OF FINANCIAL DISCIPLINE

The financialisaton of football is not simply a matter of more money flowing into the game. It refers to the reorganisation of clubs' income and expenditure structures, borrowing practices, ownership relations, and competitive strategies in line with financial-market logic. Within this framework, the football club becomes not merely an organisation pursuing sporting success, but an economic actor inclined to spend tomorrow's revenues today, deepen long-term fragility for short-term performance, and defer financial risk through rescue mechanisms. Financialisaton, then, is best understood as the reconstitution of football's institutional rationality around debt, investment, asset value, brand, and expectations of rescue (Franck, 2013; Morrow, 2014; Rohde & Breuer, 2016).

One of the most striking features of European professional football is the coexistence of chronic losses and high survival rates. Many clubs run persistent deficits, accumulate debt, and operate in conditions of technical fragility, yet do not exit the system. Under ordinary capital discipline, firms generating continuous losses and growing debt would be expected to leave the market. In football, however, survival rates remain extraordinarily high even as losses become chronic. Football's economic structure therefore cannot be explained solely through models such as win maximisation or non-profit utility. The crucial question is why the budget constraint does not harden, or why insolvency pressure does not fully operate (Storm & Nielsen, 2012; Franck, 2013).

Here the soft budget constraint approach is especially illuminating. The more clubs assume that losses will not push them out of the system, and that some rescue mechanism may intervene, the more their spending decisions are shaped accordingly. Expectations of future revenue no longer define the real limit of present expenditure. Club executives may assume that last-minute support from owners, creditors, or public authorities will be available, producing a departure from ordinary business rationality in transfer and wage spending. Excessive expenditure is therefore not merely poor management; the institutionalisation of rescueability creates a structure that rationalises overspending (Storm & Nielsen, 2012; Franck, 2013).

Combined with football's competitive logic, this deepens financialisaton still further. Title races, qualification for European competitions, relegation threats, and revenue differentials across leagues all push clubs towards ever greater investment. Overinvestment in football is therefore structural rather than exceptional. The critical issue is why it does not stop at a certain point. Competitive pressure alone cannot explain this. What matters is the expectation that deficits produced by overinvestment can later be covered by external resources. Football thus resembles less a conventional arms race than a zombie race in which even actors close to insolvency continue to compete. Clubs take risks beyond their own cash-generating capacity, yet these risks are treated as deferrable because of systemic importance, brand value, or deep social embeddedness (Franck, 2013; Storm & Nielsen, 2012).

The sources of rescue are multiple. Public authorities may keep clubs afloat through deferred tax debts, facilitated credit, debt forgiveness, or local support. Private benefactors or majority shareholders may do the same by repeatedly covering deficits. In both cases, the pressure that "if you lose money, you exit" is weakened. Especially in the case of large clubs, their weight in terms of local identity, regional belonging, and political visibility turns them into institutions that cannot, in practice, be allowed to fail. The club's social significance thus becomes a justification for suspending financial discipline, while the financial risk of a socially embedded institution is spread, directly or indirectly, onto others (Storm & Nielsen, 2012; Franck, 2013).

The clearest institutional response to this structural problem has been Financial Fair Play (FFP). At its core lies the idea that clubs should live within their means. The regulation requires that, over a given monitoring period, relevant expenses must not exceed relevant income beyond a specified threshold. Its purpose is to prevent clubs from expanding wage and transfer expenditure based on unlimited rescue expectations and to harden the budget constraint. Yet the regime does not require absolute equilibrium. It allows acceptable deviation, leaves limited room for specific forms of equity injection, and excludes some expenditures, such as those on stadiums, infrastructure, youth development, and community projects, from the relevant expense calculation. FFP therefore does not target all investment but seeks to curb sporting personnel and transfer inflation not covered by football-generated revenue.

FFP is therefore not simply a salary-cap system. Its aim is less to equalise competition directly than to limit competition financed through losses. At the theoretical level, it seeks to correct managerial incentives by replacing wage budgets based on rescue expectations with revenue generation and more sustainable management. Yet major problems emerge in implementation. The treatment of relevant income and expenses, the adjustment of related-party transactions to fair value, and the partial mismatch between break-even calculations and conventional financial statements all create room for interpretation. In addition, insufficient emphasis on cash flow, the nature of sanctions, loopholes allowing circumvention, the possibility of creative accounting, and the risk of clubs being doubly penalised both financially and sporting-wise all constitute major lines of criticism. FFP is thus not only a regime of financial discipline, but also a governance technology reshaping football's logic of accounting and reporting (Morrow, 2014).

Concrete cases show that FFP does not produce equal outcomes for all clubs in practice. In 2018, UEFA excluded AC Milan from European competitions for breaching break-even requirements, though the process was later reframed through CAS intervention and new settlement mechanisms. Similarly, Manchester City received a two-season European ban and a financial penalty in 2020, yet CAS overturned most of the sanction and reduced the fine. By contrast, sanctions proved far more destructive for more fragile clubs: the ban imposed on Málaga was upheld by CAS, while Dnipro was excluded by UEFA in 2016 for failing to meet its financial obligations. In Turkey, comparable dynamics have sometimes appeared not as direct UEFA sanctions, but through the reconstitution of club identity after financial collapse. Göztepe's return to professional football in 2008 through the competitive rights of Aliağa Belediyespor shows that financial discipline does not always erase a club's historical identity; it may instead reproduce that identity on a different institutional basis. Thus, while FFP appears to impose the same formal regime on all clubs, in practice it generates marked asymmetries between the legal defence capacity and institutional resources of large clubs and the limited room for manoeuvre available to smaller or more fragile clubs.

Another dimension of financialisaton lies in ownership structures. Analyses of Europe's elite clubs show that revenue performance is strongly linked not only to national and international sporting success but also to brand value, while sporting success itself is largely driven by team investment. One of the principal factors increasing team investment appears to be private majority investors. The private investor thus becomes a strategic actor accelerating the revenue-success-brand cycle, recoding sporting performance in terms of market value, brand expansion, and investment capacity. The widening gap in revenue growth between elite clubs follows from the same process: top clubs are becoming richer and expanding more rapidly than others (Rohde & Breuer, 2016).

Not all ownership models, however, produce identical outcomes. In the English case, publicly listed clubs appear stronger than privately owned clubs in terms of financial health, liquidity, and debt indicators, whereas clubs owned by foreign private investors enjoy an advantage over domestically privately owned clubs in sporting performance. Foreign capital may therefore strengthen short-term competitiveness, but often at the cost of higher indebtedness and weaker financial structure. The stock-market model offers a relatively more disciplined framework, yet the dominant tendency in recent years has been a move away from it and towards greater weight for private investors. Football is thus increasingly treated as an investment object that transforms sporting success into financial and symbolic returns (Wilson et al., 2013; Rohde & Breuer, 2016).

In sum, the financialisaton of football does not simply mean that clubs become wealthier. It means growth through debt, risk-taking based on expectations of rescue, concentration of ownership, the transformation of brand value into a revenue strategy, and the conversion of financial regulation into a technical-accounting field of power. Sporting competition is increasingly determined by investment capacity and financial resilience, while the club's social significance frequently serves as a justification for deferring financial discipline. This is the crucial point from a social-policy perspective: football is no longer merely an entertainment industry, but a terrain of struggle over who bears risk, who appropriates gains, and under which property regime social value is redistributed (Storm & Nielsen, 2012; Franck, 2013; Morrow, 2014; Wilson et al., 2013).

For this reason, the financialisaton of football does not mean only that clubs borrow more, attract investment, or come under financial oversight. It also raises directly the question of how far the club's social character can still be preserved. As financial-market logic grows stronger, the club's priorities shift away from community, representation, and public belonging towards continuity of revenue flows, protection of brand value, and management of investment risk. Under such conditions, even if the football club is not reduced entirely to an ordinary firm, its decommodifying dimensions are systematically marginalised.

3. MEDIA RIGHTS, MEDIA CAPITALISM, AND THE RISE OF DIGITAL PLATFORMS

In football's neoliberal transformation, media rights have become one of the principal mechanisms restructuring the game's institutional order. Understanding football's political economy therefore requires more than examining club balance sheets or sponsorship deals. What matters is how football is packaged as content, how it circulates across platforms, and under what regimes of ownership and access that circulation is organised. In modern football, a broadcasting right is not simply permission to show a match on screen, but a form of property that produces value, limits access, segments audiences, and re-hierarchises the game's social circulation according to market logic (Boyle & Haynes, 2004; Hutchins & Rowe, 2012).

At the centre of this transformation lies football's shift from shared public-service content to a strategic foundation of private, subscription-based media markets.

For much of the twentieth century in Europe, live and highlights-based football circulated within public-service broadcasting. Deregulation weakened this model, and commercial free-to-air broadcasters, followed by satellite, cable, digital, and pay-TV platforms, repositioned football as a driver of new markets. Football thus ceased to be merely a sports product and became central to media corporations' strategies of customer acquisition, subscription retention, and platform loyalty. From the 1990s onwards, the viability of new media networks increasingly depended first on securing content and then on securing customers; within this equation, football emerged as the strongest content type in the European context (King, 2016; Boyle & Haynes, 2004).

What matters here is not simply football's high viewing capacity, but its status as a live, uncertain, non-deferrable, and non-substitutable media product. Unlike fictional content, the result of a match is unknown in advance. Live broadcasting therefore remains one of the highest-value forms of content in the face of time-shifted or fragmented consumption. This has made football especially attractive for advertising, subscription, and exclusive-access models. Yet this attraction derives not only from the nature of the game. Football's historical embeddedness in European urban culture makes it an even more powerful commodity for broadcasters. Football was centralised by television and digital platforms not only because it suited those media, but because it already carried strong social resonance (King, 2016; Hutchins & Rowe, 2012).

Within this framework, the rise of media rights accelerated football's transition from public access to paid access. The shift from free-to-air broadcasting to subscription and pay-per-view appeared to offer greater choice, but in practice tied access more closely to purchasing power. The fragmented environment created by digital television and later by internet-based distribution did not make football more democratic. On the contrary, content divided into rights windows—live broadcasting, highlights, club channels, mobile clips, internet streaming, radio, archive footage, and interactive services—was transformed into separately priced assets allocated across different platforms. Football broadcasting thus ceased to be a singular public experience and became attached to a windowed, layered regime of consumption (Boyle & Haynes, 2004; Hutchins & Rowe, 2012).

One of the clearest examples of this transformation is the Premier League broadcasting regime in England. Sky's acquisition of live broadcasting rights in 1992 marked a decisive rupture in football's shift away from public-service broadcasting towards subscription-based pay-TV growth. Thereafter, rights values rose dramatically, while access to live matches moved behind pay platforms and free access became largely confined to highlights programmes and the limited matches covered by listed-events rules. The literature shows that the Premier League's pay-TV-centred growth not only expanded media revenues but also restructured the public experience of watching football by binding it to a layered regime of access (Evens & Lefever, 2011; Boyle, 2015; Geey, 2007).

This fragmentation was accompanied by the unbundling of rights. Live broadcasting, highlights packages, pay-per-view, video-on-demand, digital radio, internet streaming, mobile messaging services, and short video clips became rights categories that could be separated, marketed independently, and resold. At first glance, this promised higher revenues for rights holders and greater choice for viewers. In practice, however, it represented a more refined technique of value extraction within media capitalism, since value was generated not only from the match itself, but from the repeated commodification of the same content across different formats. A single football match could thus circulate simultaneously as a television broadcast, mobile product, online stream, clip service, and archive asset across multiple circuits of profit (Boyle & Haynes, 2004; Hutchins & Rowe, 2012).

Yet this process did not produce a more open media environment. The spread of the internet and digital devices offered clubs and leagues, in theory, the possibility of bypassing traditional broadcasters. Globally visible clubs developed web portals, club television channels, mobile applications, and online viewing services to reach supporters directly, creating opportunities both to attract sponsors and to build their own media infrastructures. At the same time, however, clubs' direct production of content could conflict with leagues' centralised agreements, while leagues' digital expansion could clash with broadcasters' expectations of exclusivity. Digitalisation thus created the possibility of disintermediation while simultaneously producing new forms of centralisation and control (Boyle & Haynes, 2004; Hutchins & Rowe, 2012).

For this reason, the key struggle in the digital age concerns less who produces content than who controls it. As leagues and clubs develop their own digital ecosystems, the exclusivity of traditional television agreements may erode. Large broadcasters therefore seek to acquire internet, mobile, and other digital rights alongside television rights within the same package; in some cases, they purchase digital rights they do not intend to use simply to prevent rivals from doing so. This practice of rights warehousing suppresses digital-market development, limits competition, and raises barriers to entry. The promise of digital plurality thus often turns into a more concentrated form of monopolistic control in the hands of large corporations (Hutchins & Rowe, 2012).

Another consequence is that media-rights revenues have deepened inequalities within football. Revenues rose after deregulation and digitalisation, but not evenly across clubs. Big-city clubs and elite teams with global brand status benefited disproportionately from the new regime. Where individual sales models were strong, large clubs signed highly lucrative contracts while smaller clubs remained dependent on weaker and secondary revenue sources. Even where collective selling continued, large clubs extracted larger shares thanks to bargaining power, visibility, and international demand. The media-rights market has therefore functioned less as a neutral mechanism supporting sporting competition than as an apparatus reinforcing existing hierarchies and widening financial gaps among clubs (King, 2016; Hutchins & Rowe, 2012).

This inequality is also visible in the public dimension of broadcasting regimes. Football's migration from public broadcasting to private and pay-based platforms has challenged both the audience share and the cultural legitimacy of public-service broadcasters. The increasing transfer of such socially significant content to paid networks has altered sport's place within public culture. The issue is which social groups can access the game simultaneously and without barriers. As public broadcasting weakens, football's capacity to function as a shared social experience is eroded, while a new form of media citizenship emerges that differentiates audiences by purchasing power, subscription preferences, and levels of technological equipment (Boyle & Haynes, 2004).

At the same time, football has ceased to be merely content used by broadcasters and has become a nodal point in the convergence of media, telecommunications, and information technology. Television, the internet, mobile networks, and gaming consoles no longer operate as separate media, but as integrated platforms distributing the same content across different devices. In contemporary media capitalism, football is transformed into content simultaneously streamed, repackaged, enhanced through interactivity, and circulated across multiple screens. The underlying logic is the shift from a single screen to multiple screens, and from a single revenue channel to a multi-channel revenue architecture. Yet this transition tends to work not in viewers' favour, but in favour of large corporations exercising property-based control over content (Hutchins & Rowe, 2012; Boyle & Haynes, 2004).

The debate on media rights, then, cannot be treated as merely technical or sectoral. What is at stake is the social regime within which football circulates. If football is a component of public culture, subjecting it entirely to exclusive and high-priced access models is also problematic from the standpoint of social policy. In that case, what is excluded is not only low-income supporters, but football's very capacity to produce shared time, shared memory, and shared access. For media corporations, however, football is one of the most efficient means of converting common interest into profit. Under such conditions, the media-rights regime constitutes one of the clearest arenas of conflict between football's public value and the property logic of media capitalism.

4. STADIUMS, URBAN ACCUMULATION AND MEGA-EVENTS

The neoliberal transformation of football has turned the stadium from a physical site of play into a central instrument in the reorganisation of urban space. It is best understood not simply as an architectural or sporting structure, but as a nodal point of spatial accumulation through which access is regulated, belonging produced, rent intensified, and public resources reallocated. On the one hand, it is the material carrier of supporters' collective memory, sense of place, and everyday rituals. On the other, modern stadium investment increasingly operates through surveillance, separation, pricing, and environmental revaluation. This dual character makes football space important for social policy, because the issue is not merely sports infrastructure, but for whom public space is reconstituted and at what social cost (Bale, 1993; Horne & Manzenreiter, 2006; Zimbalist, 2016).

The history of the stadium makes this tension clear. Modern sports space has long had a semi-public character: it appears publicly accessible, yet entry is limited by price, property, and control. Large stadiums developed alongside the enclosure of sport, ticketed spectating, and the class segmentation of crowds. More expensive seated sections were allocated to wealthier spectators, while wider standing terraces were assigned to working-class audiences, so that urban inequalities were reproduced within the stadium itself. In this sense, the stadium has never been a neutral public space but has functioned from the start as a spatial map of social stratification (Bale, 1993).

Yet the stadium is not only a space of control. Traditional inner-city grounds also generate a sense of place for supporters. This derives not only from the physical structure itself, but from the time, traces, habits, and collective memories accumulated within it. Worn terraces, the walk to the match along familiar streets, surrounding shopkeepers, sounds, smells, and practices transmitted across generations all turn the stadium into a lived social space.[1] Demolition or relocation therefore signifies not simply a change of facility, but the erosion of supporters' attachment to the city, their memories, and their symbolic sense of home. A new stadium may be safer, more comfortable, and more efficient, yet designs that exceed the human scale, become standardised, and detach themselves from their surroundings often produce placelessness rather than place (Bale, 1993).

At the same time, neoliberal urban transformation increasingly replaces the traditional inner-city ground with multipurpose complexes on the urban periphery, surrounded by parking and integrated with shopping and entertainment. This shift cannot be explained solely through security or transport concerns. The stadium is repackaged from a singular match venue into a spatial arrangement governed by real-estate value, retail consumption, automobile access, and the distribution of investment risk. Rather than remaining part of the city's social fabric, it becomes an element of entrepreneurial urban policy and an entertainment district. In this model, spontaneous publicness weakens, while controlled circulation and regulated consumption are strengthened (Bale, 1993).

Mega-events accelerate this spatial transformation still further. Events such as the Olympics and the World Cup are not merely sporting competitions, but spectacles through which cities and nations enter global circulation, generate media visibility, and legitimise major infrastructural projects. They should therefore be understood as processes that play an active role in the reconstitution of urban modernity in contemporary capitalist societies. What makes them "mega" is not only scale, but the assumption that they produce major consequences for the host city, region, or country and function as global showcases through intensive media circulation (Horne & Manzenreiter, 2006).

For this reason, mega-events are best interpreted less through economic rationality than through entrepreneurial politics and growth coalitions. The recurrent promise is that they will increase investment, tourism, employment, and international visibility while leaving a legacy. Yet the literature shows that benefits are often exaggerated, while costs, environmental effects, and opportunity costs are underestimated. Much of the research conducted beforehand is also produced on behalf of interested actors. The problem, then, is not simply miscalculation, but who benefits, who is excluded, and which social costs are rendered invisible under the discourse of general benefit. The tension between growth-machine logic and social redistribution lies at the centre of mega-event debates (Horne & Manzenreiter, 2006).

These promises are persuasive because sports investment offers a powerful symbolic solution, especially for cities marked by deindustrialisation, declining city centres, or pressure from global competition. A stadium or mega-event is presented as a lever that will place the city on the world stage, attract investment, and reverse decline. Empirical findings, however, suggest a much more cautious picture. Sport's share in the urban economy is often limited; much of the employment created is low-paid, temporary, and concentrated in the service sector; and a significant portion of spectator spending merely displaces expenditure that would otherwise have taken place elsewhere in the city. A new stadium or major event therefore often fails to generate the expected net welfare gains and may even divert public resources from more urgent social needs (Zimbalist, 2016; Horne & Manzenreiter, 2006).

Long-term costs are among the most problematic aspects of mega-events. When facilities built or transformed for a few weeks of competition fail to find adequate use afterwards, maintenance expenses, operating costs, debt servicing, and land opportunity costs remain public burdens for years. The large stadiums built for the Brazil World Cup in cities with lower-tier teams or weak local demand illustrate this vividly. These outcomes also reflected choices made at the expense of alternative urban needs such as sanitation, transport, and other forms of social infrastructure. The post-event idle stadium is therefore not merely a wasted investment, but a concrete symbol of unrealised alternative public expenditure (Zimbalist, 2016).

The Brazilian case also shows that the costs of mega-events become visible in the labour regime of preparation itself. Workers on World Cup projects engaged in numerous strikes in response to low wages, long hours, inadequate health and food conditions, and deficiencies in occupational safety; union-based reports described this process in terms of precarisation and over-exploitation of labour. The succession of fatal accidents on stadium construction sites further exposed the destructive effects of FIFA's timetable and delivery pressures on occupational health and safety. The social cost of mega-events must therefore be assessed not only in terms of public debt and idle infrastructure, but also through the living and working conditions of the labour on which such projects depend (Comitê Popular, 2012).

Just as important is the profoundly asymmetrical financial relationship between the host country and the global institutions organising the event. In the case of the World Cup, while part of the operating budget may be covered by the organiser, the main burden of transport, communication, stadium, and general infrastructure investment is left to the host country. By contrast, highly profitable revenue streams such as broadcasting, sponsorship, and licensing remain largely under the control of global governing bodies. The host assumes high fixed costs and long-term risks, while the most lucrative revenues are appropriated by transnational sports-governance structures. The mega-event is therefore not only an urban issue, but also a distributive one (Zimbalist, 2016).

Even so, it would be wrong to treat all such cases as absolute failure. Some examples, such as Barcelona, have generated gains through transport infrastructure, seafront redevelopment, or international visibility. Yet even here, the quality of employment created, the social distribution of benefits, and the long-term effects in whose favour they operate remain contested. Even supposedly successful cases are often associated with low-wage and short-term employment, real-estate valorisation, and selective spatial renewal. The key question is therefore not whether an event produces any benefit, but what kind of benefit, for whom, and at what cost (Horne & Manzenreiter, 2006).

The framework of stadiums, urban accumulation, and mega-events thus makes visible the spatial face of football's financialisaton. The tension between the historic ground that produces a sense of place and the placeless entertainment complex, the imbalance between public investment and private gain, and the gap between the rhetoric of urban spectacle and actual social costs all bring football directly into the field of social-policy debate. What is at stake is not merely the location of a sports facility or the success of an event, but how urban resources are allocated, how public benefit is defined, and for which groups collective life becomes more accessible or more exclusionary. This is why football's spatial economy remains one of the clearest terrains on which the tension between welfare and accumulation is played out.

5. FOOTBALL'S DECOMMODIFYING POTENTIAL AND ITS LIMITS

Football can perform a decommodifying function only under institutional and social conditions; otherwise, it may become a low-cost substitute mechanism that does not remedy structural inequalities but merely obscures them. The key question, therefore, is not whether football is inherently good, but under what conditions it can generate a form of social participation that limits market logic (Coalter, 2007; Collins & Kay, 2003; Spaaij et al., 2014).

The starting point for this discussion lies in the increasingly instrumental use of sport within social policy. Since the 1990s, sport has shifted from a *sport for all* approach towards a *sport for good* approach, ceasing to be treated as a public activity to be developed and instead becoming tied to external goals such as reducing crime, improving health indicators, enhancing educational attainment, alleviating youth unemployment, or promoting social cohesion. This shift has made sport's public value more visible but has also forced it to justify itself through external performance criteria. In this context, the distinction between *sport plus* and *plus sport* is crucial: in the former, sport itself remains central; in the latter, sport becomes an instrument for other social ends. The problem is not that the second approach is always wrong, but that football's social value comes to be recognised only insofar as it produces external outputs. Decommodifying potential is thus displaced from a basis in public rights and participation towards a language of performance and utility (Coalter, 2007; Spaaij et al., 2014).

For this reason, the first point to remember in any discussion of social inclusion is that access to football is already unequal. Poverty, class, gender, age, geography, ethnicity, and disability are not variables added from outside the sporting field after the fact; they are among the fundamental determinants of participation. Poverty lies at the centre of sports exclusion; low-income groups have more limited access to organised sport because of membership, equipment, transport, and time costs; and exclusion is produced not only materially but also through cultural and institutional mechanisms. In football, then, decommodification begins by asking how these inequalities of access can be reduced. The claim to create a social sphere outside the market gains meaning only once it is acknowledged that participation is, in practice, constrained by relations of income, status, and recognition (Collins & Kay, 2003; Spaaij et al., 2014).

At the same time, football's decommodifying potential is not purely theoretical. Particularly for migrants, refugees, displaced populations, and disadvantaged neighbourhoods, football can generate a social bond outside the market. Debates on social capital are illuminating here. The football club may function as a bonding space in which social networks damaged by war, migration, and poverty can be rebuilt. It can bring people together around a meaningful, purposeful, and enjoyable shared experience, and can partially suspend the exclusion felt in other areas of everyday life. Research on Somali refugees, for example, shows that football strengthens relations within the same community, reweaves fragmented networks, and serves for some participants as a kind of family, community, and refuge. In this sense, football can produce a sphere of coexistence and recognition that cannot be reduced to a commodity (Spaaij, 2012).

Yet this potential is not automatic, and when exaggerated becomes analytically misleading. The same research shows that bonding social capital is stronger, whereas bridging and linking social capital—those forms that provide access to broader institutional resources—remain much weaker. Ties with the host society often remain limited, while discrimination and hostility may reinforce group boundaries rather than transcend them. Moreover, access to resources and high-status positions within the club is not equally distributed; gender, age, ethnic hierarchies, and socio-economic position continue to matter. The fact that football produces community does not mean that it is inherently inclusive. Alongside the decommodifying experience of shared play, what matters is who is included in that experience, who is left outside it, and to which resources it is connected (Spaaij, 2012).

A central contribution of the critical literature is to show that the social benefits of football and sport often circulate less as empirically demonstrated outcomes than as normative expectations. The idea that sport is a cure for all social ills has strong political appeal because it offers a low-cost, visible, and positively coded repertoire of solutions. Yet research shows that the evidential basis for many such claims is weak; that many programmes measure outputs without adequately investigating processes, mechanisms, and enabling conditions; and that no linear relationship can be assumed between mere participation and broader social outcomes. Football does not become inclusive simply because it is played. What matters is the pedagogical, organisational, and communal relations within which it is experienced. Decommodifying potential should therefore be sought not in football itself, but in how football is organised (Coalter, 2007).

From this perspective, more critical approaches clarify why many sport-based social interventions remain limited. The dominant view treats sport as a natural vehicle for building character by fostering self-esteem, discipline, leadership, confidence, and life skills. Seen in this way, football becomes not a means of transforming structural inequalities, but a way of readapting marginalised groups to the existing order.

This approach renders invisible the historical, political, and class-based sources of poverty and exclusion by reducing the problem to individual behaviour, motivation, or skill deficits. As a result, football programmes may function less as engines of social change than as apparatuses of discipline and adaptation that reproduce social hierarchies. Put differently, a new form of governmentality may be established under the language of decommodification (Hartmann & Kwauk, 2011).

Similarly, development-oriented critiques show that football and sport are often articulated with a neoliberal imagination of citizenship. Especially in the context of the Global South, sport-based development programmes may seek to turn marginalised individuals into subjects suited to the norms of competitive capitalism, rather than interrogating the material and historical relations that produce inequality. In this framework, football is transformed from a space of solidarity and self-determination into an instrument for producing proper conduct, the right lifestyle, and successful individuals. By contrast, the critical approach argues that genuine decommodification is possible only through a rethinking both of football itself and of the development imaginary surrounding it: the issue is not simply to produce more programmes, but to break pedagogies that naturalise inequality, incorporate communities' own knowledge and experience into the process, and reconstruct the field of sport on the basis of self-determination (Darnell, 2013; Hartmann & Kwauk, 2011).

For this reason, football's value within social policy lies in its ability, when combined with broader public rights, to create a terrain of participation that partially suspends market logic. Football alone does not solve problems of housing, education, health, or employment. But when linked to these fields, it can generate a complementary common space that strengthens people's participation in social life. Youth-friendly clubs, low-cost access, local community support, connections with parents and schools, culturally responsive programme design, and forms of participation tailored to need are decisive in this respect. Football's decommodifying effect arises not from simply escaping the market, but from being reframed through principles of public responsibility, community embeddedness, and equal access (Collins & Kay, 2003; Coalter, 2007; Spaaij et al., 2014).

Football has the capacity to foster social inclusion and generate welfare effects. But this capacity is neither intrinsic, automatic, nor unlimited. Within a financialised football order, the discourse of social inclusion can operate in two opposite directions: it can either strengthen the game's dimensions of community, belonging, and public participation, thereby generating a decommodifying countertendency, or it can serve as a compensatory showcase that renders structural inequalities invisible. From the standpoint of social policy, the real question is under what institutional conditions football reduces market dependency, and under what conditions it instead reinforces the legitimacy of the financialised order. The conclusion is clear: football can open a decommodifying horizon only when organised in rights-based forms, publicly supported, collectively owned by communities, and structured in ways that do not individualise inequality. Otherwise, it remains a supplementary mechanism that softens the social costs of financialisation without eliminating them.

6. INEQUALITY, COMMODIFICATION, AND THE EXCLUSION OF SUPPORTERS: REPRESENTATION, RESISTANCE, AND DEMOCRATIC ALTERNATIVES

In football, commodification and financialisation are often discussed through broadcasting revenues, sponsorship, indebtedness, club valuations, or investor profiles. From a social-policy perspective, however, the central issue is how these transformations reorganise supportership along social and political lines. Financialisation does not simply mean that clubs generate more revenue; it also reshapes who counts as the club's legitimate constituency, who is recognised as a legitimate supporter, who can still find a place in the stadium, and whose voice is heard in decision-making. Supporter exclusion is therefore not a secondary cultural effect, but a constitutive outcome of contemporary football's financialised structure. High prices, customerisation, one-way communication, the weakening of local belonging, and governance organised around investor logic are all expressions of the same process (Brown, 2008; Cleland, 2010; Kennedy & Kennedy, 2013).

A first manifestation of this process is the shift in the club-supporter relationship from reciprocity and membership to customerhood. The traditional supporter relates to the club not solely through consumption, but through local history, community, loyalty, and mutual attachment. In the hyper-commodified order of football, by contrast, the supporter is increasingly treated as a revenue-generating market segment, and loyalty is measured through merchandise, subscriptions, broadcasting packages, and matchday spending. Attachment is thus recognised less as a public and moral bond than through the capacity to consume. The supporter is transformed not only economically, but politically: the customer is expected to spend, not to participate in governance or assert rights over the club. Financialisation therefore does not merely incorporate supporters into the market; it simultaneously excludes them from governance (Giulianotti, 2002; Cleland, 2010; Kennedy & Kennedy, 2013).

Supporter exclusion, however, cannot be reduced to ticket prices or physical access to the stadium. It is also a question of representation. Clubs have historically depended on the material and symbolic support of fans and, in many cases, on the assistance of local communities. Yet this support has rarely been transformed into lasting rights of representation. Empirical findings show that supporters experience their relationship with the club along a continuum of inclusion and exclusion, and that attachment and satisfaction tend to be higher where clubs develop two-way dialogue, forums, representative mechanisms, and institutional openness. Where one-way communication prevails, supporters are more likely to feel unheard and to view the club as no longer accountable to them. Exclusion in this sense is not a by-product of market relations, but an expression of democratic deficiency and monopolisation in governance (Cleland, 2010).

Nor does this process render supporters wholly passive. When financialisaton and customerisation reach certain thresholds, even groups that may once have appeared politically passive can develop channels of collective subjectivation. Fanzines, supporter forums, independent supporters' associations, digital platforms, and organised protests are therefore not merely forms of communication, but repertoires of political intervention directed against the reduction of the supporter to a customer. Supportership must thus be understood not only as emotional loyalty, but also as a form of citizenship practice claiming a right to shape the club's future. While financialisaton seeks to turn the supporter into a consumer, practices of resistance seek to pull the club back towards community, representation, and accountability. This tension is one of the clearest expressions, within supportership, of the broader opposition between decommodification and financialisaton (Cleland, 2010; Kennedy & Kennedy, 2013).

The deeper theoretical point is that football clubs cannot be reduced entirely to ordinary firms. They are, on the one hand, economic organisations measured through brand value, investment return, and competitive capacity; on the other, social institutions carrying history, locality, memory, and community. Supporters' reactions against commercial transformation should therefore not be dismissed as mere nostalgia. What is being contested is the subordination of the club's social and moral character to the logic of capital accumulation. The many intermediate positions that do not reject commercialisation altogether, yet resist defining the club solely in economic terms, arise from precisely this tension. The insistence that the club is not simply a company is itself a decommodifying claim: the club's social value cannot be equated with its market price (Kennedy & Kennedy, 2013; Millward, 2011).

This tension finds one of its clearest expressions in supporter ownership and democratic club initiatives. The case of F.C. United of Manchester is not merely a story of protest, but a concrete example of the institutional principles on which football can be reorganised in decommodifying ways. The reaction to the Glazer takeover did not remain a boycott; it developed into a club model based on one-member-one-vote, non-profit orientation, accessible prices, encouragement of youth and local participation, and an explicit commitment to limiting commercial logic. "Our club, our rules" is therefore not simply an emotional slogan, but a political claim about how football should be owned, governed, and directed. Here, the supporter is repositioned not as a customer, but as a founding subject and collective owner. In this sense, F.C. United remains one of the clearest examples of democratic decommodification within football (Brown, 2008).

This erosion of community-centred football is not unique to England. Barcelona's historically community-oriented and publicly legitimised identity, articulated around the slogan *Més que un club*, has also unravelled under commercial restructuring. A club that once treated the refusal of shirt sponsorship as an ethical marker later turned to paid sponsorships and, through the Spotify agreement, opened both shirt and stadium naming rights to global brand partnership. The placement of VIP seats at the centre of revenue strategy through the Personal Seat License model in the new Camp Nou project, together with continued insistence on the European Super League line, further indicates this shift. *Més que un club* may not have become meaningless, but it has increasingly moved from a founding principle of community-based exceptionalism to a symbolic legacy used to legitimise financialised restructuring (Kassing, 2019).

Yet such alternatives should not be romanticised. Supporter ownership does not mean complete escape from the market. Alternative clubs must still generate revenue, maintain facilities, remain competitive, and secure institutional sustainability. Nor is "community" a fixed or always inclusive category; new distinctions and exclusions around authenticity, loyalty, and "real" supportership may also emerge there. Debate around F.C. United has reflected this ambiguity: some have viewed it as a democratic and communal initiative, others as disloyalty to the parent club. Democratic supporter alternatives are therefore not an absolute solution to financialisaton, but contradictory yet important interventions aimed at limiting it, reframing it, and reconstructing football's social character (Brown, 2008; Millward, 2011).

The institutionalisation of supporter representation and participation is therefore the normative conclusion of this discussion. Supporters' Trusts, supporter forums, elected representative mechanisms, and two-way dialogue all seek to transform the club from a pure object of consumption into, at least partly, a negotiable community institution. Yet for such structures to become genuinely decommodifying, they must move beyond symbolic consultation and become binding and accountable. It is not enough for club management merely to speak with supporters; supporters must also be able to influence the club. Otherwise, the language of participation is reduced to an instrument for managing customer satisfaction. From a social-policy perspective, the crucial threshold lies here: the democratisation of football means not only cheaper access, but the reconstitution of the club as accountable to its community (Cleland, 2010; Kennedy & Kennedy, 2013).

Inequality and supporter exclusion in football are not secondary effects of financialisation, but forms of its social organisation. Customerisation, pricing, loss of representation, and cultural alienation are expressions of the process through which the club is redefined away from being a community entity and towards the logics of investment and brand. The resistance that develops in response is not merely nostalgic defence, but a decommodifying countermove aimed at democratising football and defending its public and community-based character. The central issue, therefore, is not only to diagnose the inequalities produced by commodification, but to consider which institutional forms might draw football back towards representation, access, and collective ownership. Although football is a field in which financialisaton is dominant, it still contains decommodifying possibilities through supporter ownership, democratic governance, and community-based accountability.

CONCLUSION

This study argues that contemporary football should be understood not merely as a commercialised entertainment industry, but as a contradictory social field in which decommodifying tendencies and financialising dynamics operate simultaneously. As the analysis has shown, the neoliberal transformation of football has tied supportership, media circulation, club governance, stadium space, and social inclusion more tightly to market logic. Debt, investment, brand value, broadcasting rights, paid access, mega-events, and the customerisation of supporters are all expressions of this financialisaton. In this respect, the dominant tendency in contemporary football is clear: the social value of the club is increasingly redefined through financial performance, revenue flow, and investment.

Yet football does not become a wholly ordinary commodity. Clubs remain institutions shaped by history, locality, memory, symbolic ownership, and community attachment. Demands for representation, struggles over access and publicness, the conditional value of social inclusion programmes, the stadium's sense of place, and democratic supporter ownership all show that football's decommodifying potential has not disappeared, even if it is often constrained or reabsorbed by financialised structures.

From a social-policy perspective, the key issue is therefore to identify the conditions under which football can sustain access, participation, representation, and collective ownership rather than deepen inequality. Football's decommodifying scope depends on equal access, community embeddedness, democratic governance, recognition of supporters as stakeholders, and stronger public responsibility. The central question is thus which institutional forms can preserve football's social and public character against thc growing dominance of financialisaton.

REFERENCES

Bale, J. (1993). *Sports, Space and The City*. Routledge. beIN Sports Türkiye. (2026). *Fenerbahçe stadının taşınması mümkün değildir*. https://beinsports.com.tr/haber/fenerbahce-stadinin-tasinmasi-mumkun-degildir

Boyle, R. (2015). Battle for control? Copyright, football and European television in the digital age. *International Journal of Digital Television*, *6*(1), 79–95.

Boyle, R., & Haynes, R. (2004). *Football in the New Media Age*. Routledge., DOI: 10.4324/9780203600467

Brown, A. (2008). 'Our club, our rules': Fan communities at FC United of Manchester. *Soccer and Society*, *9*(3), 346–358. DOI: 10.1080/14660970802008967

Cleland, J. (2017). The English Premier League in a global context. In Elliott, R., & Maguire, J. M. (Eds.), *The English Premier League: A socio-cultural analysis* (pp. 70–83). Routledge., DOI: 10.4324/9781315636696-6

Cleland, J. A. (2010). From passive to active: The changing relationship between supporters and football clubs. *Soccer and Society*, *11*(5), 537–552. DOI: 10.1080/14660970.2010.497348

Coalter, F. (2007). *A wider role for sport*. Routledge. DOI: 10.4324/9780203014615

Collins, M. F., & Kay, T. (2003). *Sport and Social Exclusion*. Routledge. DOI: 10.4324/9780203167267

Comitê Popular da Copa e Olimpíadas do Rio de Janeiro. (2012). *Mega-events and human rights violations in Rio de Janeiro: Dossier of the People's Committee for the World Cup and Olympics*. Rio on Watch.https://rioonwatch.org/wp-content/uploads/2013/05/2012-World-Cup-Olympics-Dossier-English.pdf

Darnell, S. C. (2013). *Sport for development and peace: A critical sociology*. Bloomsbury.

Evens, T., & Lefever, K. (2011). Watching the Football Game: Broadcasting Rights for the European Digital Television Market. *Journal of Sport and Social Issues*, *35*(1), 33–49. DOI: 10.1177/0193723510396665

Franck, E. P. (2013). Financial Fair Play in European Club Football—What is it All About? SSRN *Electronic Journal*. https://doi.org/DOI: 10.2139/ssrn.2284615

Geey, D. (2007). The legality of football broadcasts in the UK and the lack of choice for publicans in the Premier League broadcasting market. *Entertainment and Sports Law Journal*, *5*(1), 1–10. DOI: 10.16997/eslj.76

Giulianotti, R. (2002). Supporters, Followers, Fans, and Flaneurs: A Taxonomy of Spectator Identities in Football: A Taxonomy of Spectator Identities in Football. *Journal of Sport and Social Issues*, *26*(1), 25–46. DOI: 10.1177/0193723502261003

Giulianotti, R., & Robertson, R. (2004). The globalization of football: A study in the glocalization of the 'serious life'. *The British Journal of Sociology*, *55*(4), 545–568. DOI: 10.1111/j.1468-4446.2004.00037.x PMID: 15663424

Giulianotti, R., & Robertson, R. (2012). Mapping the global football field: A sociological model of transnational forces within the world game. *The British Journal of Sociology*, *63*(2), 216–240. DOI: 10.1111/j.1468-4446.2012.01407.x PMID: 22670645

Hartmann, D., & Kwauk, C. (2011). Sport and Development: An Overview, Critique, and Reconstruction. *Journal of Sport and Social Issues*, *35*(3), 284–305. DOI: 10.1177/0193723511416986

Hill, J. S., & Vincent, J. (2006). Globalisation and sports branding: The case of Manchester United. *International Journal of Sports Marketing & Sponsorship*, *7*(3), 61–78. DOI: 10.1108/IJSMS-07-03-2006-B008

Horne, J., & Manzenreiter, W. (2006). An Introduction to the Sociology of Sports Mega-Events. *The Sociological Review*, *54*(2), 1–24. DOI: 10.1111/j.1467-954X.2006.00650.x

Hutchins, B., & Rowe, D. (2012). *Sport Beyond Television*. Routledge. DOI: 10.4324/9780203120415

Kassing, J. W. (2019). "Mes que un club" and an empty Camp Nou: A case study of strategic ambiguity and Catalan nationalism at Football Club Barcelona. *International Journal of Sport Communication*, *12*(2), 260–274. DOI: 10.1123/ijsc.2018-0097

Kennedy, P., & Kennedy, D. (2013). *Football Supporters and the Commercialisation of Football: Comparative Responses across Europe*. Routledge.

King, A. (2016). *The European Ritual*. Routledge.

Millward, P. (2011). *The Global Football League*., DOI: 10.1057/9780230348639

Morrow, S. (2014). *Financial fair play: Implications for football club financial reporting*. Institute of Chartered Accountants of Scotland.

Niemann, A., Brand, A., & Weber, R. (2024). *Football Fandom and Identity in the 21st Century: Europe on Their Minds*. Springer Nature Switzerland., DOI: 10.1007/978-3-031-40631-7

Rohde, M., & Breuer, C. (2016). Europe's Elite Football: Financial Growth, Sporting Success, Transfer Investment, and Private Majority Investors. *International Journal of Financial Studies*, *4*(2), 2–20. DOI: 10.3390/ijfs4020012

Spaaij, R. (2012). Beyond the playing field: Experiences of sport, social capital, and integration among Somalis in Australia. *Ethnic and Racial Studies*, *35*(9), 1519–1538. DOI: 10.1080/01419870.2011.592205

Spaaij, R. F. J., Jeanes, R., & Magee, J. (2014). *Sport and social exclusion in global society*. Routledge. DOI: 10.4324/9780203066584

Storm, R. K., & Nielsen, K. (2012). Soft budget constraints in professional football. *European Sport Management Quarterly*, *12*(2), 183–201. DOI: 10.1080/16184742.2012.670660

Wilson, R., Plumley, D., & Ramchandani, G. (2013). The relationship between ownership structure and club performance in the English Premier League. *Sport, Business and Management*, *3*(1), 19–36. DOI: 10.1108/20426781311316889

Zimbalist, A. S. (2016). *Circus maximus: The economic gamble behind hosting the Olympics and the World Cup*. Brookings Institution Press. DOI: 10.5040/9780815751618

ENDNOTE

1 This sense of place is experienced concretely in the ordinary supporter's matchday routine. For a Fenerbahçe supporter, going to Kadıköy means more than watching a 90-minute match; it is a ritual extending from the walk to the stadium by ferry, metro, or Marmaray, to gatherings in and around Yoğurtçu Park, to encounters with shopkeepers and crowds in the market district, and to the recurring routes followed before and after the game. For this reason, although some criticise Chobani Stadium's location within the city on grounds of transport, traffic, and capacity, supporters do not see the issue as merely technical. Responding to renewed relocation debates in early 2026, Supreme Council President Şekip Mosturoğlu stated that moving the stadium was not possible and that the site was directly tied to the club's historical labour and memory of ownership (beIN Sports Türkiye, 2026). This is precisely what

underlies supporters' reaction: the stadium is not simply a venue for matches, but the material carrier of collective memory, neighbourhood attachment, and intergenerational routines of supportership.

Chapter 17
The Role of Sport Within Social, Legal, and Welfare Systems

Çiğdem Gökduman
http://orcid.org/0000-0003-3104-2409
Bartin University, Turkey

Hasan Aslan
http://orcid.org/0000-0003-3935-4124
Bartin University, Turkey

ABSTRACT

This chapter examines the transformation of sport from a relatively autonomous field of competition and entertainment into a multidimensional social, legal, and welfare domain. It analyzes how professionalization, commercialization, globalization, and media integration have increased the importance of labor rights, social security, and athlete welfare. The chapter particularly focuses on athletes' uncertain legal status, social risks, and working conditions within different welfare regimes, including Germany, the United Kingdom, Turkey, and China. Finally, it argues that athletes should be recognized as non-standard workers and that sport governance should adopt a welfare-oriented and rights-based approach grounded in social justice and sustainable social protection.

DOI: 10.4018/979-8-2600-3174-2.ch017

1. THE SOCIAL LAW PERSPECTIVE AND THE ROLE OF SPORT WITHIN THIS FRAMEWORK

People engage in sports activities for a wide variety of reasons, including health, fitness, relaxation, body awareness, entertainment, socialization, recognition, prestige, adventure, risk-taking, and pushing their personal limits (Heinemann, 2005). Due to this multidimensional structure, sports have been primarily addressed over the years through the lenses of performance, competition, entertainment, and organizational autonomy; it has largely been regarded as a distinct or exceptional domain governed by its own internal norms, institutional practices, and disciplinary mechanisms. Such an approach has laid the groundwork for the development of the understanding that sports partially lie outside the direct scope of general legal frameworks (Foster, 2012). Indeed, as a reflection of this approach, in many countries, sports-related relationships have been shaped not by the direct application of general legal doctrines, but rather within the framework of federation rules, club practices, informal regulations, and sector-specific traditions. This situation has led to the legal dimensions related to labor law, social protection, and public welfare remaining underdeveloped for a long time (Gardiner, 2012).

However, as we approach the present day, this approach has become increasingly unsustainable. Over the past thirty to forty years, sports have undergone profound structural transformations. These transformations in the field of sports have been shaped by a convergence of multifaceted factors, including the rise of professionalization in sports, the deepening of commercialization processes, the influence of globalization dynamics, the integration of sports with the media, the intensification of athlete mobility, and the growing economic weight of the sports industry. All these developments necessitate the repositioning of sports not merely as a sporting activity but within a broader legal and social framework (Gammelsaeter & Anagnostopoulos, 2022; Weatherill, 2017). Indeed, while sports were once perceived as a local activity that occasionally garnered government attention over the course of more than a century, today it has transformed into a global phenomenon that captures the attention of presidents, prime ministers, and monarchs. As sports have gained strategic importance on a global scale, states' awareness of sports, regulatory interest, and capacity for intervention have also increased significantly (Houlihan, 2002).

Consequently, sports today are not merely a voluntary leisure activity or a pursuit with cultural value. They are also a field of work, a means of generating income, an arena of physical risk, a realm of institutional dependency, and a domain of socio-economic vulnerability. This transformation necessitates that sports be reexamined not as an isolated sphere, but as a domain deeply embedded within the social fabric.

Social law encompasses the legal and institutional mechanisms aimed at protecting individuals against the social and economic risks arising from their participation in the workforce and their position within the social structure. Within this framework, labor law, social security law, social assistance systems, occupational health and safety, anti-discrimination norms, and public policies aimed at safeguarding social justice and human dignity fall within the scope of social law. The fundamental purpose of social law is not merely to ensure contractual order or protect private autonomy; rather, it is to address structural inequalities and protect vulnerable groups against market dependency, insecurity, and exclusion (Eichenhofer, 2015; International Labour Organization (ILO), 2026; Razavi, 2022). Therefore, when sports are examined from a social law perspective, they should be evaluated not merely as a domain of competition and institutional governance, but as a multidimensional field where rights, obligations, risks, inequalities, and protective mechanisms are both produced and distributed.

This perspective is of utmost importance in the context of sports. This is because the sports sector embodies the classic asymmetries that social law seeks to address. Athletes, coaches, referees, and other sports workers often operate under conditions such as short career spans, uncertain income structures, institutional dependency, the risk of injury, unequal bargaining power, and limited social protection. Although sports may appear to be a prestigious and attractive field from the outside, its internal dynamics can involve issues such as informality, uninsured work, low wages, and inadequate protection against risks such as career-ending injuries, illness, maternity, disability, and unemployment. For this reason, sports has become a field that must be analyzed not only through organizational or disciplinary frameworks but also through the normative language of social law (Gökduman, 2023; Gökduman et al., 2025).

1.1. The Scope of Social Law and Its Conceptual Importance in the Context of Sports

At the core of social law lies the recognition that individuals are not abstract and entirely autonomous actors; rather, they are vulnerable actors shaped by economic dependence, institutional power, and social needs. For this reason, social law deems legal intervention necessary in situations where market logic or contractual freedom alone cannot ensure justice. Within this framework, social law assumes both a protective and a redistributive function. Its protective aspect safeguards individuals against exploitation and risks, while its redistributive aspect aims to ensure access to social rights and services throughout the life cycle (Hennessy, 2023; Mayrhofer, 2025).

When this approach is applied to the field of sports, it brings about a significant analytical shift. Sports are no longer viewed merely as an autonomous domain with its own set of rules, but also as a sphere where social risks and legal statuses are defined (O'Leary et al., 2025). In this context, the following questions take on particular importance: Under what conditions do athletes work? What social risks are they exposed to? Are they protected in cases of injury, illness, maternity, disability, or retirement? How are income security and career continuity ensured? What is the legal status of athletes vis-à-vis clubs, federations, and other stakeholders? Are they employees or independent contractors?

These questions demonstrate that the world of sports is not a homogeneous field and that different groups have varying levels of protection. For example, while elite athletes competing in top-tier professional leagues enjoy certain safeguards, female athletes, amateurs, semi-professionals, and athletes in lower leagues may face significant gaps in protection. Consequently, a social justice approach brings to light the internal inequalities within the sports sector.

1.2. Sports as a "Special Domain" and Its Resistance to Legal Regulation

For many years, sports have been regarded as an autonomous domain governed by its own rules; this approach is rooted in the fact that sports have historically developed through private organizations such as clubs and federations, are defined by cultural values such as fair play, belonging, and competition, and are dominated by the concept of amateurism. Within this framework, the economic and legal dimensions of sports remained in the background for a long time, and in some legal systems, the reluctance of judicial bodies to intervene in the technical structure of sports further reinforced this perception. Nevertheless, sports has not been a domain entirely outside the law; it has developed its own distinctive normative order through elements such as disciplinary rules, transfer systems, doping regulations, and internal dispute resolution mechanisms within federations. However, this framework has often fallen short in comprehensively addressing issues that intersect with fundamental rights areas such as labor, health, social security, and equality (Kamenecka-Usova et al., 2025; Panagiotopoulos, 2016; Serby, 2017).

Today, however, the transformation of sports into an economic sector has eroded this concept of autonomy. Athletes now generate significant economic value, operate within a framework of institutional dependence, and are exposed to high risks. For this reason, the notion of viewing sports as a purely private sphere is increasingly losing its validity.

1.3. The Relationship Between Sports and Labor Law

Modern sports share many similarities with traditional employment relationships. The fact that athletes operate under specific instructions, generate economic value through performance, and work within organizational structures has brought the issue of evaluating sports within the scope of labor law to the forefront. In this context, the legal status of athletes emerges as a decisive factor; for if they are recognized as employees, they would be able to benefit from fundamental protective mechanisms such as wages, job security, working hours, and social rights. However, uncertainties regarding athletes' legal status persist in many countries, leading to significant losses of rights. Furthermore, while contracts in the sports sector may appear formally equitable, in reality, this equality is limited when considering the power imbalances between the parties. Therefore, the social law perspective offers an approach that goes beyond contractual freedom to account for the structural dependency relationships in which athletes find themselves (De Keyzer, 2023; O'Leary et al., 2025; SUPIOT, 2020).

Indeed, when the organizational structure of sports activities is examined, it becomes evident that many athletes actually experience the fundamental elements of an employment relationship. In terms of the fundamental principles of work execution, athletes who are economically and organizationally dependent on their clubs, federations, or sports organizations largely experience the elements of "performance of work," "subordination," and "wages"—classic components of an employment contract—in a manner similar to that of workers. Similarly, the athlete's primary source of income is often derived from their main activity—sports—and the level of income earned is directly linked to their athletic performance, productivity, and professional continuity. In this regard, athletics should be regarded not merely as a voluntary activity but also as a labor-based professional form of work.

1.4. The Relationship Between Sports and Social Security Law

Although athletes operate in a field that inherently involves a high level of physical and psychological risk, they often lack social security protection commensurate with these risks (Gökduman, 2023). Factors such as sports injuries, the short and intermittent nature of careers, and income instability increase athletes' vulnerability to social risks and make the need for social security even more apparent.

In this context, although sports injuries are often viewed as a natural part of athletic activity, they are not sufficiently defined or comprehensively regulated under occupational risk provisions in most legal systems. Similarly, athletes' access to retirement, disability, and health benefits is often limited; this situation leaves athletes facing significant social risks not only during their active careers but also after their careers end (Gökduman, 2023; Gökduman et al., 2025).

Therefore, sports must be addressed in a systematic and comprehensive manner within the framework of social security law. Given the nature and intensity of the risks faced by athletes, it is clear that the social security mechanisms to be developed in this field are not a privilege but a necessary protective measure in line with the principles of social justice and equality. In this regard, sports stands out as a unique field of work with its own specific risk structure, deserving of special consideration within social security systems.

1.5. The Role of Sports in Social Policy

Sports play a multifaceted and two-way role within the context of social policy. While it is positioned as a tool that enhances social welfare, supports social integration, and strengthens public health, it must also be viewed as a field that generates and redistributes various social risks within its own structure. In this regard, sports is not merely an instrument of social policy but also a policy area requiring direct intervention (Seltmann, 2026).

In traditional approaches, sports policies have largely been shaped around the axes of performance, international success, and competitiveness. However, this approach often relegates fundamental aspects of the sports production process—such as athletes' well-being, working conditions, and social security—to a secondary role (De Bosscher et al., 2021; Westerbeek & Eime, 2021). Yet the structural risks athletes face necessitate addressing sports from a social policy perspective.

In this context, sports policies must be restructured to move away from a narrow focus on athletic performance alone and adopt a rights-based and people-centered approach. Athletes' access to social protection systems, the improvement of working conditions, support for career continuity, and increasing the participation of disadvantaged groups in sports should be among the core priorities of social policy in the sports sector. In this way, sports can be repositioned not merely as a tool for generating social benefits, but as a field that must be organized in accordance with the principles of social justice, equality, and well-being.

1.6. The Relationship Between Sports and Social Law at the Global Level

The professionalization and commercialization of sports on a global scale have necessitated a reassessment of athletes' legal status and levels of protection. As sports have evolved into an economic sector, athletes' position within production processes has become more visible; this has increased the need for legal protection regarding their working conditions, social rights, and the risks they face. Indeed, discussions regarding the social protection of athletes have intensified in the international literature and policy documents. However, the fragmented nature of existing regulations, uncertainties regarding legal status, and institutional differences in implementation significantly limit athletes' access to an effective and inclusive social protection system (Fiege, 2025). Moreover, the globalization and commercialization of sports competitions, along with athletes' growing role as key actors in this field, are giving rise to new challenges and regulatory needs from the perspective of different countries' legal systems (Oleksii, 2025: 95).

In this context, sports should be viewed not merely as a cultural or recreational activity, but also as a field of work that generates multifaceted social risks and requires the management of these risks. Athletes' short and precarious career structures, their exposure to high physical and psychological risks, and their often uncertain legal statuses necessitate an examination of this field from a social law perspective. The social law approach evaluates the protection of athletes not as a privilege-based regulation but within the framework of the principles of social justice and equality; it contributes to the construction of a more inclusive, sustainable, and people-centered structure in the sports sector.

2. WELFARE REGIMES AND THE GOVERNANCE OF SPORT

The most common definition of welfare regimes is Esping-Andersen's 1990 classification of the welfare state. According to him, social rights and the stratification of the welfare state are based on qualitative differences between the state, the market, and the family: (i) Liberal regimes associated with means-tested assistance, modest universal transfers, or a modest social insurance system; (ii) Corporatist regimes where market efficiency and the value of commodification are not prioritized, rights are based on status and class, where private insurance is marginal, and which are strongly committed to preserving the church and, consequently, the traditional family structure; and (iii) regimes where social democracy is the dominant force, which, rather than tolerating a dichotomy between the state and the market or between the working class and the middle class, promote equality at the highest standards, do not promote equality at minimum standards, where a social insurance system covering all working groups constrains the market, socializes the costs of family life by providing direct transfers to children, and enhances the capacity for individual independence—these are the three fundamental models (Esping-Andersen, 1990: 26–28).

Over time, certain additions have been made to this widely accepted three-country model. For example, in 1992, Leibfried proposed a fourth model to Esping-Andersen's three-country model, which included the Latin Rim countries (Heinemann, 2005). According to him, although the southern countries of Western Europe (Spain, Portugal, Greece, and to some extent Italy and France) had adapted to the EU by the 1980s, they had established their own distinct welfare regimes. It has been noted that this regime, which in some respects resembles the Anglo-Saxon model, emphasizes mandatory entry into the labor market. On the other hand, while their constitutions strongly emphasize the "modern welfare state," it is also observed that traditional welfare traditions linked to the Catholic Church continue to be upheld (Leibfried, 1996).

Like Leibfried, Ferrera (1996) has also applied the Southern Model of Welfare to Italy, Spain, Portugal, and Greece. According to him, these countries feature a fragmented and corporatist income protection system that combines generous pension benefits with significant coverage gaps; partially universalist practices in the health sector; and, in the welfare sphere, low levels of state intervention alongside patronage and clientelistic relationships. In his study on social assistance, Gough (1996) classified Turkey, along with Italy, Spain, Portugal, and Greece, within the Southern European Welfare Regime. According to him, social assistance in these countries is low or virtually nonexistent, representing a divergence from the rest of Europe. There is no minimum income security; while categorical assistance exists for the elderly, local discretionary powers take precedence for other segments of the population.

Welfare regimes are systems that explain how the state protects individuals against social risks, how resources are distributed, and through which institutional mechanisms social policies are implemented. For this reason, welfare regimes encompass not only social security systems but also a broad range of policy areas such as education, health, employment, family policies, and leisure services. In modern societies, sports have evolved beyond being merely a cultural or recreational activity; they have become a multifaceted public policy domain that contributes to physical and psychological well-being, supports social integration, strengthens public health, and creates employment. Consequently, the organizational structure, financing, access framework, and governance of sports cannot be considered independently of the overarching logic of the welfare regime adopted by a country. For a country's welfare regime not only determines in which areas and to what extent the state intervenes in social life but also shapes how sports are positioned as a public good, a market product, or a social right (Ibsen et al., 2022).

2.1. The Concept of the Welfare State and Its Relationship to Sports

In its broadest sense, the concept of the welfare state refers to the division of responsibilities among the state, the market, and the family. This division determines the level of protection individuals receive against social risks and their access to social services. Sports policies are also shaped within this tripartite structure. In some countries, the state serves as the primary financier and regulator of sports; in others, market actors and the private sector may play a more decisive role. In yet other systems, local governments and civil society organizations assume significant roles (Seltmann, 2026).

In addition to areas such as education, culture, youth, and labor market policies, sports policy also falls within the scope of the welfare state. This is because the state is responsible for ensuring that all members of society enjoy a minimum level of physical well-being and economic security, and that everyone can participate in the social and cultural life of society according to their abilities, interests, and preferences. The welfare state integrates individuals into social and cultural life by (i) providing equal access to life opportunities for all members of society and (ii) ensuring equality in the distribution of material goods and services to guarantee a minimum standard of living (Heinemann, 2005). In this context, sports fulfill three fundamental functions within welfare regimes:

First, there is the function of social integration. Sports are viewed as a tool that brings together different social groups, strengthens a sense of social belonging, and reduces social exclusion. Sports are considered an important avenue for social participation, particularly for young people, immigrants, and disadvantaged groups (Höglund & Bruhn, 2024; Spaaij, 2012).

Second, there is the public health function. Promoting physical activity is recognized as a key policy tool in the fight against obesity, chronic diseases, and mental health issues. For this reason, many welfare states have made sports and exercise an integral part of their health policies (Warburton & Bredin, 2019; World Health Organization (WHO), 2020).

Third, it serves the function of job creation. The sports sector provides a wide range of employment opportunities through professional athletes, coaches, managers, healthcare personnel, media workers, and various support services. In this regard, sports is directly linked to economic development and labor markets (Andreff, 2011).

These three functions demonstrate that sports is not merely an individual activity but also a public policy domain.

2.2. Typology of Welfare States and Sports Policies

The concept of the welfare state emerged in Western societies in the post-World War II era. At the same time, an increasing number of governments have become actively involved in the formulation of sports-related policies. Public authorities began providing subsidies to voluntary sports organizations, while national and local governments became active providers of sports by organizing sports programs and hosting prestigious sporting events (Scheerder, et al., 2017).

On the other hand, sports policies may vary across different welfare regimes. For example, in his study, Heinemann (2005) examined the relationship between welfare regimes and sports systems in six European countries (Denmark, the United Kingdom, Germany, France, Italy, and Spain). The study demonstrates how the welfare state maintains its distinct position and influence over sports even when sports and welfare systems in these countries have different historical origins and are based on different ideologies and organizational structures.

Welfare regimes have a direct impact on the financing, organization, and level of protection for athletes.

2.2.1. Sports and the Protection of Athletes in the German Welfare System

The Bismarckian welfare system is based on a social insurance framework and refers to a system in which rights are largely contingent on employment status. Germany is one of the most typical examples of this model (Pennings, 2022). In Germany, general social rights are regulated by the German Social Code. When examined from the perspective of athletes, there are no general provisions nor any sport-specific legal regulations that specifically affect the social protection or employment relationships of elite athletes (Mittag et al., 2025).

On the other hand, Germany's state sports policy is shaped by the Federal Ministry of the Interior (BMI) and the 16 state governments. While the BMI is responsible for elite sports, the development of grassroots sports falls under the jurisdiction of the state governments. The non-governmental sector is represented by the German Olympic Sports Confederation (DOSB), which acts as the umbrella organization advocating for the interests of its member organizations before the state and the public. To ensure adequate national representation and success in international sports competitions, the BMI collaborates with the DOSB (Breuer & Nowy, 2017). Elite athletes participating in the Olympics are required to sign an athlete agreement. This document automatically expires on the final day of the Olympics. While the agreement outlines the athlete's rights and obligations, the DOSB covers the costs associated with the Olympics (Mittag et al. 2022).

In accordance with a resolution of the German Bundestag, public-private partnerships are being established to improve the level of retirement benefits for athletes after they reach retirement age. Elite athletes who hold the roster/support status designated by the German Sport Aid Foundation (DSH)—a private organization responsible for the development and promotion of national elite sports—receive up to €250 per month in public support for a retirement plan they have signed with a private insurance company (Fiege, 2025: 247). The German Sport Aid Foundation has been supporting elite athletes since 1967. All German elite athletes who are members of the national team can benefit from this private organization's financial and non-financial support (career training, mentoring, workshops, etc.). In principle, all athletes in Olympic and Paralympic sports are eligible for support from the

German Sport Aid Foundation. However, a decision may be made not to provide financial support for certain sports. This applies to some professional sports where athletes can generate sufficient income from their contracts with clubs. Decisions are made separately for each sport, with distinctions made across different disciplines and gender categories (e.g., men's soccer: youth and senior; women's soccer: senior; men's ice hockey, men's handball, etc.) (Mittag, et al., 2022).

Germany is home to nearly 86,000 sports clubs with 28.8 million members (BMI, 2026). By placing particular value on a sense of community and social interaction, these clubs distinguish themselves from commercial sports providers. An increasing number of sports clubs are collaborating with other social service providers—such as schools, other sports clubs, kindergartens, and health insurance companies—to offer sports programs. These clubs make a significant contribution to the population's health services. More than one-third of the clubs offer programs aimed at health promotion, prevention, and rehabilitation. This includes services provided for people with disabilities and chronic illnesses (Breuer & Feiler, 2015).

In Germany, public sector employment opportunities are also available to athletes. A significant number of athletes are employed by various ministries and serve the country through organizations such as the armed forces or the police. There are approximately 800 positions available for athletes in the armed forces. Athlete-soldiers are generally exempt from military duties so they can focus on their athletic development. The German Federal Police also offers a dual-career model for athletes in 21 selected sports, primarily winter sports. Up to 160 athletes can participate in the program. In addition, athletes have the opportunity to work in customs and state police forces (Mittag et al., 2022). Athletes not enrolled in such public programs may qualify as self-employed (depending on their level of taxable income), or their legal status may stem from activities outside their sports careers (e.g., student, employee, or unemployed). Athletes generally have access to general welfare services that are not specific to them. (i) Athletes under the age of 18 residing in Germany receive the monthly universal Child Benefit, (ii) an additional pregnancy-related allowance for pregnant athletes eligible for Citizen's Benefit, (iii) Citizen's Benefit for athletes who are seeking employment and capable of working, (iv) lifelong compensation for athletes performing voluntary or temporary military service in the event of injury, (v) a stipend in the event of illness, (vi) health insurance for elite athletes, (vii) means-tested basic income for individuals aged 67 and over who lack sufficient income and assets, (viii) a pension, rehabilitation, and integration assistance for the disabled and those with disabilities, (ix) a survivor's pension and death grant for the surviving spouse and children after death—these are some of the benefits (Mittag et al., 2025).

The government assumes a regulatory and supportive role rather than intervening directly. Athletes' social security rights, however, depend largely on their legal status.

While professional athletes are covered by social insurance to a certain extent, the level of protection for amateur and semi-professional athletes may be more limited (Coalter, 2007; Palier, 2010).

In summary, the civil society-based organizational structure of sports in Germany is quite robust. Sports policies are largely implemented through well-established club structures, volunteer-based associations, and federations (Houlihan, 2007). Sports clubs are viewed not merely as institutions where athletic activities take place, but also as important social tools that support social integration. This structure ensures that sports are positioned as a functional mechanism within the welfare system, strengthening social participation, promoting solidarity, and enhancing social cohesion.

2.2.2. Sports and the Protection of Athletes in the United Kingdom's Welfare System

The Beveridge-type welfare system is based on a structure that relies heavily on taxation and emphasizes the provision of universal services. The United Kingdom is one of the key examples of this model. In this system, sports policies operate within a framework where state-supported programs and market mechanisms work in tandem. Sports are strongly linked to public health policies. Increasing physical activity is among the top priorities for safeguarding public health (McCrone, 2025; Meir & Fletcher, 2020; Sessa, 2020). The UK welfare model features a dual structure. Healthcare services are provided universally through the NHS, but many income-related benefits are tied to employment history and National Insurance records. This situation creates challenges for elite athletes, who often operate outside standard employment structures and may face fragmented income arrangements, limited formal contracts, or grant-based support systems (Cattaneo, 2025).

There is no specific legislation in UK law governing the social protection of athletes (Cattaneo, 2025), however, the status of sport in the country has evolved from an underfunded, strategically neglected sector on the periphery of the government's agenda in the early 1990s to a source of social cohesion and national pride, and a partner in achieving the government's broader social, political, and economic objectives by the 2010s. UK Sport is the government agency responsible for elite sports and funds sports disciplines in the Olympic and Paralympic Games program through the World Class Programme; both agencies allocate their funds according to predetermined targets, and failure to meet these targets may result in the withdrawal or reduction of funding. The Department for Culture, Media and Sport is the public body responsible for implementing the "sport for all" policy and assisting in achieving objectives related to elite-level sporting success. On the other hand, many small clubs lack real power and have only limited resources. (Girginov, 2017).

UK Sport offers grants known as the Athlete Performance Award (APA) and the Personal Development Award (PDA). The APA aims to help high-performance athletes cover living expenses and professional development costs, while the PDA is designed to support goals such as education and career-focused development. Additionally, athletes under the World Class Programme receive individual coaching and mentoring services in areas such as career development, mental health and well-being, education, financial health, and learning and development; health insurance is also provided under the Athlete Medical Scheme (UK Sport, 2026). However, the Athlete Agreement signed under the World Class Programme does not constitute an employment contract, and the public grant under the APA does not confer employment status (Cattaneo, 2025). Due to this legal status, the athletes in question are excluded from the protective mechanisms provided by labor law.

In the United Kingdom, elite athletes may also be included in the Army Elite Sport Programme. To qualify, they must be employed by the military as enlisted personnel or officers and demonstrate their talent as elite athletes. Their primary obligation is to serve as soldiers in the military (O'Learly, et al. 2025: 258–259). Social protection provided through public sector employment—unlike in Germany—involves first being employed as a soldier and then qualifying for the elite athlete program based on demonstrated success (Fiege, 2025: 243). Athletes serving in the British Armed Forces are eligible for the Armed Forces Pension Scheme (AFPS). This plan is a fully government-funded, contribution-free occupational pension scheme based on career average earnings and length of service. Military athletes have full access to military pension benefits, including automatic pension accrual and early retirement options under certain conditions. The AFPS provides a level of pension security unmatched by other segments of the UK's athlete population and represents a significant exception to the general uncertainty surrounding retirement planning in elite sport. Beyond this, elite athletes have no statutory or automatic pension entitlement simply by virtue of being selected for the national team or an elite program, nor is there an incentive mechanism for a voluntary national plan (Cattaneo, 2025: 91).

The level of commercialization in sports is quite high in the United Kingdom, and professional sports are largely driven by market actors. This situation can lead to certain inequalities emerging between elite sports and mass sports.

In summary, as in Germany, the state in the UK has delegated the responsibility to protect athletes' social rights to private (sports) organizations; since widespread neoliberal athlete pension plans are in place, elite athletes do not have equal access to basic social protection provisions like other citizens or workers (Fiege, 2025: 247). In general, social protection rights consist of general social security rights (Cattaneo, 2025).

2.2.3. Sports and the Protection of Athletes in the Turkish Welfare Regime

Mixed welfare regimes are systems that incorporate both Bismarckian and Beveridge-type characteristics. Turkey can be classified under this model.

In Turkey, sports have evolved beyond being merely an individual pursuit or a social activity; it has become an institutional field directly shaped by public policies, supported by the state, and promoted through various means. In this context, financial resources are allocated to sports federations, and efforts are made to strengthen sports infrastructure through legal, administrative, and institutional regulations (Karagöz, 2025). The governance structure of sports in Turkey is largely centralized, and the state's role in policy-making, resource allocation, and institutional coordination processes is quite prominent. Sports policies are primarily implemented through public institutions and federations. However, in recent years, parallel to the growth of the sports economy, the influence of the private sector, sponsorship mechanisms, and market actors on the sports sector has been observed to be increasing (Tinaz et al., 2014).

The Labor Code does not apply to the employment relationships of athletes; instead, the Civil Code and federation rules apply. When comparing the provisions of the Labor Code and the Civil Code, the Civil Code establishes more general rules governing employment relationships. For example, while the Labor Code provides job security for workers who meet certain conditions, the Civil Code does not recognize such a right. Similarly, the notice periods required for the termination of indefinite-term employment contracts and the duration of annual leave are shorter under the Civil Code and do not provide the same level of protection as the Labor Code. As Öztuna (2015) notes, athletes are also deprived of the right to severance pay, which is an important right for workers.

The social security coverage for athletes in Turkey presents a heterogeneous picture. While top-level professional athletes have certain safeguards and may be included in mandatory insurance coverage, significant gaps in protection persist for amateur and semi-professional athletes. This situation indicates that the social law dimension of sports has not yet been fully institutionalized and that status-based inequalities among athletes continue to exist (Social Security Institution, 2026).

Indeed, in 1997, a voluntary "community insurance" model was proposed to provide insurance coverage for amateur athletes; however, this initiative achieved only limited coverage and failed to become a permanent institution. This regulation was repealed during the 2008 social security reform process (Karagöz, 2025: 134–136). Consequently, there is currently no independent insurance model specifically tailored for athletes within the Turkish social insurance system, which is mandatory. This situation creates significant gaps, particularly regarding long-term social risks such as old age, disability, unemployment, loss of income, and livelihood security after retirement; it makes it difficult for individuals to pursue sports as a sustainable "primary profession."

On the other hand, when evaluated in terms of non-contributory social protection mechanisms, it is evident that both the central government and local governments provide various services (Sözer, 2020). According to the Municipalities Law, municipalities "may, when necessary, provide sports equipment to young people to promote sports, offer in-kind and monetary assistance to amateur sports clubs and provide the necessary support, organize all kinds of amateur sports competitions, and award prizes—by decision of the municipal council—to students, athletes, technical managers, and coaches who achieve outstanding success or win awards in domestic and international competitions." However, any decisions made in this regard must not exceed the specified limits of budget revenues. The central government, on the other hand, grants a "sportsman's honorary allowance" to Turkish athletes who achieve success individually or as part of a team in Olympic, World, and European championships, and provides a monthly allowance to the family members of such athletes in the event of their death. Additionally, the title of "State Athlete" is granted to successful athletes who have not received a lifetime ban for offenses such as violence, match-fixing, or doping in sports. Athletes holding this title are entitled to use VIP lounges and obtain a special stamped passport.

On the other hand, cash prizes may be awarded to athletes or teams who place in competitions such as the Olympic Games, Paralympic Games, World and European Championships, Deaflympics, Universiade, and Mediterranean Games, either as a lump sum or in installments. Additionally, athletes selected for the national team are insured under a special insurance system against all types of accidents, illnesses, and injuries from the start of pre-competition training camps until they return to their residence after the competition. The Ministry of Youth and Sports trains a specified number (8,000) of athletes to prepare for the Olympics, and provides these athletes with sports-related nutrition, housing, and travel expenses, as well as a monthly allowance. National athletes may be appointed as physical education teachers provided they meet all requirements except for the condition of passing the public service selection exam, which is required to become a public servant in Turkey.

However, the limitations of public social security mechanisms and the failure of the current system to adequately address risks specific to the sports sector have increased the need for alternative protection mechanisms for athletes. In parallel with this development, private insurance practices have become increasingly widespread in Turkey over the past decade, driven by the dynamics of globalization and the influence of neoliberal policy trends. From the athletes' perspective, it is observed that private insurance solutions against economic, physical, and occupational risks arising from sports activities have become more prominent. Indeed, as noted by

Kocaoğlu (2023), athlete liability insurance, athlete life insurance, athlete accident insurance, athlete health and illness insurance, and athlete group insurance are among the primary private insurance applications developed in this field. On the other hand, as noted by Aydın and colleagues (Aydın, et al. 2017: 1881), soccer clubs are required to obtain private insurance through companies designated by the federation to cover potential risks such as accidents, injuries, disability, and death for professional soccer players. However, the study also found that, despite this requirement, 55.7% of the football players surveyed did not have any private insurance.

2.2.4. Sports and the Protection of Athletes in the Chinese Welfare Regime

East Asian welfare regimes refer to structures in which the state assumes a strong and guiding role in economic and social spheres, while social security systems are more limited and selective in nature compared to Western European models. China stands out as one of the most notable examples of this model in the realm of sports. Indeed, sports have long been an integral part of the Chinese state's policy agenda. In particular, the steady rise in elite sports achievements over the past few decades, hosting major events such as the Olympic Games, China's increasing interaction with international sports organizations, and developments in the processes of professionalization and commercialization of sports have further heightened the strategic importance of sports within public policies (Zheng, et al., 2018). In China, during the mid-1980s, alongside the reform of the urban economic system and the development of a market economy, the social security system was restructured, with a focus on pension, health, and unemployment insurance. Subsequently, the responsibilities of the social security system began to be shared among the state, local governments, institutions, and individuals (Sheng, 2017). In this context, social security policies have undergone significant developments over the past 40 years in line with social and economic changes. In recent years, China—which can be described as a hybrid of three welfare regimes—has established a cooperative health system covering the rural population, social health insurance for urban residents without income, a social pension system, and others (Gencer, 2017).

In China, sports are largely organized under state control, with a particular emphasis on elite sports policies. Olympic success and international competition are among the primary motivations driving sports policies. This situation leads to the use of sports as a tool for national prestige and political power (Chen & Hou, 2025; García & Smokvina, 2025; Ma & Ji, 2024). To this end, the country published Olympic Strategies in 1995 and 2001 (Ling and Hong, 2014). The 1995 "Physical Culture and Sports Law" of the People's Republic of China, the primary regulatory framework in the sports sector, does not define professional sports or athletes, nor does it distinguish between amateur and professional athletes. These legal gaps result in a fragmented regulatory framework implemented through local government regulations, internal rules of sports federations, and the application of general labor law (Oleksii, 2025).

China's rise in the sports arena in recent years has made it a major player in global sports competition. In particular, its rivalry with the United States at the Olympics demonstrates that sports can also be used as a geopolitical tool. According to data from the International Olympic Committee (IOC, 2026), China, which tied with the United States for the most gold medals at the 2024 Paris Olympics, ranks second behind the United States in total medal count. A similar pattern has been observed in the Summer Olympics since the 2008 Beijing Games.

Although China has achieved success on the international stage, it faces some criticism regarding the social protection of its athletes. For example, due to the decentralized nature of regulations in China, there is a reliance on decisions made by local authorities and sports federations; this leads to heterogeneity in legal regulations across different regions and sports disciplines (Oleksii, 2025). On the other hand, as Sheng (2017) notes, while China's most successful athletes generally do not worry about their livelihoods, the majority of grassroots athletes have weak safeguards. Similarly, there are policy gaps in the management of social security funds, workplace accident prevention and rehabilitation, disability protection, and other areas, and fraud in the insurance fund is a fundamental criticism of the system. As Ling and Hong (2014) noted, unlike top-tier athletes who can find employment opportunities in sports management, coaching, physical education teaching, the media or film industry, or overseas jobs after retirement; other athletes—including some world champions—may end up working in ordinary jobs (factory work, security guarding, dancing, street vending, etc.). Some elite athletes, meanwhile, struggle with unemployment and disability.

Generally speaking, different welfare systems directly influence the priorities and implementation methods of sports policies. In Bismarckian systems, sports are primarily club-based and focused on social participation, whereas in the Beveridge model, the dimensions of public health and public service take center stage. In mixed systems, the state's decisive role operates in tandem with market dynamics. In the East Asian model, elite sports and international success goals are the determining factors. These differences also have significant impacts on athletes' working conditions, social security rights, and career trajectories. For example, while athletes in some systems enjoy more comprehensive social security rights, these rights may remain limited in others. Consequently, the governance of sports reflects not only sports policies but also the overall structure of welfare regimes. This underscores once again why it is necessary to examine sports from a social law perspective (Chen & Hou, 2025; Tinaz et al., 2014; Whiting et al., 2025).

3. ATHLETES AS NON-STANDARD WORKERS IN WELFARE REGIMES

The transformation that sports has undergone in recent years has fundamentally reshaped the nature of sports participation. In this context, while sports are associated with performance, competition, and public visibility, they increasingly exhibit labor characteristics that challenge traditional legal classifications. In this context, athletes should no longer be analyzed merely as participants in voluntary or recreational activities, but rather as workers operating under non-standard and often precarious conditions within broader welfare regimes (O'Leary et al., 2025; Seltmann, 2026).

The concept of "non-standard work" refers to forms of employment that deviate from the traditional model of full-time, permanent employment with social protection. This category includes temporary contracts, part-time work, freelance work, informal employment, and other forms of work characterized by instability and limited social protection. Athletes largely fall into this category across various sports and levels of participation. While athletes' working conditions encompass elements such as economic dependence, institutional oversight, and exposure to high risks, they simultaneously lack the stability and protective mechanisms associated with standard employment (Aykaç & Kaya, 2024).

3.1. Structural Characteristics of Athletes' Labor

One of the most distinctive features of athletes' labor is its inherently temporary nature. Unlike traditional career paths, athletic careers are typically short, intermittent, and highly uncertain. Contracts are mostly fixed-term, renewed based on performance, and can end abruptly due to injury, a decline in performance, or organizational decisions. This transience creates structural vulnerability by forcing athletes to constantly seek new opportunities in an extremely competitive and uncertain environment (Gökduman, 2023).

Another closely related factor is career fragility. Athletic careers are not only short-lived but also heavily dependent on factors beyond the athletes' control. Injuries, coaching staff changes, organizational restructuring, and market dynamics can suddenly alter the course of a career. Even in the absence of injuries, performance-based evaluation systems create constant pressure and insecurity. While experience typically leads to greater stability in many professions, athletic careers often reach their peak early and experience a rapid decline. This situation limits the ability to build financial security and make long-term plans.

Another critical aspect is the situation that can be described as the "high-risk–short-term paradox." Athletes operate in environments that involve significant physical and mental risks, such as acute injuries, chronic health issues, psychological stress, and burnout. However, these high-risk conditions are often combined with careers that are short-term and do not provide long-term security. This paradox further underscores the need for effective social protection mechanisms, especially when considering that the effects of these risks extend beyond the active athletic career and impact life after sports.

3.2. Unprotected Dependency: The Legal Uncertainty of Athletes

Although athletic activity shares characteristics with labor, athletes often occupy an uncertain legal position within welfare systems. In many cases, they are neither fully recognized as workers nor considered entirely independent actors. This intermediate or undefined status has significant implications regarding access to rights and protective mechanisms. In this context, athletes generally operate under conditions of institutional dependency. They work under the direction of coaches, adhere to specific programs, are subject to strict performance and behavioral rules, and contribute to the production of economic and symbolic value for clubs and federations. These elements point to a relationship of dependency similar to an employment relationship. However, legal classification often fails to reflect this reality.

This situation gives rise to a problem that could be described as "unprotected dependency." While athletes are subject to obligations similar to those in employment relationships, they are unable to benefit from rights such as social insurance, job security, or collective bargaining. This situation is particularly pronounced in lower leagues, at the semi-professional level, and in less commercialized sports.

From a social law perspective, this uncertainty poses a serious problem. This is because social law aims to protect individuals who are economically dependent and at risk. The fact that athletes cannot be clearly categorized under any legal framework may result in their exclusion from this protective framework.

3.3. Non-Standard Work and Exposure to Social Risks

Non-standard forms of work are generally associated with increased social risks, and this is clearly evident in the sports sector. Athletes face multi-layered risks.

First and foremost is the risk of income insecurity. Athletes' incomes are often irregular, performance-based, and unevenly distributed. While a small number of elite athletes earn high incomes, the vast majority live on fluctuating and limited incomes. This situation makes it difficult to access social security systems that rely on regular income and uninterrupted premium payments.

Second, there are occupational injuries and health risks. Sports activities themselves involve physical risks. Injuries are often not exceptional but rather a natural part of performance. Nevertheless, social security systems do not always adequately recognize or cover these risks.

Third, there is the risk of career termination and transition. Athletic careers typically end at a young age. This makes it difficult for athletes to re-enter the labor market without sufficient education, experience, or social security savings.

Fourth, there are social and structural inequalities. Female athletes face additional challenges such as lower income, less contractual security, and inadequate maternity protection. Similarly, athletes in less visible sports or individuals from disadvantaged groups may experience multi-layered exclusion. These risks demonstrate that athletes' labor is not only non-standard but also embedded within a structure of deep vulnerability.

4. CONCLUSION: POLICY IMPLICATIONS FOR WELFARE-ORIENTED SPORTS GOVERNANCE

As demonstrated in the previous sections, sports can no longer be viewed solely as a field focused on performance, competition, and success. The economic, institutional, and social transformation of sports has turned this field into a structure where significant social risks are generated and redistributed. Athletes' working conditions, career durations, income structures, and the physical and psychological risks they face necessitate a reevaluation of sports within the context of social law and welfare policies. In this framework, the governance of sports must be shaped not only through organizational efficiency and athletic success but also in accordance with the principles of social protection, equality, and welfare.

A well-being-focused approach to sports governance requires redefining sports as a public policy domain. Under this approach, sports are viewed not merely as a means of producing elite performance, but also as a domain in which individuals' social rights must be safeguarded. In this context, sports policies must prioritize athletes' well-being, social security, and the management of risks they face throughout their lifetimes.

4.1. Recognizing Sports as a Social Risk Area

The first step in a well-being-focused approach is the explicit acknowledgment that sports, by its very nature, is a field that involves social risks. Sports activities entail multifaceted risks such as injury, illness, career termination, income insecurity, and psychological pressure. These risks demonstrate that sports cannot be evaluated solely on the basis of individual choice or voluntary participation.

In this context, sports should be addressed in a manner similar to other risk areas discussed in the social policy literature. Just as occupational risks have been identified for industrial workers, healthcare workers, or other professional groups, and appropriate protective mechanisms have been developed for them, a similar approach must be adopted for athletes. As long as the risk-generating nature of sports is overlooked, the structural vulnerabilities faced by athletes will remain invisible.

4.2. The Principle of Equal Social Protection for Athletes

Athletes' demands for social protection are often misinterpreted as demands for special privileges. In reality, what athletes are seeking is equal access to the fundamental social rights granted to other groups of workers. Therefore, one of the core principles of welfare-oriented sports governance is the equal and effective inclusion of athletes in social protection systems.

In this context, athletes' fundamental social rights—such as:

- Access to health insurance
- Coverage under workers' compensation and occupational disease provisions
- Access to maternity, disability, and retirement benefits
- Protection against income loss and unemployment

—must be guaranteed.

This approach is based on protecting athletes based on the risks they face, regardless of their legal status. In this way, by moving beyond the debate over whether athletes are "workers," the scope of social protection can be expanded.

4.3. The Life Cycle Approach and the Post-Career Period

One of the most significant challenges athletes face is the short and intermittent nature of their careers. For this reason, well-being-focused sports policies must focus not only on the active athletic period but on the entire life cycle of athletes.

In this context:

- Supporting athletes through education
- Developing dual-career policies
- Supporting the transition to post-career employment
- Managing psychological and social adaptation processes

stand out as key policy areas.

This approach aims to protect athletes not only during their competitive careers but also in their lives after retirement. In this way, sports can become a domain where individuals can plan their lives in a sustainable manner.

4.4. Corporate Responsibility and Multi-Stakeholder Governance

Well-being-focused sports governance is not an area solely under the responsibility of the state. Due to the nature of sports, numerous stakeholders must assume responsibility. The state, federations, clubs, the private sector, and international organizations are key components of this process.

In this context:

- The government must strengthen its regulatory and supervisory role
- Federations must develop policies that protect athletes' rights
- Clubs must improve athletes' working and living conditions
- International organizations must assume a role in setting standards and providing guidance

This multi-stakeholder structure will ensure that sports are managed in a more inclusive and sustainable manner.

4.5. Rights-Based and Harmonized Sports Policies

Given the impact of different welfare regimes on sports policies, each country must develop solutions tailored to its own institutional structure. However, these differences should not serve as an excuse for neglecting athletes' fundamental rights.

Therefore, regardless of welfare regimes:

- Establishing minimum social protection standards
- Creating a universal rights framework for athletes
- Ensuring policy harmonization at the international level

emerge as key objectives.

This approach is particularly important given the global nature of sports. The international mobility of athletes makes the portability and protection of social rights even more critical.

4.6. General Assessment: Redefining Sport

In conclusion, sport has become a multidimensional policy area in modern welfare states. Thanks to its functions—such as social integration, public health, and employment—sport has emerged as a key component of welfare regimes. However, sport's ability to fulfill these functions depends on addressing the inequalities and gaps in protection within the sector itself. Therefore, the governance of sports must be approached not only with a focus on performance and success but also through a framework grounded in social justice and rights. In this context, welfare regimes provide a critical analytical framework for understanding how sports are organized and to what extent athletes are protected. Strengthening sports' place within the social legal framework is one of the fundamental conditions for creating a more inclusive and sustainable sports system. The key finding of this study is that sports can no longer be evaluated solely as a realm of performance and competition. Sports is also an arena where social risks are concentrated and where individuals require protection against these risks.

In this context, the social protection demanded for athletes is not a privilege; it is a fundamental right. Ensuring that athletes are protected to the same extent as other groups of workers is essential both for social justice and for a sustainable sports system.

A well-being-focused approach to sports governance requires re-examining sports from a human-centered perspective. This approach aims to transform sports into a field that not only produces success but also ensures the well-being of individuals.

REFERENCES

Andreff, W. (2011). Some comparative economics of the organization of sports: Competition and regulation in north American vs. European professional team sports leagues. *The European Journal of Comparative Economics, 8*(1), 3–27.

Aydın, U., Canbey Özgüler, V., Kocabaş, F., Yalız Solmaz, D., Katırcı, H., Demirkaya, S., Yüce, A. & Etci, H. (2017). Türkiye'de Profesyonel Sporcuların Çalışma Koşulları ve Örgütlenme Eğilimleri. *Çalışma ve Toplum, 4*, 1873–1912.

Aykaç, M., & Kaya, S. (2024). İşgücü Piyasasında Yaşanan Dönüşümler: Standart Dışı İstihdam ve Çalışan Yoksulluğu İlişkisi. *Sosyoekonomi, 32*(62), 413–453. DOI: 10.17233/sosyoekonomi.2024.04.20

BMI. (2026). Topics: Sport. https://www.bmi.bund.de/EN/topics/sport/sport-node .html#:~:text=In%20Germany%2C%20sport%20participation%20is,spirit%2C%20 fair%20play%20and%20tolerance

Breuer, C., & Feiler, S. (2015). *Sport Development Report 2013/2014. Analysis of the situation of sports clubs in Germany*. Sportverlag Strauß.

Breuer, C., & Nowy, T. (2017). Germany: Autonomy, Partnership and Subsidiarity. In J. Scheerder, A. Willem & E. Claes (Eds.), *Sport Policy Systems and Sport Federations: A Cross-national Perspective*, Palgrave Mcmillan.

Cattaneo, A. (2025). 4.5. United Kingdom. In J. Mittag, L. Fiege, M. Seltmann, L. Hofmann, V. Smokvina, P. Zembura, L. Haas & A. Cattaneo (Authors), *Elite Athletes' Social Protection in Olympic Sports in Europe: An Evaluation of the Status Quo*, Erasmus+ SOPROS (Project 101090790), German Sport University Cologne. DOI: 10.25847/sopros.01.2025

Chen, S., & Hou, T. (2025). Sport policy cultures. In *Handbook on Sport and Culture* (pp. 366–381). Edward Elgar Publishing., DOI: 10.4337/9781035339983.00042

Coalter, F. (2007). *A wider social role for sport: Who's keeping the score?* Routledge. DOI: 10.4324/9780203014615

De Bosscher, V., Shibli, S., & De Rycke, J. (2021). The societal impact of elite sport: positives and negatives: introduction to ESMQ special issue. *European Sport Management Quarterly, 21*(5), 625–635. DOI: 10.1080/16184742.2021.1955944

De Keyzer, F. (2023). The employment status of the sportsperson: The Belgian case. *European Labour Law Journal, 14*(3), 438–447. DOI: 10.1177/20319525231165847

Eichenhofer, E. (2015). Social security as a human right: A European perspective. In *Research Handbook on European Social Security Law* (pp. 3–31). Edward Elgar Publishing., DOI: 10.4337/9781782547334.00011

Esping-Andersen, G. (1990). *The Three Worlds of Welfare Capitalism*. Princeton University Press.

Ferrera, M. (1996). The 'Southern Model' of Welfare in Social Europe. *Journal of European Social Policy*, *6*(1), 17–37. DOI: 10.1177/095892879600600102

Fiege, L. (2025). The social protection of Olympic elite athletes in Europe: A human right trapped between international commitment and domestic institutionalisation? *The International Sports Law Journal*, *25*(4), 234–256. DOI: 10.1007/s40318-025-00323-x

Foster, K. (2012). *Is There a Global Sports Law?* DOI: 10.1007/978-90-6704-829-3_2

Gammelsaeter, H., & Anagnostopoulos, C. (2022). Sport management: Mission and meaning for a new era. *European Sport Management Quarterly*, *22*(5), 637–642. DOI: 10.1080/16184742.2022.2100918

García, B., & Smokvina, V. (2025). The Chinese Model of Sport Empowered and Restrained in the New Era. In *The European Model of Sport Myth or Reality?* (p. 15). Routledge., DOI: 10.4324/9781032665153

Gardiner, S. W. R., B. S., & N. U. (2012). *Sports law*. Routledge.

Gencer, H. (2017). *How to Classify the Chinese Welfare State*. University of Bremen SOCIUM Research Center on Inequality and Social Policy.

Girginov, V. (2017). UK: England – National Governing Bodies of Sport and Government Agencies. In J. Scheerder, A. Willem & E. Claes (Eds.), *Sport Policy Systems and Sport Federations: A Cross-national Perspective*, Palgrave Mcmillan.

Gökduman, Ç. (2023). *Fiili Profesyonel Sporcuların Sosyal Güvenlik Hakları Üzerine Bir Araştırma*. Akdeniz Üniversitesi Sosyal Bilimler Enstitüsü.

Gökduman, Ç., Temel, C., & Alper, Y. (2025). *Social Security Practices for Professional Athletes*. DOI: 10.21203/rs.3.rs-5753949/v1

Gough, I. (1996). Social Assistance in Southern Europe. *South European Society & Politics*, *1*(1), 1–23. DOI: 10.1080/13608749608454714

Heinemann, K. (2005). Sport and the Welfare State in Europe. *European Journal of Sport Science*, *5*(4), 181–188. DOI: 10.1080/17461390500344347

Hennessy, R. (2023). Exploring the Role of Social Protection Interventions in Preventing Child Labour: Reinforcing the Case for a Human Rights-Based Model of Intervention. *Journal of Human Rights Practice, 15*(1), 262–283. DOI: 10.1093/jhuman/huac064

Höglund, F., & Bruhn, A. (2024). Sport-based interventions' – A tool for suburban social integration? *Nordic Social Work Research, 14*(1), 32–44. DOI: 10.1080/2156857X.2022.2062430

Houlihan, B. (2002). *Sport, Policy and Politics: A Comparative Analysis*. Routledge., DOI: 10.4324/9780203160640

Houlihan, B., & G. M. (2007). *Comparative elite sport development. In Comparative elite sport development*. Routledge.

Ibsen, B., Nichols, G., Piątkowska, M., Nagel, S., Llopis-Goig, R., & Elmose-Østerlund, K. (2022). What can explain the differences between European countries' public policies for sports clubs? *International Journal of Sport Policy, 14*(3), 435–451. DOI: 10.1080/19406940.2022.2052148

International Labour Organization (ILO). (2026). *Social Protection*. Https://www.Ilo.Org/Topics-and-Sectors/Social-Protection

International Olympic Committee. (2026). Paris 2024 Medal Table. https://www.olympics.com/en/olympic-games/paris-2024/medals

Kamenecka-Usova, M., Korde, Z., Zidens, J., Luika, S., Agapova, O., Palkova, K., & Martinsone, K. (2025). Research patterns in sports law and sports governance: A scopus bibliometric study. *Frontiers in Sports and Active Living, 7*, 1590858. Advance online publication. DOI: 10.3389/fspor.2025.1590858 PMID: 40735413

Karagöz, E. (2025). Türkiye'de Sporcuların Sosyal Güvenliği: Statü ve Uygulama Tartışmaları. *Hukuk Fakültesi Dergisi, 11*(2), 125–146.

Kocaoğlu, G. (2023). *Türk Hukukunda Sporcuların Sigortalanması*. Kadir Has Üniversitesi Lisansüstü Eğitim Enstitüsü.

Leibfried, S. (1996). Towards a European Welfare State. In Jones, C. (Ed.), *New Perspectives on the Welfare State in Europe*. Routledge.

Ling, Z., & Hong, F. (2014). After the Glory: Elite Athletes' Re-employment in China. *The International Journal of the History of Sport, 31*(6), 635–651. DOI: 10.1080/09523367.2013.878498

Ma, D., & Ji, L. (2024). Challenges in Reforms of Chinese Elite Sports: Towards a New Development Mode. In *The Mediating Power of Sport* (pp. 183–203). Emerald Publishing Limited. DOI: 10.1108/S1476-285420240000021011

Mayrhofer, M. (2025). The concept of vulnerability and its relation to the concepts of inequality and discrimination – a review article. *International Journal of Human Rights*, *29*(9), 1589–1618. DOI: 10.1080/13642987.2025.2488938

McCrone, P. (2025). *Contemporary Issues in Health and Social Care Policy and Practice. In Health and Social Care Funding across the OECD*. Routledge.

Meir, D., & Fletcher, T. (2020). The physical education and sport premium: Social justice, autonomy and school sport policy in England. *International Journal of Sport Policy*, *12*(2), 237–253. DOI: 10.1080/19406940.2019.1673790

Mittag, J., Fiege, L., Seltmann, M., & Hofmann, K. (2025). 4.2. Germany. In J. Mittag, L. Fiege, M. Seltmann, L. Hofmann, V. Smokvina, P. Zembura, L. Haas & A. Cattaneo (Authors), *Elite Athletes' Social Protection in Olympic Sports in Europe: An Evaluation of the Status Quo*, Erasmus+ SOPROS (Project 101090790), German Sport University Cologne. DOI: 10.25847/sopros.01.2025

Mittag, J., Seltmann, M., & Fiege, L. (2022). 3. Central Europe. In J. Mittag, M. Seltmann, L. Fiege, L. O'Leary, P. Zembura, V. Smokvina, L. Haas & T. Santos (Authors), *Fact Report: Understanding the Employment Relations of Athetes in Olympic Sports in Europe*, Erasmus+ Programme.

O'Leary, L., Seltmann, M., & Smokvina, V. (2025). Elite Athletes and Worker Status. *Industrial Law Journal*, *54*(2), 248–277. DOI: 10.1093/indlaw/dwae025

Oleksii, N. (2025). Legal Status of a Professional Athlete: Normative Definition and Problems of Regulation, *Visegrad. Journal of Human Rights*, *2*(2), 94–99. DOI: 10.61345/1339-7915.2025.2.14

Öztuna, B. (2015). Türk Sporcularının Sosyal Güvenliği. *International Journal of Science Culture and Sport, Special Issue*, (3), 805–808.

Palier, B. (2010). *A long goodbye to Bismarck?: the politics of welfare reforms in continental Europe*. Amsterdam University Press. DOI: 10.1017/9789048512454

Panagiotopoulos, D. P. (2016). Physical Activities-Legal Horizon and Sports Regulation as Lex Specialis: Lex Sportiva. *The Open Sports Sciences Journal*, *9*(1), 35–42. DOI: 10.2174/1875399X01609010035

Pennings, F. (2022). *European social security law*. Intersentia.

Razavi, S. (2022). Making the Right to Social Security a Reality for All Workers. *The Indian Journal of Labour Economics : The Quarterly Journal of the Indian Society of Labour Economics, 65*(2), 269–294. DOI: 10.1007/s41027-022-00378-6 PMID: 35911186

Scheerder, J., Claes, E., & Willem, A. (2017). Does It Take Two to Tango? The Position and Power of National Sport bodies Compared to Their Public Authorities. In Scheerder, J., Willem, A., & Claes, E. (Eds.), *Sport Policy Systems and Sport Federations: A Cross-national Perspective*. Palgrave Mcmillan. DOI: 10.1057/978-1-137-60222-0_1

Seltmann, M. (2026). Different worlds of athlete welfare? A social policy perspective on elite sport in six European countries. *International Journal of Sport Policy, 18*(1), 125–152. DOI: 10.1080/19406940.2025.2583977

Serby, T. (2017). Sports corruption: Sporting autonomy, Lex Sportiva and the rule of law. *ESLJ, 15*(1).

Sessa, G., Occhini, G., Milani, C., Marini, G., & Sarro, A. (2020). A public health Italian ethical movement to sustain the beveridge model: Health promotion and equity. *European Journal of Public Health, 30*(5, Supplement_5), 166–1284. DOI: 10.1093/eurpub/ckaa166.1284

Sheng, K. (2017). Analysis on the Social Security System of Retired Athletes in China. *Advances in Economics. Business and Management Research, 32*, 218–221.

Sözer, A. N. (2020). *Türk Sosyal Hukuku* (2nd ed.). Beta.

Spaaij, R. (2012). Beyond the playing field: Experiences of sport, social capital, and integration among Somalis in Australia. *Ethnic and Racial Studies, 35*(9), 1519–1538. DOI: 10.1080/01419870.2011.592205

Sport, U. K. (2026). Athlete Support. https://stories.uksport.gov.uk/support-for-athletes/

Supiot, A.SUPIOT. (2020). The tasks ahead of the ILO at its centenary. *International Labour Review, 159*(1), 117–136. DOI: 10.1111/ilr.12164

Tinaz, C., Turco, D. M., & Salisbury, P. (2014). Sport policy in Turkey. *International Journal of Sport Policy, 6*(3), 533–545. DOI: 10.1080/19406940.2014.893247

Warburton, D. E. R., & Bredin, S. S. D. (2019). Health Benefits of Physical Activity: A Strengths-Based Approach. *Journal of Clinical Medicine, 8*(12), 2044. DOI: 10.3390/jcm8122044 PMID: 31766502

Weatherill, S. (2017). *Principles and practice in EU sports law*. Oxford University Press.

Westerbeek, H., & Eime, R. (2021). The Physical Activity and Sport Participation Framework—A Policy Model Toward Being Physically Active Across the Lifespan. *Frontiers in Sports and Active Living*, *3*, 608593. Advance online publication. DOI: 10.3389/fspor.2021.608593 PMID: 34027402

Whiting, S., Abu-Omar, K., Gelius, P., Firmino-Machado, J., Rakovac, I., & Mendes, R. (2025). Physical activity policy implementation and physical activity levels in the European Union: Are we on track to close the gap between policy and practice? *Health Policy (Amsterdam)*, *151*, 105200. DOI: 10.1016/j.healthpol.2024.105200 PMID: 39550929

World Health Organization (WHO). (2020). *WHO guidelines on physical activity and sedentary behaviour*.

Zheng, J., Chen, S., Tan, T.-C., & Lau, P. W. C. (2018). Sport Policy in China (Mainland). *International Journal of Sport Policy*, *10*(3), 469–491. DOI: 10.1080/19406940.2017.1413585

Compilation of References

Abanoz, E. I., & Soyer, F. (2018). Sporun toplumsal değerler üzerindeki etkisi hakkında bir çalışma. *Uluslararas Insan Bilimleri Dergisi*, *15*(1), 309–318. DOI: 10.14687/jhs.v15i1.4951

Abberley, P. (1987). The concept of oppression and the development of a social theory of disability. *Disability, Handicap & Society*, *2*(1), 5–19. DOI: 10.1080/02674648766780021

Acker, J. (2020). Gendered organizations and intersectionality: Problems and possibilities. *Equality, Diversity and Inclusion*, *39*(1), 3–18. DOI: 10.1108/EDI-11-2019-0340

Adamson, B., Adamson, M., Clarke, C., Richardson, E. V., & Sydnor, S. (2022). Social justice through sport and exercise studies: A manifesto. *Journal of Sport and Social Issues*, *46*(5), 407–444. DOI: 10.1177/01937235221099150

Adriaanse, J. (2016). Gender diversity in the governance of sport associations: The Sydney scoreboard global index of participation. *Journal of Business Ethics*, *137*(1), 149–160. DOI: 10.1007/s10551-015-2550-3

Ağazade, S. (2025). An analysis of the Turkish sports industry based on data from the sports activities sector. In Günay, N. (Ed.), *Proceedings of the Turkish Sports Congress: From the Founding of the Republic to the Turkish Century* (25–27 April 2024). Turkish Historical Society Publications. https://ttk.gov.tr/wp-content/uploads/2025/10/46-Seymur-Agazde.pdf DOI: 10.37879/978-975-17-6294-8.2025.1015

Akın, Y. (2005). Ana hatları ile Cumhuriyet döneminde beden terbiyesi ve spor politikaları. *Toplum ve Bilim*, *103*, 53–92.

Alcock, P., & Erskine, A. May, May, M. (2002). The Blackwell Dictionary of Social Policy, Oxford: Blackwell Publishing.

Alev, A., Alemdar, U., Alemdar, B., Yaman, S., & Sığırtmaç, Y. (2021). Türk spor yönetiminin dünden bugüne yapısal analizi: Yeni kamu yönetimi ve yönetişim yaklaşımları açısından bir değerlendirme. *Beden Eğitimi ve Spor Bilimleri Dergisi, 23*(2), 103–124.

Ali, A. E., Millington, R., Darnell, S. C., & Smith, T. (2024). Policy vs. practice in sport and climate change: The perspectives of key actors in global sport and international development. *Frontiers in Sports and Active Living, 6*, 1297739. Advance online publication. DOI: 10.3389/fspor.2024.1297739

Allport, G. W. (1954). *The nature of prejudice.* Addison-Wesley.

Alshikhy, T., O'Sullivan, H., Polkinghorne, M., & Gennings, E. (2025). The role and impact of sporting mega-events in the context of soft power. *Encyclopedia, 5*(1), 31. DOI: 10.3390/encyclopedia5010031

Altan, Ö. Z. (2007). Sosyal Politika. Eskişehir: Anadolu Üniversitesi Yayınları Yayını No: 1744.

Altan, Ö. Z. (2009). Sosyal Politika Dersleri. Eskişehir: Anadolu Üniversitesi Yayınları Yayın No: 1987.

Altındağ, S. (2017). Engelli bireylerin toplumsal uyum süreçlerinde sporun rolü. *Toplum ve Sosyal Bilimler Dergisi, 6*(2), 30–45.

Amis, J., Slack, T., & Berrett, T. (1999). Sport sponsorship as distinctive competence. *European Journal of Marketing, 33*(3/4), 250–272. DOI: 10.1108/03090569910253044

Amnesty International. (2023, February 14). *Saudi Arabia: FIFA's award of the World Cup to Saudi Arabia is blatant sportswashing*. https://www.amnesty.org/en/latest/news/2023/02/saudi-arabia-fifas-award-of-the-world-cup-to-saudi-arabia-is-blatant-sports-washing/

Anderson, B. (1983). *Imagined communities: Reflections on the origin and spread of nationalism.* Verso.

Anderson-Butcher, D., Iachini, A., & Riley, A. (2021). Social work and youth sport. *Child & Adolescent Social Work Journal, 38*(4), 359–365. DOI: 10.1007/s10560-021-00777-6 PMID: 34075276

Andreff, W. (2011). Some comparative economics of the organization of sports: Competition and regulation in north American vs. European professional team sports leagues. *The European Journal of Comparative Economics, 8*(1), 3–27.

Andrews, D., & Silk, M. (2012). *Sport and neoliberalism: Politics, consumption, and culture* (p. 316).

Andrews, D. L., Batts, C., & Silk, M. (2014). Sport, glocalization and the new Indian middle class. *International Journal of Cultural Studies, 17*(3), 259–276. DOI: 10.1177/1367877913487531

Andrews, D. L., & Silk, M. L. (2018). *Sport and neoliberalism: Politics, consumption, and culture.* Temple University Press., DOI: 10.2307/j.ctvr43k8s

Anney, V. N. (2014). Ensuring the quality of the findings of qualitative research: Looking at trustworthiness criteria. [jeteraps]. *Journal of Emerging Trends in Educational Research and Policy Studies, 5*(2), 272–281.

Anorim, L., Cavalcanti, G., & Cruz, R. (2023). The choice of scaling technique matters for classification performance. *Applied Soft Computing, 133.* Advance online publication. DOI: 10.1016/j.asoc.2022.109924

Antonie, A., Begović, M., & Petracovschi, S. (2024). Sport policy in Romania. *Sports Law. Policy and Diplomacy Journal, 2*(2), 17–35.

Aracı, H. (1999). *Öğretmen ve Okullarda Beden Eğitimi.* Bağırgan Yayınevi.

Arıkan, Ç. (2001). Aile ve özürlülük: 'Görme Özürlüler Derneği' üye özürlü aileleri üzerine bir araştırma. *Ufkun Ötesi Bilim Dergisi, 1*(1), 45–60.

Atalay, A. (2017). Spor yönetimi açısından Türk spor politikalarına eleştirel bir bakış. *Spor Bilimleri Araştırmaları Dergisi, 2*(2), 52–65.

Aydın, U., Canbey Özgüler, V., Kocabaş, F., Yalız Solmaz, D., Katırcı, H., Demirkaya, S., Yüce, A. & Etci, H. (2017). Türkiye'de Profesyonel Sporcuların Çalışma Koşulları ve Örgütlenme Eğilimleri. *Çalışma ve Toplum, 4*, 1873–1912.

Aydın, A. D., Demir, H., & Yetim, A. (2007). Türk spor politikalarında öngörülen hedeflerin gerçekleşme düzeylerinin belirlenmesi üzerine bir araştırma: GSGM örneği. *Beden Eğitimi ve Spor Bilimleri Dergisi, 1*(2), 87–96.

Aydın, A. D., Turgut, M., & Bayırlı, R. (2007). Spor kulüplerinin halka açılmasının Türkiye'de uygulanan modeller açısından incelenmesi. *Gazi Üniversitesi Ticaret ve Turizm Eğitim Fakültesi Dergisi, 1*, 59–70.

Aydos, O. S. (2013). Sporcu sözleşmesinin feshi [Termination of athlete contracts]. Ankara Üniversitesi Hukuk Fakültesi Dergisi [Ankara University Faculty of Law Journal], 62(3), 643–690.

Aykaç, M., & Kaya, S. (2024). İşgücü Piyasasında Yaşanan Dönüşümler: Standart Dışı İstihdam ve Çalışan Yoksulluğu İlişkisi. *Sosyoekonomi, 32*(62), 413–453. DOI: 10.17233/sosyoekonomi.2024.04.20

Aykın, A. G., & Bilir, F. P. (2013). Hükümet programları ve spor politikaları. *Çukurova Üniversitesi Sosyal Bilimler Enstitüsü Dergisi, 22*(2), 239–254.

Aysoy, M. (2008). *Hayatı Paylaşmak İçin "Engel Çok"*. Açı Kitaplar.

Ayvaz, Z. (2022). Erken Cumhuriyet Türkiyesinde uygulanan öjenik politikaların spora yansıması: Beden Terbiyesi Kanunu üzerine bir inceleme. *Journal of Sport Sciences Research*, *7*(1), 174–196. DOI: 10.25307/jssr.1116251

Baade, R. A., & Matheson, V. A. (2006). Have public finance principles been shut out in financing new stadiums for the NFL? *Public Finance and Management*, *6*(3), 284–320. DOI: 10.1177/152397210600600301

Bailey, R. (2005). Evaluating the relationship between physical education, sport and social inclusion. *Educational Review*, *57*(1), 71–90. DOI: 10.1080/0013191042000274196

Balcı, S. (2019). Engellilerin sosyal dışlanma algılarının bazı sosyodemografik değişkenlere göre incelenmesi. *Tıbbi Sosyal Hizmet Dergisi*, *0*(14), 59–79. DOI: 10.46218/tshd.1139360

Bale, J. (1993). *Sports, Space and The City*. Routledge. beIN Sports Türkiye. (2026). *Fenerbahçe stadının taşınması mümkün değildir.* https://beinsports.com.tr/haber/fenerbahce-stadinin-tasinmasi-mumkun-degildir

Ball, K., Carver, A., Downing, K., Jackson, M., & O'Rourke, K. (2015). Addressing the social determinants of inequities in physical activity and sedentary behaviours. *Health Promotion International*, *30*(Suppl 2), ii18–ii19. DOI: 10.1093/heapro/dav022 PMID: 25855784

Barengo, N. C., & Alkhatib, A. (2022). Editorial: Physical activity, health equity and health related outcomes. *Frontiers in Public Health*, *10*, 828108. DOI: 10.3389/fpubh.2022.828108 PMID: 35284398

Barr, A. N. (1992). *Economic theory and the welfare state: a survey and interpretation*. LSE.

Barton, L. (1993). The Struggle for Citizenship: The Case of Disabled People. *Disability, Handicap & Society*, *8*(3), 235–248. DOI: 10.1080/02674649366780251

Bay, H., & İnneci, A. (2017). The taxation of wage income in Türkiye from the perspective of tax justice. *International Journal of Public Finance*, *2*(2), 196–219. DOI: 10.30927/ijpf.327776

Beck, U. (1992). *Risk society: Towards a new modernity*. SAGE Publications.

Bedir, E., Özaydın, M. M. ve Metin, B. (2013). Sosyal Politika 1. Eskişehir: Anadolu Üniversitesi, Açıköğretim Fakültesi Yayınları, No: 1589

Begović, M. (2020). The development of sport policy in Montenegro. *International Journal of Sport Policy*, *12*(2), 321–330. DOI: 10.1080/19406940.2020.1719186

Beierlein, C., Werner, C. S., Brähler, E., & Zick, A. (2023). An integrated approach to the conceptualisation and measurement of social cohesion. *Social Indicators Research*, *167*(1–3), 147–172. DOI: 10.1007/s11205-023-03110-z

Bekik, M. E. (2025). Social Policy Developments. In *The Ottoman Empire In The Context Of The Tanzimat And Islahat Edicts. Türkiye ve Dünyada Sosyal Politika* (pp. 1–17). Yaz Yayınları.

Bergsgard, N. A., Bratland-Sanda, S., Giulianotti, R., & Tangen, J. O. (Eds.). (2020). *Sport, outdoor life and the Nordic world.* Routledge. DOI: 10.4324/9781003009047

Bergsgard, N. A., Houlihan, B., Mangset, P., Nødland, S. I., & Rommetvedt, H. (2007). *Sport policy: A comparative analysis of stability and change*. Elsevier.

Bhoi, N., & Acharya, S. K. (2024). Health status of particularly vulnerable tribal groups (PVTGs) of Odisha: A narrative review. *Journal of Health, Population and Nutrition*, *43*(1), 176. DOI: 10.1186/s41043-024-00671-8 PMID: 39478584

Blachnicka-Ciacek, D., & Trąbka, A. (2024). 'Football was the key': The role of sports in facilitating migrants' belonging and inclusion in Poland. *Leisure Studies*, *43*(6), 932–945. DOI: 10.1080/02614367.2022.2088834

Bloyce, D. ve Smith, A. (2010). *Sport policy and development: An introduction*. Routledge.

BMI. (2026). Topics: Sport. https://www.bmi.bund.de/EN/topics/sport/sport-node.html#:~:text=In%20Germany%2C%20sport%20participation%20is,spirit%2C%20fair%20play%20and%20tolerance

Boehl, W. R., & Ignácio, M. C. (2023). Talent in top-flight football: Concept, recruitment and predictive models for identification. In Wojda, T. (Ed.), *Technology in sports - Recent advances, new perspectives and application.*, DOI: 10.5772/intechopen.1002431

Bonoli, G. (2005). The politics of the new social policies: Providing coverage against new social risks in mature welfare states. *Policy and Politics*, *33*(3), 431–449. DOI: 10.1332/0305573054325765

Borgers, J., Pilgaard, M., Vanreusel, B., & Scheerder, J. (2018). Can we consider changes in sports participation as institutional change? A conceptual framework. *International Review for the Sociology of Sport, 53*(1), 84–100. DOI: 10.1177/1012690216639598

Bourdieu, P. (1986). The forms of capital. In J. Richardson (Ed.), *Handbook of Theory and Research for the Sociology of Education*. Greenwood Press.

Bourdieu, P. (1984). *Distinction: A Social Critique of the Judgement of Taste*. Harvard University Press.

Bourdieu, P. (1986). The forms of capital. In Richardson, J. G. (Ed.), *Handbook of theory and research for the sociology of education* (pp. 241–258). Greenwood.

Boykoff, J. (2022). Toward a theory of sportswashing: Mega-events, soft power, and political conflict. *Sociology of Sport Journal, 39*(4), 342–351. DOI: 10.1123/ssj.2022-0095

Boyle, R. (2015). Battle for control? Copyright, football and European television in the digital age. *International Journal of Digital Television, 6*(1), 79–95.

Boyle, R., & Haynes, R. (2004). *Football in the New Media Age*. Routledge., DOI: 10.4324/9780203600467

Bozkurt, M. N. (2010). Spor hukuku uyuşmazlıklarının çözümünde Milletlerarası Spor Tahkim Mahkemesi [The Court of Arbitration for Sport in the resolution of international sports disputes] [Ankara Bar Journal]. *Ankara Barosu Dergisi, 2*, 165–190.

Bradburn, N. M. (1969). *The Structure of Psychological Well-Being*. Aldine Publishing Company.

Bradbury, J. C., Coates, D., & Humphreys, B. R. (2023). The impact of professional sports franchises and venues on local economies: A comprehensive survey. *Journal of Economic Surveys, 37*(4), 1389–1431. DOI: 10.1111/joes.12533

Brannagan, P. M., Grix, J., & Norrito, A. (2026). Demystifying sportswashing: An assemblage theory perspective on authoritarian states' investment in global sport. *British Journal of Politics and International Relations, 28*(1), 144–164. DOI: 10.1177/13691481251352321

Breuer, C., & Nowy, T. (2017). Germany: Autonomy, Partnership and Subsidiarity. In J. Scheerder, A. Willem & E. Claes (Eds.), *Sport Policy Systems and Sport Federations: A Cross-national Perspective*, Palgrave Mcmillan.

Breuer, C., & Feiler, S. (2015). *Sport Development Report 2013/2014. Analysis of the situation of sports clubs in Germany.* Sportverlag Strauß.

Breuer, C., Wicker, P., Dallmeyer, S., & Ilgner, M. (2018). *Die Lebenssituation von Spitzensportlern und -Sportlerinnen in Deutschland.* Bundesinstitut für Sportwissenschaft.

Brown, A. (2008). 'Our club, our rules': Fan communities at FC United of Manchester. *Soccer and Society*, *9*(3), 346–358. DOI: 10.1080/14660970802008967

Bruce, T. (2016). New rules for new times: Sportswomen and media representation in the third wave. *Sex Roles*, *74*(7–8), 361–376. DOI: 10.1007/s11199-015-0497-6

Bruening, J. E., & Dixon, M. A. (2019). Work-family conflict in coaching: A top-down perspective. *Journal of Sport Management*, *33*(1), 1–15. DOI: 10.1123/jsm.2018-0054

Buğra, A., & Keyder, Ç. (2006). The Turkish welfare regime in transformation. *Journal of European Social Policy*, *16*(3), 211–228. DOI: 10.1177/0958928706065593

Bull, M., & Whittam, G. (2021). Sustainable value creation? Entrepreneurial orientations in the football industry. *International Journal of Entrepreneurial Behaviour & Research*, *27*(1), 27–44. DOI: 10.1108/IJEBR-07-2020-0498

Bundesministerium des Innern. (2026). Reform Athletenförderung. Accessed April 2026. Available at: https://www.bmi.bund.de/DE/themen/sport/nationale-sportpolitik/spitzensportreform/athletenfoerderung Case C-415/93, European Court of Justice, Union Royale Belge des Sociétés de Football Association and others v. Bosman and others, ECLI:EU:C:1995:463.

Burton, L. J. (2015). Underrepresentation of women in sport leadership: A review of research. *Sport Management Review*, *18*(2), 155–165. DOI: 10.1016/j.smr.2014.02.004

Çalışkan, N. (2020). Engelli bireylerin fiziksel sağlıklarına sporun etkileri. *Toplum ve Sağlık Dergisi*, *7*(1), 27–34.

Canniford, R., & Hill, T. (2022, January 17). *Sportswashing: How mining and energy companies sponsor your favourite sports to help clean up their image.* The Conversation. https://theconversation.com/sportswashing-how-mining-and-energy-companies-sponsor-your-favourite-sports-to-help-clean-uptheir-image-173589

Case C-650/22, Court of Justice of the European Union (Diarra), 2024.

Cattaneo, A. (2025). 4.5. United Kingdom. In J. Mittag, L. Fiege, M. Seltmann, L. Hofmann, V. Smokvina, P. Zembura, L. Haas & A. Cattaneo (Authors), *Elite Athletes' Social Protection in Olympic Sports in Europe: An Evaluation of the Status Quo*, Erasmus+ SOPROS (Project 101090790), German Sport University Cologne. DOI: 10.25847/sopros.01.2025

Cem, Ç. (2012). *Profesyonel Futbolcu Transfer Sözleşmesi* [Professional Footballer Transfer Contracts]. Oniki Levha Publishing.

Çeribaş, D. (2020). The taxation of athletes' wages in Türkiye. *Hacettepe Law Faculty Journal*, *10*(2), 555–583. https://doi.org/10.32957/hacettepehdf.761172

Chakraborty, S. (2024). Rethinking tribes in India through context of tribe-caste Continuum: Negotiation of identity and exploration of Hypervisibility among Siddi Tribe. *International Journal of Developmental Research*, *14*(12), 67270–67280.

Chen, S., & Hou, T. (2025). Sport policy cultures. In *Handbook on Sport and Culture* (pp. 366–381). Edward Elgar Publishing., DOI: 10.4337/9781035339983.00042

Choi, Y. D., Jo, S. H., & Ok, G. (2019). Evolution of the sports for all policy in National Sports Promotion Plan in South Korea, 1962–2017. *The International Journal of the History of Sport*, *36*(9–10), 876–891. DOI: 10.1080/09523367.2019.1675643

Çınarlı, S., & Ersöz, G. (2010). Recommendations regarding sponsorship and tax regulations in terms of the development of sports services for people with disabilities. Journal of the Institute of Social Sciences. *Süleyman Demirel University*, (12), 141–156. https://izlik.org/JA38NX95DD

Clays, E., Lidegaard, M., De Bacquer, D., Van Herck, K., De Backer, G., Kittel, F., De Smet, P., & Holtermann, A. (2014). The Combined Relationship of Occupational and Leisure-Time Physical Activity With All-Cause Mortality Among Men, Accounting for Physical Fitness. *American Journal of Epidemiology*, *179*(5), 559–566. DOI: 10.1093/aje/kwt294 PMID: 24305575

Cleland, J. (2017). The English Premier League in a global context. In Elliott, R., & Maguire, J. M. (Eds.), *The English Premier League: A socio-cultural analysis* (pp. 70–83). Routledge., DOI: 10.4324/9781315636696-6

Cleland, J. A. (2010). From passive to active: The changing relationship between supporters and football clubs. *Soccer and Society*, *11*(5), 537–552. DOI: 10.1080/14660970.2010.497348

Coakley, J. (2017). Sports in society: Issues and controversies. McGraw: Hill Education.

Coakley, J. (2011). Youth Sports: What Counts as "Positive Development?". *Journal of Sport and Social Issues, 35*(3), 306–324. DOI: 10.1177/0193723511417311

Coakley, J. (2021). *Sports in society: Issues and controversies* (13th ed.). McGraw-Hill Education.

Coalter, F. (2007). *A wider social role for sport: Who's keeping the score?* Routledge. DOI: 10.4324/9780203014615

Coalter, F. (2013). *Sport for development: What game are we playing?* Routledge. DOI: 10.4324/9780203861257

Coalter, F. (2015). Sport-for-change: Some thoughts from a sceptic. *Social Inclusion (Lisboa), 3*(3), 19–23. DOI: 10.17645/si.v3i3.222

Coalter, F. (2017). Sport for social inclusion: Evidence-based policy and practice. *Social Inclusion (Lisboa), 5*(2), 141–149. DOI: 10.17645/si.v5i2.852

Coates, D., & Humphreys, B. R. (2008). Do economists reach a conclusion on subsidies for sports franchises, stadiums, and mega-events? *Econ Journal Watch, 5*(3), 294.

Coleman, J. S. (1988). Social capital in the creation of human capital. *AJS; American Journal of Sociology, 94*(Supplement), S95–S120. DOI: 10.1086/228943

Collins, M. F. (2003). *Sport, physical activity and social exclusion*. Routledge. DOI: 10.4324/9780203167267

Collins, M. F. (2004). Sport, physical activity and social exclusion. *Journal of Sports Sciences, 22*(8), 727–740. DOI: 10.1080/02640410410001712430 PMID: 15370484

Collins, P. H. (2019). *Intersectionality as critical social theory*. Duke University Press., DOI: 10.1215/9781478007098

Comeau, G. S. (2013). The evolution of Canadian sport policy. *International Journal of Sport Policy, 5*(1), 73–93. DOI: 10.1080/19406940.2012.694368

Comitê Popular da Copa e Olimpíadas do Rio de Janeiro. (2012). *Mega-events and human rights violations in Rio de Janeiro: Dossier of the People's Committee for the World Cup and Olympics*. Rio on Watch.https://rioonwatch.org/wp-content/uploads/2013/05/2012-World-Cup-Olympics-Dossier-English.pdf

Connell, J. (2018). Fiji, rugby and the geopolitics of soft power. Shaping national and international identity. *New Zealand Geographer, 74*(2), 92–100. DOI: 10.1111/nzg.12184

Connell, R. (2009). *Gender in world perspective* (2nd ed.). Polity Press.

Cooky, C., & Antunovic, D. (2020). “This isn’t just about us”: Articulations of feminism in media narratives of athletes’ activism. *Communication & Sport*, *8*(4–5), 692–711. DOI: 10.1177/2167479519896360

Cooky, C., Messner, M. A., & Musto, M. (2021). “It’s dude time!” A quarter century of excluding women’s sports in televised news. *Communication & Sport*, *9*(1), 3–34. DOI: 10.1177/2167479519892930

Council of Europe. (2021). Recommendation CM/Rec(2021)5 of the Committee of Ministers to Member States on the Revised European Sports Charter (2021), Article 14. Available at: https://www.coe.int/en/web/sport/the-european-sports-charter

Crenshaw, K. (2017). *On intersectionality: Essential writings*. The New Press., DOI: 10.2307/j.ctt1ggjjnm

Crompton, J. L. (2006). Economic Impact Studies: Instruments for Political Shenanigans? *Journal of Travel Research*, *45*(1), 67–82. DOI: 10.1177/0047287506288870

Crowther, D., Singh, R., Singh, A., & Rani, S. (2024). Assessing the Impact of Artificial Intelligence on Healthcare Sector for Enhancing Sustainability. In Singh, R., Shafik, W., Crowther, D., & Kumar, V. (Eds.), *Transforming Healthcare Sector Through Artificial Intelligence and Environmental Sustainability. Approaches to Global Sustainability, Markets, and Governance*. Springer., DOI: 10.1007/978-981-97-9555-0_1

ÇSGB. (n.d.). https://www.csgb.gov.tr/poco-pages/asgari-ucret/ (Accessed Date:02/05/2026)

Çubuk, A. (1979). *Sosyal Politika*. Ankara İktisadi ve Ticari İlimler Akademisi Yayını.

Da Costa, L. P., & Miragaya, A. (2002). *Worldwide experiences and trends in sport for all*. Meyer & Meyer Sport.

Darnell, S. C. (2012). *Sport for development and peace: A critical sociology*. Bloomsbury Academic., DOI: 10.5040/9781849665896

Datta, R. (2022, April 18). How Odisha's Kalinga Institutes provide free education to tribal children in remote areas. *India today*. https://www.indiatoday.in/magazine/happiness-quest/story/20220418-how-odisha-s-kalinga-institutes-provide-free-education-to-tribal-children-in-remote-areas-1934626-2022-04-08

De Bosscher, V., Shibli, S., & De Rycke, J. (2021). The societal impact of elite sport: positives and negatives: introduction to ESMQ special issue. *European Sport Management Quarterly*, *21*(5), 625–635. DOI: 10.1080/16184742.2021.1955944

De Castro, S. B. E., De Souza, J. V. M., De Camargo, P. R., & Mezzadri, F. M. (2025). Government budget and priorities for sports in Brazil (2004-2020). *Managing Sport and Leisure, 30*(3), 487–505. DOI: 10.1080/23750472.2023.2196529

De Keyzer, F. (2023). The employment status of the sportsperson: The Belgian case. *European Labour Law Journal, 14*(3), 438–447. DOI: 10.1177/20319525231165847

Değer, R. (2022). The Development of the Sports Economy in Turkey and State Support. *Scientific Journal of Finance and Financial Law Studies, 2*(1), 61-70. https://izlik.org/JA76NH54DY (Accessed Date:02/03/2026)

Deloitte. (2024). *The rise of women's sports: Unlocking commercial growth.* Deloitte Insights.

Deloitte. (2024). *Women's sports revenue forecast.* Deloitte Insights.

Department of Education. (2016). *K to 12 physical education curriculum guide.* Republic of the Philippines.

Department of Health. (2020). *Philippine physical activity guidelines.* Republic of the Philippines.

Devecioğlu, S. (2005). Türkiye'de spor sektörü stratejilerinin geliştirilmesi. *Verimlilik Dergisi, 2005*(2), 117–134.

Devecioğlu, S., Çoban, B., Karakaya, Y. E., & Karataş, Ö. (2012). Türkiye'de spor kulüplerinin şirketleşmeye yönelimlerinin değerlendirilmesi. *SPORMETRE Beden Eğitimi ve Spor Bilimleri Dergisi, 10*(2), 35–42. DOI: 10.1501/Sporm_0000000218

Dewasiri, N. J., Singh, R., Ranasinghe, A., Dsilva, J., & Shaikh, M. I. (2026). Industry 5.0 for a Climate-Resilient South Asia: A Human-Centric Approach to Net-Zero Futures. In Singh, R., Filho, W. L., & Kumar, V. (Eds.), *Data-Driven Sustainability: Harnessing Technology for A Greener Future and Environmental Resilience. World Sustainability Series.* Springer., DOI: 10.1007/978-3-032-13412-7_23

Diener, E. (1984). Subjective Well-Being. *Psychological Bulletin, 95*(3), 542–575. DOI: 10.1037/0033-2909.95.3.542 PMID: 6399758

Dietl, H., Lang, M., & Werner, S. (2009). Social welfare in sports leagues with profit-maximizing and/or win-maximizing clubs. *Southern Economic Journal, 76*(2), 375–396. DOI: 10.4284/sej.2009.76.2.375

Doğu, H. M. (2020). E-spor ve e-spor hukuku'nda sporcu sözleşmeleri [E-sports and athlete contracts in e-sports law]. *Ankara Üniversitesi Hukuk Fakültesi Dergisi, 69*(2), 443–453. DOI: 10.33629/auhfd.848644

Donnelly, P. (2008). Sport and human rights. *Sport in Society*, *11*(4), 381–394. DOI: 10.1080/17430430802019326

Dorfman, E. (2009). History of the lifeworld: From husserl to merleau-ponty. *Philosophy Today*, *53*(3), 294–303. DOI: 10.5840/philtoday200953317

Dowling, F. (2024). Is sport's 'gateway for inclusion' on the latch for ethnic minorities? A discourse analysis of sport policy for inclusion and integration. *International Review for the Sociology of Sport*, *59*(2), 239–257. Advance online publication. DOI: 10.1177/10126902231198864

Duval, A., & van Maren, O. (2017). The labour status of professional football players in the European Union: Unity in/and/or diversity? *European Labour Law Journal*, *8*(3), 258–278. DOI: 10.1177/2031952517716279

Eather, N., Wade, L., Pankowiak, A., & Eime, R. (2023). The impact of sports participation on mental health and social outcomes in adults: A systematic review and the 'Mental Health through Sport' conceptual model. *Systematic Reviews*, *12*, 102. DOI: 10.1186/s13643-023-02264-8

Eccles, R. G., Ioannou, I., & Serafeim, G. (2020). The impact of corporate sustainability on organizational processes and performance. *Management Science*, *60*(11), 2835–2857. DOI: 10.1287/mnsc.2014.1984

Edexlive (2018, May 17). Learn the Art of Giving from one of it's most successful practitioners, Dr Achyuta Samanta, *The New Indian Express*. https://www.edexlive.com/campus/learn-the-art-of-giving-from-one-of-its-most-successful-practitioners-dr-achyuta-samanta-2875.html

Edexlive. (2020, November, 27). How Kalinga Institute of Social Sciences is providing Odisha's youth access to quality education. *The New Indian Express*. https://www.edexlive.com/news/how-kalinga-institute-of-social-sciences-is-providing-odishas-youth-access-to-quality-education-15351.html

Edugraph, (2025, April 11). KIIT recognised as Best University for Promotion of Sports at 2025 Sportstar Aces Awards. *Telegraph India*. https://www.telegraphindia.com/edugraph/campus/kiit-recognised-as-best-university-for-promotion-of-sports-at-2025-sportstar-aces-awards/cid/2093598#goog_rewarded

Eichenhofer, E. (2015). Social security as a human right: A European perspective. In *Research Handbook on European Social Security Law* (pp. 3–31). Edward Elgar Publishing., DOI: 10.4337/9781782547334.00011

Eime, R. M., Young, J. A., Harvey, J. T., Charity, M. J., & Payne, W. R. (2013). A systematic review of the psychological and social benefits of participation in sport for children and adolescents: Informing development of a conceptual model of health through sport. *The International Journal of Behavioral Nutrition and Physical Activity*, *10*(98), 98. Advance online publication. DOI: 10.1186/1479-5868-10-98 PMID: 23945179

Ekholm, D. (2016). Sport as a means of responding to social problems: Rationales of governing welfare and social change [Doktora tezi, Linköping Üniversitesi].

Ekholm, D. (2016). *Sport as a means of responding to social problems: Rationales of government, welfare and social change* (Doctoral dissertation, Linköping University).

Ekholm, D. (2016). *Sport as a means of responding to social problems: Rationales of government, welfare and social change* (Linköping Studies in Arts and Science No. 687). Linköping University.

Ekholm, D. (2019). Sport as a means of governing social integration: Discourses on bridging and bonding social relations. *Sociology of Sport Journal*, *36*(2), 152–161. DOI: 10.1123/ssj.2018-0099

Ekholm, D., & Dahlstedt, M. (2023). *Sport as social policy: Midnight football and the governing of society*. Routledge.

Ekici, S. (2002). *Türkiye'de spor federasyonlarını oluşturan fahri(gönüllü) çalışanların spor politikalarının oluşumu ve uygulamalarına yaklaşımları, Yayınlanmamış doktora tezi.* Gazi Üniversitesi Sağlık Bilimleri Enstitüsü.

Elkington, J. (1997). *Cannibals with forks: The triple bottom line of 21st century business*. Capstone.

Elsborg, P., Nielsen, G., Klinker, C. D., Melby, P. S., Christensen, J. H., & Bentsen, P. (2019). Sports-based recreation as a means to address social inequity in health: Why, when, where, who, what, and how. *BMC Public Health*, *19*(1), 1084. DOI: 10.1186/s12889-019-7428-3 PMID: 31399029

Elson, D. (2017). Recognize, reduce, and redistribute unpaid care work. *Gender and Development*, *25*(1), 9–24. DOI: 10.1080/13552074.2017.1297473

Emmenegger, P., Kvist, J., Marx, P., & Petersen, K. (2015). Three Worlds of Welfare Capitalism: The Making Of A Classic. *Journal of European Social Policy*, *25*(1), 3–13. DOI: 10.1177/0958928714556966

Emmons, R. A. (1986). Personal strivings: An approach to personality and subjective well-being. *Journal of Personality and Social Psychology, 51*(5), 1058–1068. DOI: 10.1037/0022-3514.51.5.1058

Ergür, O. K., & Köstekçi, A. (2021). Tax justice in the taxation of wage income in Türkiye: The case of athletes. *Journal of Human and Social Sciences Research, 10*(3), 2936–2951. https://doi.org/10.15869/itobiad.907247

Eriçok, R. E. (2019). The Evolution of Tax Expenditures in Turkey: 2015-2021. *Istanbul Journal of Economics, 69*(2), 321-355. https://doi.org/10.26650/ISTJECON2019-0012

Eriksen, I. M., Stefansen, K., & Smette, I. (2025). Sports participation as a reflection of social inclusion in youth: A holistic exploration of sport within young people's lives. *Sport Education and Society*, 1–12. Advance online publication. DOI: 10.1080/13573322.2025.2451354

Erkal, M. (1992). *Sosyolojik Açıdan Spor.* Kutsun Matbaa Reklam Merkezi.

Ersöz, H. Y. (2003). Doğuşundan Günümüze Sosyal Politika Anlayışı ve Sosyal Politika Kurumlarının Değişen Rolü. İstanbul Üniversitesi İktisat Fakültesi Mecmuası, 53(2), 119-144.

Erturan-Öğüt, E., & Şahin, M. Y. (2017). Problems of amateur sports clubs: An exploratory study. *Journal of Sports Sciences, 28*(2), 101–120. https://doi.org/10.17644/sbd.356710

Esping-Andersen, G. (1990). *The Three Worlds Of Welfare Capitalism.* Policy Press.

Esping-Andersen, G. (1990). *The Three Worlds of Welfare Capitalism.* Polity Press.

Esping-Andersen, G. (1990). *The three worlds of welfare capitalism.* Princeton University Press.

Esping-Andersen, G. (1999). *Social Foundations of Postindustrial Economies.* Oxford University Press. DOI: 10.1093/0198742002.001.0001

Esping-Andersen, G. (2015). Welfare regimes and social stratification. *Journal of European Social Policy, 25*(1), 124–134. DOI: 10.1177/0958928714556976

Esping-Andersen, G., Gallie, D., Hemerijck, A., & Myles, J. (2002). *Why we need a new welfare state.* Oxford University Press., DOI: 10.1093/0199256438.001.0001

European Commission. (2018). *Special Eurobarometer 472: Sport and physical activity.* Directorate-General for Education, Youth, Sport and Culture.

European Commission. (2022). *Special Eurobarometer 525: Sport and physical activity*. Directorate-General for Education, Youth, Sport and Culture.

European Institute for Gender Equality. National ministries with responsibility for sports, chromeextension://efaidnbmnnnibpcajpcglclefindmkaj/https://eige.europa.eu/sites/default/files/wmid_mapping_sp_natmin_1.pdf

Eurostat, Employed persons in sport, https://ec.europa.eu/eurostat/databrowser/view/sprt_emp_sex/default/table?lang=en&category=sprt.sprt_emp

Eurostat, General government expenditure by function (COFOG), https://ec.europa.eu/eurostat/databrowser/view/gov_10a_exp$dv_584/default/table?lang=en&category=sprt.sprt_gov

Eurostat, Mean consumption expenditure of private households on sporting goods and services by COICOP consumption purpose, https://ec.europa.eu/eurostat/databrowser/view/sprt_pcs_hbs/default/table?lang=en&category=sprt.sprt_exp

Eurostat, Perception survey results, https://ec.europa.eu/eurostat/databrowser/view/urb_percep$dv_283/default/table?lang=en&category=sprt.sprt_pcs.sprt_pcs_urb

Eurostat, Persons not participating in cultural or sport activities in the last 12 months, https://ec.europa.eu/eurostat/databrowser/view/ilc_scp06$dv_2402/default/table?lang=en&category=sprt.sprt_pcs.sprt_pcs_ilc

Eurostat, Persons participating in cultural or sport activities in the last 12 months, https://ec.europa.eu/eurostat/databrowser/view/ilc_scp03$dv_551/default/table?lang=en&category=sprt.sprt_pcs.sprt_pcs_ilc

Eurostat, Persons participating in formal voluntary activities, https://ec.europa.eu/eurostat/databrowser/view/ilc_scp23$dv_2403/default/table?lang=en&category=sprt.sprt_pcs.sprt_pcs_ilc

Eurostat, Time spent on health-enhancing (non-work-related) aerobic physical activity, https://ec.europa.eu/eurostat/databrowser/view/hlth_ehis_pe2e$dv_300/default/table?lang=en&category=sprt.sprt_pcs.sprt_pcs_pha

Eurostat, Time spent, participation time and participation rate in the main, https://ec.europa.eu/eurostat/databrowser/view/tus_00age$dv_167/default/table?lang=en&category=sprt.sprt_pcs.sprt_pcs_tus

Evans, A. B., & Pfister, G. (2021). Women in sports leadership: A systematic narrative review. *International Review for the Sociology of Sport*, *56*(3), 317–342. DOI: 10.1177/1012690220911842

Evans, A. B., & Pfister, G. (2024). Women in sports leadership: Structural barriers and opportunities. *Sport in Society*, *27*(2), 215–230. DOI: 10.1080/17430437.2023.2187654

Evans, M. D., & Knepper, H. J. (2023). Women's sports and public administration: Intertwined paths to social equity. *Administrative Theory & Praxis*, *46*(2), 107–124. DOI: 10.1080/10841806.2023.2282920

Evens, T., & Lefever, K. (2011). Watching the Football Game: Broadcasting Rights for the European Digital Television Market. *Journal of Sport and Social Issues*, *35*(1), 33–49. DOI: 10.1177/0193723510396665

Fahlén, J., & Stenling, C. (2016). Sport policy in Sweden. *International Journal of Sport Policy*, *8*(4), 515–531. DOI: 10.1080/19406940.2015.1063530

Farrelly, F. J., Quester, P. G., & Burton, R. (1997). Integrating sports sponsorship into the corporate marketing function: An international comparative study. *International Marketing Review*, *14*(3), 170–182. DOI: 10.1108/02651339710170249

Farrer, L., Marinetti, C., Cavaco, Y. K., & Costongs, C. (2015). Advocacy for health equity: A synthesis review. *The Milbank Quarterly*, *93*(2), 392–437. DOI: 10.1111/1468-0009.12112 PMID: 26044634

Ferragina, E., & Seeleib-Kaiser, M. (2011). Welfare regime debate: Past, present, futures? *Policy and Politics*, *39*(4), 583–611. DOI: 10.1332/030557311X603592

Ferrera, M. (1996). The 'southern model' of welfare in social europe. *Journal of European Social Policy*, *6*(1), 17–37. DOI: 10.1177/095892879600600102

Fiege, L. (2025). The social protection of Olympic elite athletes in Europe: A human right trapped between international commitment and domestic institutionalisation? *The International Sports Law Journal*, *25*(4), 234–256. DOI: 10.1007/s40318-025-00323-x

Fiege, L. (2025). *The social protection of Olympic elite athletes in Europe: A human right trapped between international commitment and domestic institutionalisation?* The International Sports Law Journal.

FIFA. (2025). Regulations on the Status and Transfer of Players incl. interim regulatory framework, January.

Fink, J. S. (2016). Hiding in plain sight: The embedded nature of sexism in sport. *Journal of Sport Management*, *30*(1), 1–7. DOI: 10.1123/jsm.2015-0278

Fişek, K. (1985). *100 soruda Türkiye spor tarihi*. Gerçek Yayınevi.

FIVB. (2025, December 14). Athletes take centre stage as kiit kiss centre of excellence is formalized in india. *FIVB.com.* https://www.fivb.com/athletes-take-centre-stage-as-kiit-kiss-centre-of-excellence-is-formalised-in-india/

Fonseca, X., Lukosch, S., & Brazier, F. (2019). Social cohesion revisited: A new definition and how to characterize it. *Innovation (Abingdon)*, *32*(2), 231–253. DOI: 10.1080/13511610.2018.1497480

Foster, K. (2012). *Is There a Global Sports Law?* DOI: 10.1007/978-90-6704-829-3_2

Français, S. (2015–2016). Proposition de loi visant à protéger les sportifs de haut niveau et professionnels. Rapport n° 70.

Franck, E. P. (2013). Financial Fair Play in European Club Football—What is it All About? SSRN *Electronic Journal.* https://doi.org/DOI: 10.2139/ssrn.2284615

Freeman, R. E. (1984). *Strategic Management: A stakeholder Approach.* Pitman.

Fruh, K., Archer, A., & Wojtowicz, J. (2023). Sportswashing: Complicity and corruption. *Sport, Ethics and Philosophy*, *17*(1), 101–118. DOI: 10.1080/17511321.2022.2107697

Fujiwara, D., & Kudrna, L. ve Dolan, P. (2014). Quantifying and valuing the wellbeing impacts of culture and sport. Department for Culture, Media & Sport.

Fung, A. (2006). *Empowered Participation: Reinventing Urban Democracy.* Princeton University Press.

Gaafar, A., Al-Yaaribi, A., Al Droushi, A. R., Al Kitani, M., Al Jadidi, K., & Al Maqbali, D. H.. (2025). Public-private partnerships in supporting talented athletes: Enhancing sports development in educational institutions. *International Journal of Human Movement and Sports Sciences*, *13*(4), 750–758. DOI: 10.13189/saj.2025.130410

Gammelsaeter, H., & Anagnostopoulos, C. (2022). Sport management: Mission and meaning for a new era. *European Sport Management Quarterly*, *22*(5), 637–642. DOI: 10.1080/16184742.2022.2100918

García, B., & Smokvina, V. (2025). The Chinese Model of Sport Empowered and Restrained in the New Era. In *The European Model of Sport Myth or Reality?* (p. 15). Routledge., DOI: 10.4324/9781032665153

Gardiner, S. W. R., B. S., & N. U. (2012). *Sports law*. Routledge.

Gasparini, W. (2020). Sports organisations and policies in France. In Porro, N. R., Martelli, S., & Testa, A. (Eds.), *Sport, Welfare and Social Policy in the European Union* (pp. 86–98). Routledge. DOI: 10.4324/9781351118064-8

Geertz, C. (1973). *The Interpretation of Cultures*. Basic Books.

Geey, D. (2007). The legality of football broadcasts in the UK and the lack of choice for publicans in the Premier League broadcasting market. *Entertainment and Sports Law Journal*, *5*(1), 1–10. DOI: 10.16997/eslj.76

Gencer, H. (2017). *How to Classify the Chinese Welfare State*. University of Bremen SOCIUM Research Center on Inequality and Social Policy.

Geyer, R. R. (2000). *Exploring European social policy*. Polity Press.

GİB (Revenue Administration). (2025) *Tax Expenditure Report*. https://cdn.gib.gov.tr/api/gibportal-file/file/getFileResources?objectKey=arsiv/kurumsal/Vergi_Harcamalari_Raporu_2025.pdf (Accessed: 24/05/2026)

Giddens, A. (1998). *The third way: The renewal of social democracy*. Polity Press.

Girginov, V. (2017). UK: England – National Governing Bodies of Sport and Government Agencies. In J. Scheerder, A. Willem & E. Claes (Eds.), *Sport Policy Systems and Sport Federations: A Cross-national Perspective*, Palgrave Mcmillan.

Giulianotti, R. (2002). Supporters, Followers, Fans, and Flaneurs: A Taxonomy of Spectator Identities in Football: A Taxonomy of Spectator Identities in Football. *Journal of Sport and Social Issues*, *26*(1), 25–46. DOI: 10.1177/0193723502261003

Giulianotti, R. (2011). The sport, development and peace sector: A model of four social policy domains. *Journal of Social Policy*, *40*(4), 757–776. DOI: 10.1017/S0047279410000930

Giulianotti, R. (2016). *Sport: A critical sociology* (2nd ed.). Polity Press.

Giulianotti, R., & Robertson, R. (2004). The globalization of football: A study in the glocalization of the 'serious life'. *The British Journal of Sociology*, *55*(4), 545–568. DOI: 10.1111/j.1468-4446.2004.00037.x PMID: 15663424

Giulianotti, R., & Robertson, R. (2012). Mapping the global football field: A sociological model of transnational forces within the world game. *The British Journal of Sociology*, *63*(2), 216–240. DOI: 10.1111/j.1468-4446.2012.01407.x PMID: 22670645

Gökduman, Ç. (2023). *Fiili Profesyonel Sporcuların Sosyal Güvenlik Hakları Üzerine Bir Araştırma*. Akdeniz Üniversitesi Sosyal Bilimler Enstitüsü.

Gökduman, Ç., Temel, C., & Alper, Y. (2025). *Social Security Practices for Professional Athletes*. DOI: 10.21203/rs.3.rs-5753949/v1

Gosselin, V., Boccanfuso, D., & Laberge, S. (2020). Social return on investment (SROI) method to evaluate physical activity and sport interventions: A systematic review. *The International Journal of Behavioral Nutrition and Physical Activity, 17*(1), 26. DOI: 10.1186/s12966-020-00931-w PMID: 32106872

Gough, I. (1996). Social Assistance in Southern Europe. *South European Society & Politics, 1*(1), 1–23. DOI: 10.1080/13608749608454714

Gratton, C., Shibli, S., & Coleman, R. (2005). Sport and economic regeneration in cities. *Urban Studies (Edinburgh, Scotland), 42*(5–6), 985–999. DOI: 10.1080/00420980500107045

Gratton, C., Shibli, S., & Coleman, R. (2006). The economic impact of major sports events: A review of ten events in the UK. *The Sociological Review, 54*(2_suppl, s2), 41–58. DOI: 10.1111/j.1467-954X.2006.00652.x

Gratton, C., & Taylor, P. (2000). *Economics of sport and recreation*. Spon Press.

Green, M. (2006). From "sport for all" to not about "sport" at all? Interrogating sport policy interventions in the United Kingdom. *European Sport Management Quarterly, 6*(3), 217–238. DOI: 10.1080/16184740601094936

Grix, J., & Brannagan, P. M. (2016). Of mechanisms and myths: Conceptualising states' "soft power" strategies through sports mega-events. *Diplomacy and Statecraft, 27*(2), 251–272. DOI: 10.1080/09592296.2016.1169791

Grix, J., & Brannagan, P. M. (2024). *Sports mega-events as foreign policy: Sport diplomacy, "soft power," and "sportswashing". American Behavioral Scientist.* Online First., DOI: 10.1177/00027642241262042

Grix, J., & Carmichael, F. (2012). Why do governments invest in elite sport? A polity-specific analysis. *International Journal of Sport Policy and Politics, 4*(1), 73–90. DOI: 10.1080/19406940.2011.627358

Grix, J., & Houlihan, B. (2014). Sports mega-events as part of a nation's soft power strategy: The cases of Germany (2006) and the UK (2012). *British Journal of Politics and International Relations, 16*(4), 572–596. DOI: 10.1111/1467-856X.12017

Grix, J., & Lee, D. (2013). Soft power, sports mega-events and emerging states: The lure of the politics of attraction. *Global Society, 27*(4), 521–536. DOI: 10.1080/13600826.2013.827632

Grusky, D. B., & Szelényi, S. (Eds.). (2006). *Inequality: Classic readings in race, class, and gender.* Westview Press.

Grütjen, D. (2008). The Turkish welfare regime: An example of the Southern European model? The role of the state, market and family in welfare provision. *Turkish Policy Quarterly*, *7*(1), 111–129.

Güler, E., & Yaman, M. (2023). Siyasal partiler ve spor politikaları. *New Era International Journal of Interdisciplinary Social Researches*, *8*(18), 19–34.

Gumuş, İ. (2020). Esping-Andersen and welfare regime discussions: A theoretical assessment. *Ekonomi Maliye Isletme Dergisi*, *3*(1), 101–117. DOI: 10.46737/emid.753591

Günay, F., & Enes, K. (2014). *An analysis of incentives and support provided for sports tourism. 3rd Eastern Mediterranean Tourism Congress.* Congress Date 21-04-2014 / 23-04-2014, Mersin, 92-103. https://www.researchgate.net/publication/357484948_SPOR_TURIZMINE_SAGLANAN_TESVIK_VE_DESTEKLER_UZERINE_BIR_INCELEME (Accessed Date:01/05/2026)

Günışık, E. (1990). 'Spor Psikolojisi. *Journal of Physical Education and Sports Studies*, *1*(3), 34.

Gunter, A. (2014). Mega events as a pretext for infrastructural development: the case of the All African Games Athletes Village, Alexandra, Johannesburg. In Szymańska, D., & Biegańska, J. (Eds.), *Bulletin of geography: Socio-economic series* (Vol. 23, pp. 39–52)., DOI: 10.2478/bog-2014-0003

Gürek, A. (2018). *Taxation of footballers and football clubs in Türkiye* [Master's thesis]. Istanbul Okan University. https://tez.yok.gov.tr/UlusalTezMerkezi/tezDetay.jsp?id=mWVegi4Y8dm1L-kP2wOFtA&no=x6LgKBRezeWFAQwolhPZ1w (Accessed Date:02/04/2026)

Güven, S. (2001). *Sosyal Politikanın Temelleri (3. Baskı).* Ezgi Kitabevi Yayınları.

Hallmann, K., Wicker, P., Breuer, C., & Schönherr, L. (2012). Understanding the importance of sport infrastructure for participation in different sports – findings from multi-level modeling. *European Sport Management Quarterly*, *12*(5), 525–544. DOI: 10.1080/16184742.2012.687756

Hallmann, K., Wicker, P., Breuer, C., & Schüttoff, U. (2011). Interdependency of sport supply and sport demand in German metropolitan and medium-sized municipalities – findings from multi-level analyses. *EJSS European Journal for Sport and Society*, *8*(1–2), 65–84. DOI: 10.1080/16138171.2011.11687870

Hancock, M. G., Darvin, L., & Walker, N. A. (2023). Gender equity in sport: Progress and challenges. *Sport Management Review*, *26*(3), 345–360. DOI: 10.1016/j.smr.2022.09.001

Han, J., Kamber, M., & Pei, J. (2012). *Data minin: concepts and techniques*. Morgan Kaufman Press.

Hargreaves, J. (1994). *Sporting females: Critical issues in the history and sociology of women's sports*. Routledge.

Harris, D., O'Boyle, M., Bates, E., & Buckley, C. (2018). Law of the European Convention on Human Rights (4th ed.). Oxford University Press.

Harrison, D.. (2024). Using sport and physical activity interventions to develop life skills and reduce delinquency in youth: A systematic review. *International Review of Sport and Exercise Psychology*. Advance online publication. DOI: 10.1080/1750984X.2024.2349994

Hartmann, D., & Kwauk, C. (2011). Sport and development: An overview, critique, and reconstruction. *Journal of Sport and Social Issues*, *35*(3), 284–305. DOI: 10.1177/0193723511416986

Hartmann-Tews, I. (2006). Social stratification in sport and sport policy in the European Union. *EJSS European Journal for Sport and Society*, *3*(2), 109–124. DOI: 10.1080/16138171.2006.11687784

Hassan, M. K., & Lewis, M. K. (Eds.). (2007). *Handbook of Islamic Banking*. Edward Elgar Publishing., DOI: 10.4337/9781847205414

Hasson, R. E.. (2024). Harnessing the power of sport and physical activity for social change: An interdisciplinary approach to address health equity. *Kinesiology Review (Champaign, Ill.)*, *14*(1), 23–35. DOI: 10.1123/krj.2023-0048

Heggie, V. (2016). Bodies, sport and science in the nineteenth century. *Past & Present*, *231*(1), 169–200. DOI: 10.1093/pastj/gtw004

Heinemann, K. (2005). Sport and the welfare state in Europe. *European Journal of Sport Science*, *5*(4), 181–188. DOI: 10.1080/17461390500344347

Hemerijck, A. (2017). *The uses of social investment*. Oxford University Press. DOI: 10.1093/oso/9780198790488.001.0001

Hennessy, R. (2023). Exploring the Role of Social Protection Interventions in Preventing Child Labour: Reinforcing the Case for a Human Rights-Based Model of Intervention. *Journal of Human Rights Practice*, *15*(1), 262–283. DOI: 10.1093/jhuman/huac064

Henseler, J., Wilson, B., & Westberg, K. (2011). Managers' perceptions of the impact of sport sponsorship on brand equity: Which aspects of the sponsorship matter most? *Sport Marketing Quarterly*, *20*(1), 7–21. DOI: 10.1177/106169341102000104

Hermens, N., Super, S., Verkooijen, K. T., & Koelen, M. A. (2017). A systematic review of life skill development through sports programs serving socially vulnerable youth. *Research Quarterly for Exercise and Sport*, *88*(4), 408–424. DOI: 10.1080/02701367.2017.1355527 PMID: 28796575

Higgerson, J., Halliday, E., Ortiz-Nunez, A., Brown, R., & Barr, B. (2018). Impact of free access to leisure facilities and community outreach on inequalities in physical activity: A quasi-experimental study. *Journal of Epidemiology and Community Health*, *72*(3), 252–258. DOI: 10.1136/jech-2017-209882 PMID: 29330166

Hill, J. S., & Vincent, J. (2006). Globalisation and sports branding: The case of Manchester United. *International Journal of Sports Marketing & Sponsorship*, *7*(3), 61–78. DOI: 10.1108/IJSMS-07-03-2006-B008

Himanshu (2025, December 27). KISS student Jyoshna Shabar conferred with Pradhan Mantri Rashtriya Bal Puraskar; a rising star of Indian weightlifting. *Kalinga TV.* https://kalingatv.com/odisha/kiss-universitys-sports-talent-jyotsna-shabar-receives-pradhan-mantri-rashtriya-bal-puraskar/ https://indiananthro.in/codeofethics.html

Hirschi, T. (1969). *Causes of delinquency*. University of California Press.

Hoeber, L. (2018). Exploring the gaps between meanings and practices of gender equity in a sport organization. *Gender, Work and Organization*, *25*(1), 58–74. DOI: 10.1111/gwao.12162

Hoekman, R., & Scheerder, J. (2021). Sport policy practice and outcome: Theoretical and empirical approaches. *European Journal of Sport Science*, *18*(2), 103–113. DOI: 10.1080/16138171.2021.1926772

Höglund, F., & Bruhn, A. (2024). Sport-based interventions' – A tool for suburban social integration? *Nordic Social Work Research*, *14*(1), 32–44. DOI: 10.1080/2156857X.2022.2062430

Horne, J., & Manzenreiter, W. (2006). An introduction to the sociology of sports mega-events. *The Sociological Review*, *54*(2, suppl), 1–24. DOI: 10.1111/j.1467-954X.2006.00650.x

Houlihan, B., & G. M. (2007). *Comparative elite sport development. In Comparative elite sport development*. Routledge.

Houlihan, B. (2002). *Sport, Policy and Politics: A Comparative Analysis*. Routledge., DOI: 10.4324/9780203160640

Houlihan, B., Bloyce, D., & Smith, A. (2009). Developing the research agenda in sport policy. *International Journal of Sport Policy and Politics, 1*(1), 1–12. DOI: 10.1080/19406940802681186

Houlihan, B., & Green, M. (2009). Modernization and sport: The reform of sport England and UK sport. *Public Administration, 87*(3), 678–698. DOI: 10.1111/j.1467-9299.2008.01733.x

Houlihan, B., & Green, M. (Eds.). (2011). *Routledge handbook of sports development*. Routledge.

Houlihan, B., & White, A. (2003). *The politics of sports development: Development of sport or development through sport?* Routledge. DOI: 10.4324/9780203478547

Human Rights Watch. (2024, January 17). *Saudi government uses European football to sportswash its reputation*. https://www.hrw.org/news/2024/01/17/saudi-government-uses-european-football-sportswash-its-reputation

Hutchins, B., & Rowe, D. (2012). *Sport Beyond Television*. Routledge. DOI: 10.4324/9780203120415

Hylton, K. (2009a). *"Race" and sport: Critical race theory*. Routledge.

Hylton, K. (2009b). *"Race" and Sport: Critical Race Theory*. Routledge.

Hylton, K., & Bramham, P. (2008). *Sports development: Policy, process and practice* (2nd ed.). Routledge.

Ibsen, B., Nichols, G., Piątkowska, M., Nagel, S., Llopis Goig, R., & Elmosc-Østerlund, K. (2022). What can explain the differences between European countries' public policies for sports clubs? *International Journal of Sport Policy, 14*(3), 435–451. DOI: 10.1080/19406940.2022.2052148

Ibsen, B., & Seippel, Ø. (2010). Voluntary organized sport in Denmark and Norway. *Sport in Society, 13*(4), 593–608. DOI: 10.1080/17430431003616266

İmamoğlu, S. H. (2009). An evaluation of the legal framework regarding sports sponsorship. *Ankara University Faculty of Law Journal, 58*(1), 63–94. https://doi.org/10.1501/Hukfak_0000001564

Im, Y.-J., Jung, H.-Y., & Kim, S.-G. (2026). The effects of public sports welfare programs on participants' psychological well-being recovery. *Journal of Sport and Applied Science, 10*(1), 17–23. DOI: 10.13106/jsas.2026.vol10.no1.17

Ince-Yenilmez, M.. (2025). Does gender equality in sports matter? Examining the socio-economic impact on public perceptions. *Frontiers in Public Health*. Advance online publication. DOI: 10.3389/fpubh.2025.1489000

İnci, H. (2011). *Avrupa Birliği ülkeleri ve Türkiye'de yerel yönetimlerin spora katkıları ve spor politikalarının karşılaştırılması* (Master's thesis, Sakarya University).

Indelicato, A. (2025). Does gender equality in sports matter? Examining the socio-economic impact on public perceptions. *Frontiers in Sports and Active Living*, *7*, 1537064. DOI: 10.3389/fspor.2025.1537064 PMID: 40093422

India Education diary Bureau (2023, December 13). KISS Model of Holistic Education for Tribal Children Earns Praise in Lok Sabha. *India education diary*. https://indiaeducationdiary.in/kiss-model-of-holistic-education-for-tribal-children-earns-praise-in-lok-sabha/

India education Diary Bureau. (2025, November 20). KIIT & KISS Set for a Grand Participation at Khelo India University Games 2025. *India Education Diary*. https://indiaeducationdiary.in/kiit-kiss-set-for-a-grand-participation-at-khelo-india-university-games-2025/

International Labour Organisation (ILO). (1948). Freedom of Association and Protection of the Right to Organise Convention (No. 87). https://normlex.ilo.org/dyn/normlex_en/f?p=NORMLEXPUB:12100:0:NO:P12100_INSTRUMENT_ID:312232

International Labour Organisation (ILO). (1949). Right to Organise and Collective Bargaining Convention (No. 98). https://normlex.ilo.org/dyn/normlex_en/f?p=NORMLEXPUB:12100:0:NO:P12100_INSTRUMENT_ID:312243

International Labour Organisation (ILO). (1952). C102 Social Security (Minimum Standards) Convention. https://normlex.ilo.org/dyn/normlex_en/f?p=NORMLEXPUB:12100:0:NO:P12100_INSTRUMENT_ID:312247

International Labour Organisation (ILO). (1981). Collective Bargaining Convention (No. 154). https://normlex.ilo.org/dyn/normlex_en/f?p=NORMLEXPUB:12100:0:NO:P12100_INSTRUMENT_ID:312299

International Labour Organisation (ILO). (1998). ILO Declaration on Fundamental Principles and Rights at Work. Geneva: ILO. https://www.ilo.org/declaration/lang--en/index.htm

International Labour Organisation (ILO). (2012a). Social Protection Floors Recommendation (No. 202). https://www.social-protection.org/gimi/RessourcePDF.action?id=56900

International Labour Organisation (ILO). (2012b). *International Standard Classification of Occupations (ISCO-08)* (Vol. 1). ILO.

International Labour Organisation (ILO). (2019). Issues paper for discussion at the Global Dialogue Forum on Decent Work in the World of Sport. Geneva: ILO. GDFWS/2020.

International Labour Organisation (ILO). (2020). Global Dialogue Forum on Decent Work in the World of Sport – Points of consensus. Geneva, 20–22 January 2020, Sectoral Policies Department. https://www.ilo.org/sites/default/files/wcmsp5/groups/public/%40ed_dialogue/%40sector/documents/meetingdocument/wcms_735388.pdf

International Labour Organization (ILO). (2026). *Social Protection*. Https://www.Ilo.Org/Topics-and-Sectors/Social-Protection

International Olympic Committee. (2026). Paris 2024 Medal Table. https://www.olympics.com/en/olympic-games/paris-2024/medals

Isakjee, A. (2017). Welfare state regimes: A literature review. University of Birmingham Institute for Research into Superdiversity Working Paper 18.

Jarvie, G. (2011). Sport, social division and social inequality. *Sport Science Review*, *20*(1-2), 95–109. DOI: 10.2478/v10237-011-0049-0

Jarvie, G. (2023). Sport policy in Scotland. In *Sport policy across the United Kingdom* (pp. 40–59). Routledge. DOI: 10.4324/9781003241232-3

Jayanthi, N. A., Holt, D. B.Jr, LaBella, C. R., & Dugas, L. R. (2018). Socioeconomic factors for sports specialization and injury in youth athletes. *Sports Health*, *10*(4), 303–310. DOI: 10.1177/1941738118778510 PMID: 29851549

Jespersen, L. N., Michelsen, S. I., Tjørnhøj-Thomsen, T., Svensson, M. K., Holstein, B. E., & Due, P. (2019). Living with a disability: A qualitative study of associations between social relations, social participation and quality of life. *Disability and Rehabilitation*, *41*(11), 1275–1286. DOI: 10.1080/09638288.2018.1424949 PMID: 29357697

Jones, C. (2001). A level playing field? Sports stadium infrastructure and urban development in the United Kingdom. *Environment & Planning A*, *33*(5), 845–861. DOI: 10.1068/a33158

Jürgen, M (2022), Good Governance in the Employment Relations of Athletes in Olympic Sports in Europe: Understanding Evaluating – Improving, European Commission, Physical Education and Sport at School in Europe Eurydice Report.

Juszczak, P., Tax, D., & Duin, R. (2002). Feature scaling in support vector data description. *8th Annual Conf. Of The Advanced School For Computing And Imaging*.

Kaal, H. (2021). Boundary disputes: New approaches to the interaction between sport and politics in the postwar years. *Journal of Modern European History, 19*(3), 362–379. DOI: 10.1177/16118944211014418

Kabeer, N. (2021). Gender equality, inclusive growth, and development. *World Development, 142*, 105–415. DOI: 10.1016/j.worlddev.2020.105415

Kahneman, D., & Deaton, A. (2010). High income improves evaluation of life but not emotional well-being. *Proceedings of the National Academy of Sciences of the United States of America, 107*(38), 16489–16493. DOI: 10.1073/pnas.1011492107 PMID: 20823223

Kalinga Institute of Social Sciences (KISS) – Empowering Underprivileged Tribal Children to Aim for the Sky (2020, November 5). *News Indiatimes.* https://newsindiatimes.com/kalinga-institute-of-social-sciences-kiss-empowering-underprivileged-tribal-children-to-aim-for-the-sky/

Kalinga Institute of Social Sciences (KISS). (2025). *Annual Report: Scaling the SDGs*. KISS Publications.

Kamenecka-Usova, M., Korde, Z., Zidens, J., Luika, S., Agapova, O., Palkova, K., & Martinsone, K. (2025). Research patterns in sports law and sports governance: A scopus bibliometric study. *Frontiers in Sports and Active Living, 7*, 1590858. Advance online publication. DOI: 10.3389/fspor.2025.1590858 PMID: 40735413

Kane, M. J. (2013). The better sportswomen get, the more the media ignore them. *Communication & Sport, 1*(3), 231–236. DOI: 10.1177/2167479513484579

Kang, T., & Kwon, S. Y. (2024). Development of sport policy in South Korea: Historical and institutional analysis. [Yayınevi/journal bilgisi eksik.]

Karagöz, E. (2025). Türkiye'de Sporcuların Sosyal Güvenliği: Statü ve Uygulama Tartışmaları. *Hukuk Fakültesi Dergisi, 11*(2), 125–146.

Karataş Durmuş, N. (2016). Taxation of Sports Clubs. *Journal of the Turkish Academy of Justice, 27*, 245-278. https://izlik.org/JA86CW76RB

Karstensen, J. M., Sandvik, M., & Itkonen, H. (2024). Unlocking the power of sports: An exploration of the nexus between shared place, community competence, and sense of community. International Journal of Sport Policy and Politics. Advance online publication. DOI: 10.1080/19406940.2024.2396836

Kasapoğlu, M. M., & Öçal, M. (2021). Türkiye'de spor yatırımlarının tabana yayılması politikasının sosyal adalet açısından önemi. *Yönetim ve Ekonomi Araştırmaları Dergisi, 19*(3), 173–191. DOI: 10.11611/yead.991462

Kassing, J. W. (2019). "Mes que un club" and an empty Camp Nou: A case study of strategic ambiguity and Catalan nationalism at Football Club Barcelona. *International Journal of Sport Communication, 12*(2), 260–274. DOI: 10.1123/ijsc.2018-0097

Kat, H. (2009). *Bireysel sporcularla takım sporcularının stres düzeyleri ve problem çözme becerilerinin karşılaştırılması. (Yayınlanmamış Yüksek Lisans Tezi).* Erciyes Üniversitesi Sağlık Bilimleri Ensitüsü.

Kay, T., & Bradbury, S. (2009a). Youth sport volunteering: Developing social capital? *Sport Education and Society, 14*(1), 121–140. DOI: 10.1080/13573320802615288

Kearns, C., Sinclair, G., Black, J., Doidge, M., Fletcher, T., Kilvington, D., Liston, K., Lynn, T., & Santos, G. L. (2024). 'Best run club in the world': Manchester City fans and the legitimation of sportswashing? *International Review for the Sociology of Sport, 59*(4), 479–501. DOI: 10.1177/10126902231210784

Kellett, P., Hede, A.-M., & Chalip, L. (2008). Social policy for sport events: Leveraging (relationships with) teams from other nations for community benefit. *European Sport Management Quarterly, 8*(2), 101–121. DOI: 10.1080/16184740802024344

Kelly, L. (2011). 'Social inclusion' through sports-based interventions? *Critical Social Policy, 31*(1), 126–150. DOI: 10.1177/0261018310385442

Kennedy, P., & Kennedy, D. (2013). *Football Supporters and the Commercialisation of Football: Comparative Responses across Europe.* Routledge.

Kennedy, S. S., & Rosentraub, M. S. (2000). Public-private partnerships, professional sports teams and the protection of the public's interests. *American Review of Public Administration, 30*(4), 436–459. DOI: 10.1177/02750740022064768

Keyes, C. L. (2003). *Complete mental health: An agenda for the 21th century. C. L. Keyes, & J. Haidt (Dü) içinde, Flourishing: Positive psychology and the life well-lived.* American Psychological Association.

Kidd, B. (2008). A new social movement: Sport for development and peace. *Sport in Society, 11*(4), 370–380. DOI: 10.1080/17430430802019268

Kidd, B. (2021). Sport and social movements: A global perspective. *International Review for the Sociology of Sport, 56*(6), 847–862. DOI: 10.1177/1012690220972935

Kihl, L. A. (2023). Development of a national sport integrity system. *Sport Management Review, 26*(1), 24–47. DOI: 10.1080/14413523.2022.2048548

King, A. (2016). *The European Ritual.* Routledge.

King, N. (2009). *Sport Policy and Governance: Local Perspectives* (1st ed.). Routledge., DOI: 10.4324/9780080942476

Kleiber, D. A., & Kirshnit, C. E. (2019). Sport involvement and identity formation. In *Mind-body maturity* (pp. 193–212). Taylor & Francis. DOI: 10.4324/9781315792194-14

Klenk, C., Albrecht, J. B., & Nagel, S. (2019). Social participation of people with disabilities in organized community sport. A systematic review. *German Journal of Exercise and Sport Research, 49*(4), 365–380. DOI: 10.1007/s12662-019-00584-3

Koca, C., & Hacısoftaoğlu, İ. (2011). Struggling for empowerment: Sport participation of women and girls in Turkey. In Benn, T., Pfister, G., & Jawad, H. (Eds.), *Muslim women and sport* (pp. 154–166). Routledge.

Koçak, F. (2014). Leisure constraints and facilitators: Perspectives from Turkey. *European Journal of Physical Education and Sport, 6*(4), 184–194.

Koçak, F., & Özşaker, M. (2015). Youth's preferences for the participation of recreational activities: The case of Turkey. *Kastamonu Education Journal, 23*(2), 699–712.

Kocaoğlu, G. (2023). *Türk Hukukunda Sporcuların Sigortalanması.* Kadir Has Üniversitesi Lisansüstü Eğitim Enstitüsü.

Koivunen, A., Ojala, J., & Holmén, J. (Eds.). (2021). *The Nordic economic, social and political model: Challenges in the 21st century.* Routledge. DOI: 10.4324/9780429026690

Kokko, S., Ng, K., Mehtälä, A., Villberg, J., Aira, T., Jussila, A., & Vasankari, T. (2016). An evaluation of equity and equality in physical activity policies in four European countries. *Health Promotion International, 31*(3), 567–577. DOI: 10.1093/heapro/dav001

Koray, M. (2012). *Sosyal Politika (4.baskı).* İmge Kitabevi.

Koronios, K., Psiloutsikou, M., Kriemadis, A., Zervoulakos, P., & Leivaditi, E. (2016). Sport sponsorship: The impact of sponsor image on purchase intention of fans. *Journal of Promotion Management, 22*(2), 238–250. DOI: 10.1080/10496491.2016.1121739

Krieger, J., & Nordhagen, S. E. (2025). The Scandinavian sport model. In García, B., & Smokvina, V. (Eds.), *The European model of sport: Myth or reality?* (1st ed.). Routledge., DOI: 10.4324/9781032665153-10

Kuhnle, S. (2000). The developmental welfare state in Scandinavia. UNRISD Discussion Paper.

Kumar, H., & Downward, P. (2018). Sport participation: From policy, through facilities, to users' health, well-being, and social capital. *Sport Management Review*, *21*(5), 549–562. DOI: 10.1016/j.smr.2018.01.002

Leach, M., Raworth, K., & Rockström, J. (2018). Between social and planetary boundaries. *Nature Sustainability*, *1*(12), 693–695. DOI: 10.1038/s41893-018-0181-1

Leal Filho, W., Azul, A. M., Brandli, L., Özuyar, P. G., & Wall, T. (2021). Gender equality for sustainability in higher education institutions. *Sustainability*, *13*(20), 11469. DOI: 10.3390/su132011469

Lee, S., & No, S. (2022). China's overseas financial direct investment (ODI) in European football clubs: Revisiting ODI in the context of sport industry. *Journal of Global Sport Management*, *7*(3), 391–405. DOI: 10.1080/24704067.2020.1805163

Leibfried, S. (2014). Towards a European welfare state?Jones. C (Eds), New perspectives on the welfare state in Europe (pp. 120-143). Routledge: London and New York.

Leibfried, S. (1993). Towards a European welfare state? In Jones, P. (Ed.), *New Perspectives on the Welfare State in Europe* (pp. 135–156). Routledge.

Levermore, R. (2011). Sport-for-development and the 2010 football world cup. *Geography Compass*, *5*(12), 886–897. DOI: 10.1111/j.1749-8198.2011.00460.x

Levermore, R., & Beacom, A. (Eds.). (2009). *Sport and international development*. Palgrave Macmillan. DOI: 10.1057/9780230584402

Levitas, R. (2005). *The inclusive society? Social exclusion and new labor*. Palgrave Macmillan., DOI: 10.1057/9780230511552

Ley, C.. (2025). The use of sport for social integration amongst disadvantaged populations: A systematic review. *Managing Sport and Leisure*. Advance online publication. DOI: 10.1080/14413523.2025.2603799

Ley, C., Karus, F., Wiesbauer, L., Rato Barrio, M., & Spaaij, R. (2021). Health, integration and agency: Sport participation experiences of asylum seekers. *Journal of Refugee Studies*, *34*(4), 4140–4160. DOI: 10.1093/jrs/feaa081

Liang, X., Quinton, M., Veldhuijzen van Zanten, J., Duan, Z., Zoob Carter, B., Heyes, A., Lee, M., Alharbi, A., & Chen, S. (2024). Legacies and impacts of major sporting events for communities and individuals from disadvantaged backgrounds: A systematic review. *Equality, Diversity and Inclusion*. Advance online publication. DOI: 10.1108/EDI-02-2024-0058

Lindsey, I., Kay, T., Jeanes, R., & Banda, D. (2017). Sport for development in policy, practice and research. In Lindsey, I., Kay, T., Jeanes, R., & Banda, D. (Eds.), *Localizing global sport for development* (pp. 17–51). Manchester University Press., DOI: 10.7765/9781526104991.00008

Ling, Z., & Hong, F. (2014). After the Glory: Elite Athletes' Re-employment in China. *The International Journal of the History of Sport*, *31*(6), 635–651. DOI: 10.1080/09523367.2013.878498

Liu, S., & Qi, W. (2024). Sports poverty alleviation: Concept and model innovation for the development of Chinese sports towns in the new era. *Frontiers in Sports and Active Living*, *6*, 1423767. Advance online publication. DOI: 10.3389/fspor.2024.1423767

Lord, J. E., & Stein, M. A. (2009). Social rights and the relational value of the rights to participate in sport, recreation, and play. *BU Int'l LJ*, *27*, 249.

Ma, D., & Ji, L. (2024). Challenges in Reforms of Chinese Elite Sports: Towards a New Development Mode. In *The Mediating Power of Sport* (pp. 183–203). Emerald Publishing Limited. DOI: 10.1108/S1476-285420240000021011

Madden, P. (2015). Welfare economics of "financial fair play" in a sports league with benefactor owners. *Journal of Sports Economics*, *16*(2), 159–184. DOI: 10.1177/1527002512465759

Madsen, F. (2009). *Transnational Organized Crime* (0 ed.). Routledge. DOI: 10.4324/9780203875827

Mahindru, A., Patil, P., & Agrawal, V. (2023). Role of physical activity on mental health and well-being: A review. *Cureus*, *15*(1), e33475. DOI: 10.7759/cureus.33475 PMID: 36756008

Marin, B., & Lee, C. (2020). Exploring new trends of sport business: Japanese companies' investment in ownership of foreign football clubs. *Sport in Society*, *23*(12), 2031–2054. DOI: 10.1080/17430437.2020.1817897

Mayrhofer, M. (2025). The concept of vulnerability and its relation to the concepts of inequality and discrimination – a review article. *International Journal of Human Rights*, *29*(9), 1589–1618. DOI: 10.1080/13642987.2025.2488938

McConkey, R., Dowling, S., Hassan, D., & Menke, S. (2013). Promoting social inclusion through unified sports for youth with intellectual disabilities: A five-nation study. *Journal of Intellectual Disability Research : JIDR*, *57*(10), 923–935. DOI: 10.1111/j.1365-2788.2012.01587.x PMID: 22672339

McCrone, P. (2025). *Contemporary Issues in Health and Social Care Policy and Practice. In Health and Social Care Funding across the OECD*. Routledge.

McCullough, B. P., Kellison, T. B., & Melton, E. N. (2020). Developing an environmentally sustainable sport industry. *Sport Management Review, 23*(2), 175–190. DOI: 10.1016/j.smr.2019.01.004

Meggyesy, D., & Rosner, S. (2022). Athlete activism and social justice. *Journal of Sport and Social Issues, 46*(5), 389–402. DOI: 10.1177/01937235211068789

Meier, M. (2023). Gender equality and sport development. *European Sport Management Quarterly, 23*(4), 567–584. DOI: 10.1080/16184742.2022.2037645

Meier, M., & Saavedra, M. (2020). Women and sport in Africa: Historical and contemporary perspectives. *The International Journal of the History of Sport, 37*(13–14), 1383–1400. DOI: 10.1080/09523367.2020.1846204

Meir, D., Brown, A., Macrae, E., & McGillivray, D. (2024). Country profile: Sport and physical activity policy in Scotland. *International Journal of Sport Policy, 16*(1), 181–197. DOI: 10.1080/19406940.2023.2271940

Meir, D., & Fletcher, T. (2020). The physical education and sport premium: Social justice, autonomy and school sport policy in England. *International Journal of Sport Policy, 12*(2), 237–253. DOI: 10.1080/19406940.2019.1673790

Menhas, R., & Saqib, Z. A.. (2024). Does physical activity influence health behavior, mental health, and psychological resilience under the moderating role of quality of life? *Frontiers in Psychology, 15*, 1349880. DOI: 10.3389/fpsyg.2024.1349880 PMID: 38529092

Mensah, J. (2019). Sustainable development: Meaning, history, principles, pillars, and implications for human action. *Cogent Social Sciences, 5*(1), 1653531. DOI: 10.1080/23311886.2019.1653531

Metelski, A., Jarosz, O., & Kornakov, K. (2026). Multi-club ownership: A new business model in football. *Journal of Global Sport Management*, 1–19. https://doi .org/DOI: 10.1080/24704067.2025.2459921

Millward, P. (2011). *The Global Football League.*, DOI: 10.1057/9780230348639

Ministry of Youth and Sports. (2019). Strategic plan 2019–2023. Republic of Türkiye Ministry of Youth and Sports.

Ministry of Youth and Sports. (2022). Annual activity report. Republic of Türkiye Ministry of Youth and Sports.

Miragaia, D. A., Ferreira, J. J., & Ribeiro, I. J. (2025). Can sports events contribute to public policy development strategies? *Managing Sport and Leisure*, *30*(1), 1–20. DOI: 10.1080/23750472.2022.2098172

Misener, L., & Darcy, S. (2014). Managing disability sport: From athletes with disabilities to inclusive organisational perspectives. *Sport Management Review*, *17*(1), 1–7. DOI: 10.1016/j.smr.2013.12.003

Mittag, J., Fiege, L., Seltmann, M., ... (2025). Elite athletes' social protection in Olympic sports in Europe: An evaluation of the status quo. SOPROS Evaluation Report.

Mittag, J., Seltmann, M., & Fiege, L. (2022). 3. Central Europe. In J. Mittag, M. Seltmann, L. Fiege, L. O'Leary, P. Zembura, V. Smokvina, L. Haas & T. Santos (Authors), *Fact Report: Understanding the Employment Relations of Athetes in Olympic Sports in Europe*, Erasmus+ Programme.

Mittag, J., Seltmann, M., Fiege, L., & O'Leary, L.. (2022). *Good governance in the employment relations of athletes in Olympic sports in Europe* [EMPLOYS Project Report]. University of Rijeka, Faculty of Law.

Moran, A. P., Matthews, J. J., & Kirby, K. (2011). Whatever happened to the third paradigm? Exploring mixed methods research designs in sport and exercise psychology. *Qualitative Research in Sport, Exercise and Health*, *3*(3), 362–369. DOI: 10.1080/2159676X.2011.607843

Morel, N., Palier, B., & Palme, J. (Eds.). (2012). *Towards a social investment welfare state? Ideas, policies and challenges*. Policy Press.

Morgan, H.. (2025). Sport as a catalyst for social justice and inclusion: A case study of the Gaelic Athletic Association's role in community and youth development. *Youth*, *5*(3), 70. DOI: 10.3390/youth5030070

Morris, J. (2001). Social exclusion and young disabled people with high levels of support needs. *Critical Social Policy*, *21*(2), 161–183. DOI: 10.1177/026101830102100202

Morrow, S. (2014). *Financial fair play: Implications for football club financial reporting*. Institute of Chartered Accountants of Scotland.

Mousa, S. (2020). Building social cohesion between Christians and Muslims through soccer in post-ISIS Iraq. *Science*, *369*(6505), 866–870. DOI: 10.1126/science.abb3153 PMID: 32792403

Moustakas, L. (2022). Sport for social cohesion: Transferring from the pitch to the community? *Social Sciences (Basel, Switzerland)*, *11*(11), 513. DOI: 10.3390/socsci11110513

Moustakas, L. (2024). Sport for social cohesion: A conceptual framework linking common practices and theory. *Sport in Society*, *27*(10), 1549–1567. DOI: 10.1080/17430437.2024.2304231

Moustakas, L., & Robrade, D. (2022). Sport for social cohesion: From scoping review to new research directions. *Sport in Society*. Advance online publication. DOI: 10.1080/17430437.2022.2100304

Mudd, A. L., Bal, M., van Lenthe, F. J., & Kamphuis, C. B. M. (2024). Understanding educational inequalities in sports participation through structurally based resources and individual agency: A sequential mediation analysis. *International Journal for Equity in Health*, *23*(1), 218. DOI: 10.1186/s12939-024-02303-3 PMID: 39434092

Mumcu, H. E., Mumcu, N., Kusan, O., ve Öztürk, O. (2025). İki temel politika: Herkes için spor ve elit spor politikası. EFES Spor Bilimleri Dergisi, 1(1), 20-49.

Murphy, P., & Waddington, I. (1998). Sport for all: Some public health policy issues and problems. *Critical Public Health*, *8*(3), 193–205. DOI: 10.1080/09581599808402907

Musgrave, R. A. (1987). Public Finance. In Macmillan, P. (Ed.), *The New Palgrave Dictionary of Economics* (pp. 1–11)., DOI: 10.1057/978-1-349-95121-5_1643-1

Naluang, S. (2024). The legal architecture of employment contracts for professional athletes. *Rajapark Journal*, *18*(56), 386–404.

Narin, M. (2025). Sekiz ülke politikasında sporun performanstan toplumsal refaha evriminde sosyolojik analiz. *Fenerbahçe Üniversitesi Spor Bilimleri Dergisi*, *5*(2), 3–13.

Nayak, S. (2025, October 23). Asia Rugby Emirates Sevens Trophy 2025: Indian men's team announced, 3 from KISS included. *Kalinga TV*. https://kalingatv.com/odisha/asia-rugby-emirates-sevens-trophy-2025-indian-mens-team-announced-3-from-kiss-included/

Nichols, G. (2007). *Sport and Crime Reduction: The Role of Sports in Tackling Youth Crime* (1st ed.). Routledge., DOI: 10.4324/9780203089156

Nicholson, M., & Hoye, R. (2008). *Sport and social capital*. Elsevier-Butterworth-Heinemann. DOI: 10.4324/9780080569727

Niemann, A., Brand, A., & Weber, R. (2024). *Football Fandom and Identity in the 21st Century: Europe on Their Minds.* Springer Nature Switzerland., DOI: 10.1007/978-3-031-40631-7

Nussbaum, M. C. (2003). Capabilities as fundamental entitlements: Sen and social justice. *Feminist Economics, 9*(2–3), 33–59. DOI: 10.1080/1354570022000077926

Nussbaum, M. C. (2011). *Creating Capabilities: The Human Development Approach.* Harvard University Press. DOI: 10.4159/harvard.9780674061200

Nwokolo, S. C., Singh, R., Khan, S., Kumar, A., & Luthra, S. (2023a). Africa's Awakening to Climate Action. In *Africa's Path to Net-Zero. CSR, Sustainability, Ethics & Governance.* Springer., DOI: 10.1007/978-3-031-44514-9_9

O'Connell, P. J. (1991). The Three Worlds of Welfare Capitalism. by Gøsta Esping-Anderson. *Social Forces, 70*(2), 532–534.

O'Leary, L., Seltmann, M., & Smokvina, V. (2025). Elite athletes and worker status. *Industrial Law Journal, 54*(2), 248–277. DOI: 10.1093/indlaw/dwae025

O'Malley, P. (1992). Risk, power and crime prevention. *Economy and Society, 21*(3), 252–275. DOI: 10.1080/03085149200000013

Öçal, M., ve Kutlu, Ö. (2024). İstihdamın karanlık yüzü: Ter atölyelerine (sweat-shop) insani bir bakış ve ter indeksi ile bir kıyaslama. Çalışma ve Toplum, 2024/4, 1391-1424. https://doi.org/.DOI: 10.54752/ct.1569636

Öçal, M., & Kutlu Dönmez, Ö. (2022). Ruhsal engeli olan bireylerin evsizlik sorununa insani bir bakış ve çözüm önerisi: "Önce konut yaklaşımı". *Mehmet Akif Ersoy Üniversitesi İktisadi ve İdari Bilimler Fakültesi Dergisi, 9*(3), 2006–2026. DOI: 10.30798/makuiibf.1097609

Öçal, M., & Kutlu, Ö. (2023a). A Study On Welfare And Lıvıng Condıtıons Of Dısadvantaged Groups: The Case Of Burdur Provınce. *Journal of Management and Economics Research, 21*(3), 410–425. DOI: 10.11611/yead.1333231

Öçal, M., & Kutlu, Ö. (2023b). Two Sides of the Coin in Ageing in Place: Neighbourhood Safety and Elder Abuse. In Asiamah, N. (Eds.), *Sustainable Neighbourhoods for Ageing in Place.* Springer., DOI: 10.1007/978-3-031-41594-4_5

Odisha Diary Bureau. (2025, December 16), KISS Higher Secondary School Clinches Double Title at CHSE Inter Higher Secondary Schools Rugby Championship 2025. *Odisha Diary.* https://orissadiary.com/four-kiss-tribal-girls-selected-for-u-14-india-team-for-fide-iscf-world-school-chess-championship-2026/

Odisha Diary Bureau. (2026, April 4), Four kiss tribal girls selected for u-14 india team for fide iscf world school chess championship 2026. *Odisha Diary.* https://orissadiary.com/four-kiss-tribal-girls-selected-for-u-14-india-team-for-fide-iscf-world-school-chess-championship-2026/

OECD. (2022). *Gender equality in sport: Policy frameworks and practices.* OECD Publishing., DOI: 10.1787/1f8c9f2a-

Öğüt, E. (2014). Türkiye'de spor yönetiminin neoliberal dönüşümü. *Amme İdaresi Dergisi, 47*(4), 1–26.

Okur, N. ve Erbil Erdugan, F. (2010). "Sosyal Haklar ve Özürlüler: Özürlülük Modelleri Bağlamında Tarihsel Bir Değerlendirme", II. Sosyal Haklar Ulusal Sempozyumu Bildiri Kitabı (s. 245-263), Denizli: Pamukkale Üniversitesi Yayınları.

Oldenburg, R. (1989). *The great good place: Cafes, coffee shops, bookstores, bars, hair salons and other hangouts at the heart of a community.* Paragon House.

Oleksii, N. (2025). Legal Status of a Professional Athlete: Normative Definition and Problems of Regulation, *Visegrad. Journal of Human Rights, 2*(2), 94–99. DOI: 10.61345/1339-7915.2025.2.14

Olimpics, Winner Reward, https://www.olympics.com/ioc/ioc-overview/ioc-history/ancient-olympic-games/rewards

Organisation for Economic Co-operation and Development. (2011). *How's Life? Measuring Well-being.* OECD Publishing., DOI: 10.1787/9789264121164-

Orlick, T. (2015). *In pursuit of excellence.* Human Kinetics.

Österlind, M. (2016). Sport policy evaluation and governing participation in sport: Governmental problematics of democracy and health. *International Journal of Sport Policy and Politics, 8*(3), 347–362. DOI: 10.1080/19406940.2015.1123755

Öz, E., Akçay, F. (2013) Taxation of Athletes, with a Focus on Footballers. *Journal of Tax Issues, 300*, September, 35-54

Özdemir, S. (2011).Refah devletinin gelişme ve bunalım dönemlerinde iş piyasaları. İktisat Fakültesi Mecmuası (Prof.Dr. Toker Dereliye Armağan Özel Sayısı), 55(1), 695-733.

Özdemir, H. (2019). Sosyal uyum ve spor: Engelli bireyler üzerine bir inceleme. *Sosyal Bilimlerde Güncel Araştırmalar Dergisi, 10*(1), 65–72.

Özdemir, S. (2005). Sosyal Gelişim Düzeyleri Farklı Refah Devletlerinin Sınıflandırılması Üzerine Bir İnceleme. *Sosyal Siyaset Konferansları, 49*, 231–266.

Öztuna, B. (2015). Türk Sporcularının Sosyal Güvenliği. *International Journal of Science Culture and Sport, Special Issue*, (3), 805–808.

Öztürk, P., & Koca, C. (2018). Uluslararası politika belgeleri kapsamında spor ve toplumsal cinsiyet politikaları. *Spor Bilimleri Dergisi, 29*(3), 114–130. DOI: 10.17644/sbd.364514

Özveri, M. (2024). *Bireysel İş İlişkileri Açısından Türkiye İşçi Hukuku Tarih-Öğreti-Uygulama-Eleştiri* [Turkish Labour Law in Terms of Individual Employment Relations: History, Doctrine, Practice, Critique]. 2nd ed., Vol. I). E. Ceren Özveri Education and Solidarity Foundation Publication.

Palier, B. (2010). *A long goodbye to Bismarck?: the politics of welfare reforms in continental Europe*. Amsterdam University Press. DOI: 10.1017/9789048512454

Panagiotopoulos, D. P. (2016). Physical Activities-Legal Horizon and Sports Regulation as Lex Specialis: Lex Sportiva. *The Open Sports Sciences Journal, 9*(1), 35–42. DOI: 10.2174/1875399X01609010035

Parnell, D., Millward, P., Widdop, P., King, N., & May, A. (2018). Sport policy and politics in an era of austerity. *International Journal of Sport Policy, 10*(1), 1–5. DOI: 10.1080/19406940.2018.1432672

Parrish, R. (2003). *Sports law and policy in the European Union*. Manchester University Press. DOI: 10.7228/manchester/9780719066061.001.0001

Peace, R. (2001). Social Exclusion: A Concept in Need of Definition? *Social Policy Journal of New Zealand, 16*, 17–36.

Pegoraro, A., Comeau, G. S., & Frederick, E. (2021). #LikeAGirl: Examining social media conversations surrounding women's sports. *Communication & Sport, 9*(2), 271–289. DOI: 10.1177/2167479519893332

Pegoraro, A., Comeau, G., & Frederick, E. (2022). Social media and women athletes. *Communication & Sport, 10*(2), 235–252. DOI: 10.1177/2167479520969785

Pennings, F. (2022). *European social security law*. Intersentia.

Plumley, D., Faulkner, T., & Ioannidis, G. (2025). Inside the deal: Analysing the investment strategy behind UK football club acquisitions—Sport finance and sports law in action. *International Sports Law Review*, 32–43.

Porter, M. E., & Kramer, M. R. (2019). Creating shared value. *Harvard Business Review, 89*(1–2), 62–77.

Prasad, A. (2022, July 8). KIIT & KISS: A sports hub with world-class infrastructure. *The Hindu.* https://sportstar.thehindu.com/other-sports/kalinga-kiit-kiss-odisha-sports-infrastructure-feature-alumni-stadiums/article65598333.ece

Preuss, H. (2004). Calculating the regional economic impact of the Olympic Games. *European Sport Management Quarterly*, *4*(4), 234–253. DOI: 10.1080/16184740408737479

Putnam, R. (2000). *Bowling Alone: The Collapse and Revival of American Community*. Simon & Schuster.

Putnam, R. D. (1993). *Making Democracy Work: Civic Tradition and Modern Italy*. Princeton University Press.

Putnam, R. D. (2000). Bowling alone: America's declining social capital. In *Culture and politics: A reader* (pp. 223–234). Palgrave Macmillan US.

Putnam, R. D. (2000). *Bowling alone: The collapse and revival of American community*. Simon and Schuster.

Putnam, R. D. (2000a). Bowling alone: The collapse and revival of American community. *Proceedings of the 2000 ACM Conference on Computer Supported Cooperative Work*, 357. DOI: 10.1145/358916.361990

PwC. (2023). *The rise of women's sports: Commercial trends and future opportunities*. PricewaterhouseCoopers.

PwC. (2023). *Women's sports outlook and investment trends*. PricewaterhouseCoopers.

Rai, S. M., Hoskyns, C., & Thomas, D. (2019). Depletion: The cost of social reproduction. *International Feminist Journal of Politics*, *21*(3), 381–403. DOI: 10.1080/14616742.2018.1535683

Ramsden, R., Hayman, R., Potrac, P., & Hettinga, F. J. (2023). Sport participation for people with disabilities: Exploring the potential of reverse integration and inclusion through wheelchair basketball. *International Journal of Environmental Research and Public Health*, *20*(3), 2491. DOI: 10.3390/ijerph20032491 PMID: 36767857

Rawls, J. (1971). *A theory of justice*. Harvard University Press. DOI: 10.4159/9780674042605

Rawls, J. (2020). *A Theory of Justice* (Revised Edition). Harvard University Press.

Raworth, K. (2017). *Doughnut economics: Seven ways to think like a 21st-century economist*. Chelsea Green Publishing.

Razavi, S. (2022). Making the Right to Social Security a Reality for All Workers. *The Indian Journal of Labour Economics : The Quarterly Journal of the Indian Society of Labour Economics*, *65*(2), 269–294. DOI: 10.1007/s41027-022-00378-6 PMID: 35911186

Rein, I., & Shields, B. (2007). Place branding sports: Strategies for differentiating emerging, transitional, negatively viewed and newly industrialised nations. *Place Branding and Public Diplomacy*, *3*(1), 73–85. DOI: 10.1057/palgrave.pb.6000049

Reis, C. J. O. D., & Cabral, S. (2017). Public-private partnerships (PPP) in mega-sport events: A comparative study of the provision of sports arenas for the 2014 FIFA World Cup in Brazil. *Revista de Administração Pública*, *51*(4), 551–579. DOI: 10.1590/0034-7612158071

Reiser, M., Breuer, C., & Wicker, P. (2012). The sponsorship effect: Do sport sponsorship announcements impact the firm value of sponsoring firms? *International Journal of Sport Finance*, *7*(3), 232–248. DOI: 10.1177/155862351200700303

Republic of Türkiye Official Gazette. (1971). Labour Act No. 1475.

Republic of Türkiye Official Gazette. (2003). Labour Act No. 4857.

Richard, V., Piumatti, G., Pullen, N., Lorthe, E., Guessous, I., Cantoreggi, N., & Stringhini, S. (2023). Socioeconomic inequalities in sport participation: Pattern per sport and time trends – a repeated cross-sectional study. *BMC Public Health*, *23*(1), 785. DOI: 10.1186/s12889-023-15650-7 PMID: 37118691

Riffi Acharki, E., Spaaij, R., & Nieuwelink, H. (2023). Social inclusion through sport? Pedagogical perspectives of Dutch youth sport coaches. *Sport Education and Society*, *28*(2), 144–158. DOI: 10.1080/13573322.2021.2006174

Riordan, J. (1999). *The international politics of sport in the 20th century*. Routledge.

Roberts, K. (2008). *Key Concepts in Sociology*. Macmillan Education UK.

Robeyns, I. (2017). *Wellbeing, Freedom and Social Justice: The Capability Approach Re-Examined*. DOI: 10.11647/OBP.0130

Robeyns, I. (2005). The capability approach: A theoretical survey. *Journal of Human Development*, *6*(1), 93–117. DOI: 10.1080/146498805200034266

Rogers, E. M. (2004). A prospective and retrospective look at the diffusion model. *Journal of Health Communication*, *9*(sup1, S1), 13–19. DOI: 10.1080/10810730490271449 PMID: 14960401

Rohde, M., & Breuer, C. (2016). Europe's Elite Football: Financial Growth, Sporting Success, Transfer Investment, and Private Majority Investors. *International Journal of Financial Studies*, *4*(2), 2–20. DOI: 10.3390/ijfs4020012

Rohde, M., & Breuer, C. (2017). The market for football club investors: A review of theory and empirical evidence from professional European football. *European Sport Management Quarterly*, *17*(3), 265–289. DOI: 10.1080/16184742.2017.1279203

Ryan, R. M., & Deci, E. L. (2001). On happiness and human potentials: A review of research on hedonic and eudaimonic well-being. *Annual Review of Psychology*, *52*(1), 141–166. DOI: 10.1146/annurev.psych.52.1.141 PMID: 11148302

Ryff, C. D. (1989). Happiness is everything, or is it? Explorations on the meaning of psychological well-being. *Journal of Personality and Social Psychology*, *57*(6), 1069–1081. DOI: 10.1037/0022-3514.57.6.1069

Ryff, C. D., & Singer, B. H. (2008). Know thyself and become what you are: A eudaimınic approach to psychological well-being. *Journal of Happiness Studies*, *9*(1), 13–39. DOI: 10.1007/s10902-006-9019-0

Saavedra, M. (2022). Women, sport, and development. *Sport in Society*, *25*(6), 1105–1120. DOI: 10.1080/17430437.2021.1899173

Şahan, H. (2007). *Üniversite öğrencilerinin sosyalleşme sürecinde spor aktivitelerinin rolü. (Doktora Tezi)*. Selçuk Üniversitesi Sosyal Bilimler Enstitüsü.

Samanta, A. (2021). *Art of Giving: A Way of Life*. KIIT University Press.

Samanta, A. (2024). The KISS Model of Holistic Education. In *Global Perspectives on Social Inclusion*. IGI Global.

Sam, M. P. (2009). The Public Management of Sport: Wicked problems, challenges and dilemmas. *Public Management Review*, *11*(4), 499–514. DOI: 10.1080/14719030902989565

Samuelson, P. A. (1954). The Pure Theory of Public Expenditure. *The Review of Economics and Statistics*, *36*(4), 387. DOI: 10.2307/1925895

Sandford, R., Beckett, A., & Giulianotti, R. (2022). Sport, disability and (inclusive) education: Critical insights and understandings from the Playdagogy programme. *Sport Education and Society*, *27*(2), 150–166. DOI: 10.1080/13573322.2021.1902299

Santomier, J. (2008). New media, branding and global sports sponsorship. *International Journal of Sports Marketing & Sponsorship*, *10*(1), 9–22. DOI: 10.1108/IJSMS-10-01-2008-B005

Sapancalı, F. (2005). *Sosyal Dışlanma*. Dokuz Eylül Yayınları.

Sapir, A. (2006). Globalization and the reform of european social models. *Journal of Common Market Studies, 44*(2), 369–390. DOI: 10.1111/j.1468-5965.2006.00627.x

Sauder, M. H., & DeLuca, J. R. (2023). Framing Course Content on Diversity and Inclusion: Varying Outcomes From Teaching on Disability in Sport Management. Sport Management Education Journal, 1(aop), 1-6.

Saydam, Ç. (2024). Türkiye'de spor politikaları ve İstanbul planlarında spor. *Journal of Social. Humanities and Administrative Sciences*, *7*(46), 2352–2363. DOI: 10.31589/JOSHAS.858

SBB (n.d.). *Presidency of Strategy and Budget, Twelfth Development Plan*. On-Ikinci-Kalkinma-Plani_2024-2028_11122023.pdf (Accessed Date:24/05/2026)

Schausteck De Almeida, B., Barboza Eiras De Castro, S., Mezzadri, F. M., & Lange De Souza, D. (2018). Do sports mega-events boost public funding in sports programs? The case of Brazil (2004–2015). *International Review for the Sociology of Sport*, *53*(6), 685–705. DOI: 10.1177/1012690216680115

Scheerder, J., Claes, E., & Willem, A. (2017). Does It Take Two to Tango? The Position and Power of National Sport bodies Compared to Their Public Authorities. In Scheerder, J., Willem, A., & Claes, E. (Eds.), *Sport Policy Systems and Sport Federations: A Cross-national Perspective*. Palgrave Mcmillan. DOI: 10.1057/978-1-137-60222-0_1

Schulenkorf, N. (2017). Sport for development and peace. *Journal of Sport Management*, *31*(3), 243–251. DOI: 10.1123/jsm.2016-0131

Schulenkorf, N., Sherry, E., & Rowe, K. (2016). Sport for development: An integrated literature review. *Journal of Sport Management*, *30*(1), 22–39. DOI: 10.1123/jsm.2014-0263

Seippel, Ø. (2006). Sport and social capital. *Acta Sociologica*, *49*(2), 169–183. DOI: 10.1177/0001699306064771

Seltmann, M. (2025). Different worlds of athlete welfare? A social policy perspective on elite sport in six European countries. International Journal of Sport Policy and Politics, 1–28. DOI: .DOI: 10.1080/19406940.2025.2583977

Seltmann, M., & Fiege, L. (2025). Many a little makes a mickle: Lessons from negotiating athletes' social protection for strengthening social dialogue in sport. Sports Law, Policy & Diplomacy Journal, 3(2).

Sen, A. (2000). Social exclusion: Concept, application, and scrutiny.

Sen, A. (2006). Conceptualizing and measuring poverty. *Poverty and inequality, 30*, 46.

Sen, A. (1999). *Development as freedom*. Oxford University Press.

Sen, A. (2009). *The Idea of Justice*. Harvard University Press.

Senne, J. A. (2023). Gender equity in sport funding. *Sport Management Review, 26*(2), 210–225. DOI: 10.1016/j.smr.2022.05.004

Serby, T. (2017). Sports corruption: Sporting autonomy, Lex Sportiva and the rule of law. *ESLJ, 15*(1).

Sessa, G., Occhini, G., Milani, C., Marini, G., & Sarro, A. (2020). A public health Italian ethical movement to sustain the beveridge model: Health promotion and equity. *European Journal of Public Health, 30*(5, Supplement_5), 166–1284. DOI: 10.1093/eurpub/ckaa166.1284

Seyyar, A. (2006). Özürlülere adanmış sosyal politika yazıları. Sakarya: Adapazarı Büyükşehir Belediyesi.

Sheng, K. (2017). Analysis on the Social Security System of Retired Athletes in China. *Advances in Economics. Business and Management Research, 32*, 218–221.

Sherry, E., & Coalter, F. (2009). A Wider Social Role for Sport: Who's Keeping the Score? *Sport Management Review, 12*(4), 273–274. DOI: 10.1016/j.smr.2009.05.002

Shilling, C., & Mellor, P. A. (2014). Re-conceptualizing sport as a sacred phenomenon. *Sociology of Sport Journal, 31*(3), 349–376. DOI: 10.1123/ssj.2013-0034

Singh, R., Crowther, D., & Ravesangar, K. (2024b). Harnessing Human Capital for a Sustainable Future: HR's Pivotal Role Toward Net Zero Policies. In Singh, R., & Crowther, D. (Eds.), *Transition Towards a Sustainable Future. Approaches to Global Sustainability, Markets, and Governance*. Springer., DOI: 10.1007/978-981-97-5756-5_2

Singh, R., Ravesangar, K., Narayanan, S., & Singh, K. K. H. (2024a). HRM Practices in Creating Net Zero: Supporting Organizational Sustainability. In Singh, R., Khan, S., Kumar, A., Luthra, S., & Chokshi, H. (Eds.), *Net Zero Economy, Corporate Social Responsibility and Sustainable Value Creation. CSR, Sustainability, Ethics & Governance*. Springer., DOI: 10.1007/978-3-031-55779-8_1

Şişman, Y., (2023). Engellik Alanındaki Kavramsal Karmaşanın Nedenleri ve Mevcut Durum. Üçüncü Sektör Sosyal Ekonomi, vol.58, no.3, 2444-2459.

Şişman, Y. (2017). Türkiye'de Sosyal Politika'nın Dünü, Bugünü: Hayırseverliğin Kurumsallaşması mı? Gelişmesi mi? *Optimum Ekonomi ve Yönetim Bilimleri Dergisi, 4*(2), 1–22.

Sivrikaya, K., & Demir, A. (2019). Türkiye'de 2001 yılı ve sonrasında uygulanan spor ekonomisi politikalarına yönelik bir değerlendirme. *Süleyman Demirel Üniversitesi Vizyoner Dergisi, 10*(23), 126–136. DOI: 10.21076/vizyoner.451499

Skey, M. (2023). Sportswashing: Media headline or analytic concept? *International Review for the Sociology of Sport, 58*(5), 749–764. DOI: 10.1177/10126902221136086

Skille, E. Å. (2010). Competitiveness and health: The work of sport clubs as seen by sport clubs representatives-a Norwegian case study. *International Review for the Sociology of Sport, 45*(1), 73–85. DOI: 10.1177/1012690209352395

Smoll, F. L., Smith, R. E., Barnett, N. P., & Everett, J. J. (1993). Enhancement of children's self-esteem through social support training for youth sport coaches. *The Journal of Applied Psychology, 78*(4), 602–610. DOI: 10.1037/0021-9010.78.4.602 PMID: 8407704

Sotiriadou, P., & De Haan, D. (2019). Women and leadership: Advancing gender equity policies in sport leadership through sport governance. *International Journal of Sport Policy, 11*(3), 365–383. DOI: 10.1080/19406940.2019.1577902

Sözer, A. N. (2020). *Türk Sosyal Hukuku* (2nd ed.). Beta.

Spaaij, R. (2012). Beyond the playing field: Experiences of sport, social capital, and integration among Somalis in Australia. *Ethnic and Racial Studies, 35*(9), 1519–1538. DOI: 10.1080/01419870.2011.592205

Spaaij, R., Magee, J., & Jeanes, R. (2013). Urban youth, worklessness and sport: A comparison of sports-based employability programmes in Rotterdam and Stoke-on-Trent. *Urban Studies (Edinburgh, Scotland), 50*(8), 1608–1624. DOI: 10.1177/0042098012465132

Spaaij, R., Magee, J., & Jeanes, R. (2014). *Sport and social exclusion in global society*. Routledge. DOI: 10.4324/9780203066584

Spicker, P. (2014). *Social policy: Theory and practice* (2nd ed.). Policy Press.

Sport, U. K. (2026). Athlete Support. https://stories.uksport.gov.uk/support-for-athletes/

Sports Law Center. (2026). Collective bargaining agreements in sports leagues. Justia. Accessed April 2026. Available at: https://www.justia.com/sports-law/collective-bargaining-agreements-in-sports-leagues/

Spruit, A., van der Put, C. E., van Vugt, E. S., & Stams, G. J. J. M. (2018). The effect of a sport-based intervention to prevent juvenile delinquency in at-risk adolescents. *Child Abuse & Neglect, 83*, 84–93. DOI: 10.1016/j.chiabu.2018.09.009

Stewart, B., Nicholson, M., Smith, A., & Westerbeek, H. (2004). *Australian sport-better by design?: The evolution of Australian sport policy*. Routledge. DOI: 10.4324/9780203462928

Stiftung Deutsche Sporthilfe. (2026). Die Sporthilfe-Förderung. Accessed April 2026. Available at: https://www.sporthilfe.de/athletenfoerderung/foerderkonzept/

Stiglitz, J. E., Sen, A., & Fitoussi, J. P. (2009). Report by the Commission on the Measurement of Economic Performance and Social Progress.

Storm, R. K., & Nielsen, K. (2012). Soft budget constraints in professional football. *European Sport Management Quarterly, 12*(2), 183–201. DOI: 10.1080/16184742.2012.670660

Subramanyam, V., & Rao, S. N. (2022). Cultural identity, exclusion and inclusion of tribes in India: An empirical research study in Visakha Agency of Andhra Pradesh. *Skylines of the Anthropology, 2*(2), 141–155.

Sunal, O. (2011). Sosyal Politika: Sosyal Adalet Açısından Kuramsal Bir Değerlendirme. *Ankara Üniversitesi SBF Dergisi, 66*(03), 283–305. DOI: 10.1501/SBFder_0000002223

Sunay, H. (2024). Spor ve politika ilişkisi perspektifinde Türk spor politikası. In *Yeni Türkiye: Beden Eğitimi ve Spor Özel Sayısı-I* (pp. 58–78). Yeni Türkiye Yayınları.

Sunay, H. (2024). *Spor ve Politika İlişkisi Perspektifinde Türk Spor Politikası. Yeni Türkiye (Beden Eğitimi ve Spor Özel Sayısı-I).* Yeni Türkiye Yayınları.

Supiot, A.SUPIOT. (2020). The tasks ahead of the ILO at its centenary. *International Labour Review, 159*(1), 117–136. DOI: 10.1111/ilr.12164

Sütlü, S., & Kutlu, Ö. (2025). Profile of substance individual with substance use disorders: Community-based project results. *Journal of Substance Use, 30*(5), 761–766. DOI: 10.1080/14659891.2024.2403079

T.C. Gençlik ve Spor Bakanlığı. (2012). *Ulusal gençlik ve spor politikası belgesi.* GSB.

Tak, M., Sam, M. P., & Jackson, S. J. (2018). The politics of countermeasures against match-fixing in sport: A political sociology approach to policy instruments. *International Review for the Sociology of Sport, 53*(1), 30–48. DOI: 10.1177/1012690216639748

Taylor, P., Davies, L., Wells, P., & Gilbertson, J. ve Tayleur, W. (2014). A review of the social impacts of culture and sport. Sheffield Hallam University.

Taylor-Gooby, P. (Ed.). (2004). *New risks, new welfare: The transformation of the European welfare state*. Oxford University Press. DOI: 10.1093/019926726X.001.0001

Team Sportstar. (2023, December 5). KIIT University bags Best Sports Facility award in CII Sports Business Awards 2023. *The Hindu*. https://sportstar.thehindu.com/other-sports/kiit-university-bags-best-sports-facility-award-in-cii-sports-business-awards-2023/article67606871.ece

Teke, M. S., & Karakuş, S. (2022). Sporun sosyal gelişim sürecine etkisi. *Journal of Social. Humanities and Administrative Sciences*, *8*(53), 733–736. DOI: 10.29228/JOSHAS.62508

Telepbergen, A., & Ermiş, A. (2024). Engelli Bireylerin Sosyal Yaşantıya Dahil Edilmesinde Sporun Önemi. *Optimal Zenith Spor Bilimleri Dergisi*, *1*(2), 49–56. DOI: 10.70736/jozss.2007

The Guardian. (2023, October 8) *The Guardian view on World Cup sportwashing: Money talks- and what it says is troubling*. https://www.theguardian.com/commentisfree/2023/oct/08/the-guardian-view-on-world-cup-sportwashing-money-talks-and-what-it-says-is-troubling

The Independent. (2019, August 9). *What are Man City? Premier League champions, the greatest team ever and a 'sportswashing instrument' of a foreign state*. https://www.independent.co.uk/sport/football/premier-league/manchester-city-premier-league-season-preview-champions-greatest-team-eversportswashing-abu-dhabi-a9046866.html

Thibault, L., & Harvey, J. (2013). The evolution of federal sport policy from 1960 to today. In *Sport policy in Canada* (pp. 11–35).

Till, M., Abu-Omar, K., Ferschl, S., Reimers, A. K., & Gelius, P. (2021). Measuring capabilities in health and physical activity promotion: A systematic review. *BMC Public Health*, *21*(1), 353. DOI: 10.1186/s12889-020-10151-3 PMID: 33588799

Tinaz, C., Turco, D. M., & Salisbury, P. (2014). Sport policy in Turkey. *International Journal of Sport Policy*, *6*(3), 533–545. DOI: 10.1080/19406940.2014.893247

Titmuss, R. M. (1968). *Commitment to Welfare*. Pantheon Books. DOI: 10.1111/j.1467-9515.1968.tb00093.x

Titmuss, R. M. (1974). *Social policy: An introduction*. Allen and Unwin.

Tokatlıoğlu, A. E. (2021). Cumhuriyet modernleşmesinde devletin spor üzerinden bedene bakışı ve spor politikaları. *Journal of Applied and Theoretical Social Sciences, 3*(2), 125–143. DOI: 10.37241/jatss.2021.29

Trendafilova, S., McCullough, B., Pfahl, M., Nguyen, S. N., Casper, J., & Picariello, M. (2014). Environmental sustainability in sport: Current state and future trends. *Global Journal on Advances in Pure & Applied Sciences*, *3*, 9–14.

TRIBES, I. O. S. (2023). LIVES ON THE EDGES: SCHEDULED TRIBES.

Tripathi, R. C. (2026). Revitalising indigenous sports in India: An examination of their impact on fostering social and character development of children. *Curriculum Studies in Health and Physical Education*, *17*(1), 82–93. DOI: 10.1080/25742981.2024.2400259

True, J. (2022). Gender equality and institutional reform. *Politics & Gender*, *18*(2), 345–359. DOI: 10.1017/S1743923X21000445

Tuastad, S. (2019). The Scandinavian sport model: Myths and realities. Norwegian football as a case study. *Soccer and Society*, *20*(2), 341–359. DOI: 10.1080/14660970.2017.1323738

Tugal, A., Özden, S., Türkay, H., & Şahin, O. (2025). Sport as an Investment Vehicle. *International Journal of Current Educational Research, 11*(1), 29-41. https://izlik.org/JA48PH88GR

TÜİK (Turkish Statistical Institute). (2022). *Time use survey*. TÜİK.

TÜİK. (2024) *Industry and Services Statistics*. https://biruni.tuik.gov.tr/medas/?kn=129&locale=tr (Accessed: 24/05/2026)

Turaç, G. (2024). Spor odaklı rekreasyon alanlarının toplumsal sağlık ve sosyal etkileşim üzerindeki rolü. *Beden Eğitimi ve Spor Bilimleri Dergisi*, *18*(3), 621–636. DOI: 10.61962/bsd.1588768

Uçar, A. (2016). *Türkiye'de spor ve rekreasyon politikalarının oluşumu ve bu hizmetlerin sunumu*. [Tez/kitap bilgisi eksik.]

UN. (2006). Engellilerin haklarına ilişkin sözleşme. www.un.org/disabilities/documents/natl/turkey.doc

UNESCO. (2023). *Gender equality and sport: Breaking barriers for women and girls*. UNESCO Publishing.

UNESCO. (2023). *Global report on women and sport participation*. UNESCO Publishing.

United Nations Children's Fund (UNICEF). (2019). *Getting into the game: Understanding the evidence for child-focused sport for development*. UNICEF.

United Nations Development Programme (UNDP). (2020). Human Development Report.

United Nations Educational, Scientific and Cultural Organization (UNESCO). (2015). *Quality physical education (QPE): Guidelines for policy-makers*. UNESCO.

United Nations India. (2024). *KISS: A Global Hub for Sustainable Development Goals*. UN Resident Coordinator's Office.

United Nations. (2003). *Sport for development and peace: Towards achieving the Millennium Development Goals. Report of the Inter-Agency Task Force on Sport for Development and Peace*. United Nations.

United Nations. (2003). *Sport for development and peace: Towards achieving the Millennium Development Goals*. United Nations.

United Nations. (2015). Transforming our world: The 2030 agenda for sustainable development. United Nations General Assembly Resolution A/RES/70/1.

United Nations. (2015). *Transforming our world: The 2030 agenda for sustainable development*. United Nations.

United Nations. (2023). *The Sustainable Development Goals report 2023*. United Nations., DOI: 10.18356/9789210024914

United States Court of Appeals, Johnson v. NCAA, 2024.

Unsal Yılmaz, B., & Şahin, M. (2023). Overview of sports metaphors through visual rhetoric classification in the context of the postmodern consumer culture. *Spormetre Journal of Physical Education and Sport Sciences*, *21*(3), 89–106. DOI: 10.33689/spormetre.1251664

Vanderstraeten, G. G., & Oomen, A. G. (2010). Sports for disabled people: A general outlook. *International Journal of Rehabilitation Research. Internationale Zeitschrift für Rehabilitationsforschung. Revue Internationale de Recherches de Réadaptation*, *33*(4), 283–284. DOI: 10.1097/MRR.0b013e32834012b1 PMID: 22470933

Varea-Calderón, A. D., Rejón-Guardia, F., Ramírez-Hurtado, J. M., & Berbel-Pineda, J. M. (2025). Impact and development of sport sponsorship: A three-decade bibliometric analysis (1993–2024). *Sport, Business and Management*, *15*(2), 176–203. DOI: 10.1108/SBM-09-2024-0134

Vella, S. A., Sutcliffe, J. T., Fernandez, D., Liddelow, C., Aidman, E., Teychenne, M., Smith, J. J., Swann, C., Rosenbaum, S., White, R. L., & Lubans, D. R. (2023). Context matters: A review of reviews examining the effects of contextual factors in physical activity interventions on mental health and wellbeing. *Mental Health and Physical Activity, 25*, 100520. DOI: 10.1016/j.mhpa.2023.100520

Verdot, C., & Schut, P.-O. (2012). Sport and social inclusion: The political position vs. practices. *EJSS European Journal for Sport and Society, 9*(3), 203–227. DOI: 10.1080/16138171.2012.11687897

Wacquant, L. (2009). *Punishing the poor: The neoliberal government of social insecurity*. Duke University Press.,

Walker, A., & Walker, C. (1997). *Britain divided: The growth of social exclusion in the 1980s and 1990s*. Child Poverty Action Group.

Warburton, D. E. R., & Bredin, S. S. D. (2019). Health Benefits of Physical Activity: A Strengths-Based Approach. *Journal of Clinical Medicine, 8*(12), 2044. DOI: 10.3390/jcm8122044 PMID: 31766502

Warburton, D., & Bredin, S. S. D. (2017). Health benefits of physical activity: A systematic review. *Current Opinion in Cardiology, 32*(5), 541–556. DOI: 10.1097/HCO.0000000000000437 PMID: 28708630

Washington, R. E., & Karen, D. (2001). Sport and society. *Annual Review of Sociology, 27*(1), 187–212. DOI: 10.1146/annurev.soc.27.1.187

Watson, K. (2011). D. Kahneman. (2011). *Thinking, Fast and Slow.* New York, NY: Farrar, Straus and Giroux. 499 pages. *The Canadian Journal of Program Evaluation, 26*(2), 111–113. DOI: 10.3138/cjpe.26.010

Weatherill, S. (2017). *Principles and practice in EU sports law*. Oxford University Press.

Weed, M., Coren, E., Fiore, J., Wellard, I., Chatziefstathiou, D., Mansfield, L., & Dowse, S. (2015a). The Olympic Games and raising sport participation: A systematic review of evidence and an interrogation of policy for a demonstration effect. *European Sport Management Quarterly, 15*(2), 195–226. DOI: 10.1080/16184742.2014.998695

Westerbeek, H., & Eime, R. (2021). The Physical Activity and Sport Participation Framework—A Policy Model Toward Being Physically Active Across the Lifespan. *Frontiers in Sports and Active Living, 3*, 608593. Advance online publication. DOI: 10.3389/fspor.2021.608593 PMID: 34027402

Whitaker, A. A., Baker, G., Matthews, L. J., McCombs, J. S., & Barrett, M. (2021). Socioeconomic inequities in youth participation in physical activity and sports. *International Journal of Environmental Research and Public Health, 18*(13), 7124. DOI: 10.3390/ijerph18137124 PMID: 34281061

Whiting, S., Abu-Omar, K., Gelius, P., Firmino-Machado, J., Rakovac, I., & Mendes, R. (2025). Physical activity policy implementation and physical activity levels in the European Union: Are we on track to close the gap between policy and practice? *Health Policy (Amsterdam), 151*, 105200. DOI: 10.1016/j.healthpol.2024.105200 PMID: 39550929

WHO. (2011). *World report on disability*. World Health Organization.

WHO. (2014). *Strengthening Mental Health Promotion* [Fact Sheet No. 220]. World Health Organization.

WHO. (2022). *Physical activity and women's health*. World Health Organization.

Wicker, P., & Breuer, C. (2014). Exploring the organizational capacity and organizational problems of disability sport clubs in Germany using matched pairs analysis. *Sport Management Review, 17*(1), 23–34. DOI: 10.1016/j.smr.2013.03.005

Wicker, P., Feiler, S., & Breuer, C. (2023). Gender differences in sport participation and earnings. *European Sport Management Quarterly, 23*(5), 789–807. DOI: 10.1080/16184742.2022.2041123

Wilson, R., Plumley, D., & Ramchandani, G. (2013). The relationship between ownership structure and club performance in the English Premier League. *Sport, Business and Management, 3*(1), 19–36. DOI: 10.1108/20426781311316889

Winnick, J. P., & Porretta, D. L. (2016). *Adapted physical education and sport*. Human Kinetics.

Women in Sport. (2023). *Gender equality and women's participation in sport report*. Women in Sport Foundation.

Women, U. N. (2023). *Women in sport: Towards gender equality*. United Nations.

World Bank. (2020). *Social inclusion overview*. World Bank. https://www.worldbank.org

World Bank. (2023). *Gender equality and economic development*. World Bank.

World Health Organization (WHO). (2020). *WHO guidelines on physical activity and sedentary behaviour*.

World Health Organization. (2010). *Global recommendations on physical activity for health*. WHO.

World Health Organization. (2018). Global action plan on physical activity 2018–2030.

World Health Organization. (2018). *Global action plan on physical activity 2018–2030: More active people for a healthier world*. World Health Organization.

World Health Organization. (2020). *WHO guidelines on physical activity and sedentary behaviour*. WHO.

World Health Organization. (2020). WHO guidelines on physical activity and sedentary behaviour. World Health Organization. https://www.who.int/publications/i/item/9789240015128

World Health Organization. (2022). *Global status report on physical activity 2022*. World Health Organization. https://www.who.int

World Rugby. (2025). *The Evolution of Rugby in Odisha*. World Rugby Development Series.

Xaxa, V. (2018). Isolation, inclusion and exclusion: The case of Adivasis in India. In *Adivasi rights and exclusion in India* (pp. 27–40). Routledge India.

Yates, B. T., & Marra, M. (2017). Introduction: Social return on investment (SROI). *Evaluation and Program Planning*, *64*, 95–97. DOI: 10.1016/j.evalprogplan.2016.10.013 PMID: 27866664

Yerlikaya, B. (2012). *Spor kavramında dönüşüm ve sporun bir sosyal politika aracı olarak kullanımı* (Master's thesis, Marmara University).

Yerlikaya, B. (2012). Spor kavramında dönüşüm ve sporun bir sosyal politika aracı olarak kullanımı [Yüksek lisans tezi, Marmara Üniversitesi]

Yerlikaya, B., & Öcal, A. T. (2015). Sports as a social policy tool in Turkey. *British Journal of Arts and Social Sciences*, *20*(1), 38–52.

Yetim, A., & Şenel, Ö. (2001). Türkiye'de spor yöneticisi yetiştirme faaliyetlerinin görünümü. *Milli Eğitim Dergisi*, *150*, 50–56.

Yıldırım, F. (2014). *Gri ilişkisel analiz*. Dora Publising.

Yıldırım, S. (2011). *Lisanslı olarak takım sporu ve bireysel spor yapan ile spor yapmayan ortaöğretim öğrencilerinin sosyal beceri düzeylerinin karşılaştırılması. (Yayımlanmamış Yüksek Lisans Tezi)*. Abant İzzet Baysal Üniversitesi Sosyal Bilimler Enstitüsü.

Young, K. (2019). *Sport, violence and society* (2nd ed.). Routledge. DOI: 10.4324/9781315737089

Zhang, T., Liu, H., Lu, Y., & Wang, Q. (2023). The nexus of sports-based development and education of mental health and physical fitness. *International Journal of Environmental Research and Public Health, 20*(4), 3737. DOI: 10.3390/ijerph20043737 PMID: 36834432

Zheng, J., Chen, S., Tan, T.-C., & Lau, P. W. C. (2018). Sport Policy in China (Mainland). *International Journal of Sport Policy, 10*(3), 469–491. DOI: 10.1080/19406940.2017.1413585

Zimbalist, A. S. (2016). *Circus maximus: The economic gamble behind hosting the Olympics and the World Cup*. Brookings Institution Press. DOI: 10.5040/9780815751618

About the Contributors

Mehmet Öçal completed his PhD in Labor Economics and Industrial Relations in 2022 and has been serving as an associate professor in the Department of Social Work at Burdur Mehmet Akif Ersoy University since May 2022. He received the 2022 Outstanding Achievement Award from the Council of Higher Education (YÖK) and the 2023 Prof. Dr. Cahit Talas Doctoral Thesis of the Year Award. Furthermore, in 2024, it received the best thesis award from MEMUR-SEN, and in 2025, it was awarded the best article in the field of social policy by the Social Policy Association. His academic work focuses on improving the welfare and social inclusion of disadvantaged groups.

Mehmet Öztürk, who works on disability and rehabilitation through sports, serves as the president of the Turkish Sports Toto Organization and the general director of educational services at the Ministry of Sports, in addition to his academic work.

***

Hasan Aslan completed his doctoral studies in 2024 at Pamukkale University, Social Sciences Institute, Türkiye, with a dissertation titled "The Outlook on Elderly Poverty in Türkiye and the Role of Old-age Pensions in Elderly Poverty Prevention." He previously earned his master's degree from the same institute in 2018 with a thesis titled "International Seasonal Agricultural Migration: The Case of Artvin." He received his bachelor's degree in 2013 from Pamukkale University, Department of Labour Economics and Industrial Relations. He has been serving as an Assistant Professor since 2026. Prior to this position, he worked as a Lecturer between 2019 and 2026. In addition to his academic roles, Dr. Aslan has held several administrative positions. He served as the Vice Director of a Vocational School from 2023 to 2025 and as the Head of the Department of Property Protection and Security from 2019 to

2022. Before transitioning fully into academia, he worked as a Revenue Specialist at the Ministry of Finance between 2015 and 2019.

Ozal Cicek completed his PhD program at Suleyman Demirel University, Institute of Social Sciences, Department of Labour Economics and Industrial Relations in 2019 with his dissertation titled "The Impacts of the Privatization of Sugar Mills in Turkey on the Productive Class and the Pursuit of Alternative Models". In 2019, his doctoral study was deemed "commendable" in the doctorate category within the scope of the Prof. Dr. Cahit Talas Social Policy Award. He continues his studies as an associate professor at Suleyman Demirel University, Faculty of Economics and Administrative Sciences, Department of Social Work. His academic interests include labor markets, industrial relations, social policies, and new cooperatives.

Julius I. De Guzman is a dedicated educator with 20 years of experience in teaching specialize in Physical education and MAPEH he graduated from pamantasan ng lungsod ng Maynila with a degree in bachelor in physical education (BPE)and finish his master at St. Paul university Manila under the program of Master of Arts in curriculum design development and supervision major in MAPEH. served as MAPEH coordinator for two years at fort bonifacio high school assigned as deped ncr palaro officials in basketball (2018-2023)currently affiliated as path fit instructor at UST under the Institute of physical education and athletics (IPEA) in which awarded as one of the highest student evaluation SY 22-23 serve as speaker and trainer for basketball at the municipality of Sampaloc quezon under the program of IPEA sports:love care and share (may 17-19 2024) member of IAPES

Rosalie I. Dela Cruz is an accomplished educator with 11 years of teaching experience. She currently serves as the Program Chair of the Bachelor of Science in Exercise and Sports Science (BSESS) at the College of Human Kinetics in the University of Makati. Dedicated to the advancement of sports education, she is also a module writer in sports and a passionate dance specialist, inspiring students to excel in both academic and athletic pursuits. Her commitment to holistic learning and her expertise in physical education continue to contribute significantly to the university's mission of nurturing well-rounded individuals.

Ariel S. Dela Cruz, Ed.D., is a distinguished academic leader and a seasoned educator with a career spanning over 15 years in physical education and sports development. He currently serves as the Head of the Physical Education Department and concurrent Sports Development Coordinator at the Technological Institute of the Philippines (T.I.P.), Manila, where he provides strategic direction and oversight for the institution's physical education and sports programs. Dr. Dela Cruz brings a wealth of experience from his long tenure at T.I.P. Quezon City (2009-2023) and his impactful role as a Teacher and Coach at Dr. Juan Nolasco High School. His dual experience in both higher education and secondary school settings has equipped him with a comprehensive understanding of student development across different age groups. As a coach for baseball and softball, he has demonstrated exceptional mentorship, fostering discipline, teamwork, and a drive for excellence among his student-athletes. His leadership is firmly grounded in a robust academic foundation. He earned his Doctor of Education, Major in Educational Management, from Governor Andres Pascual College in 2023, complementing his Bachelor's and Master's degrees in Physical Education from Polytechnic University of the Philippines (PUP) and Bulacan State University (BulSU), respectively. This advanced qualification in educational management underpins his ability to design effective curricula, develop faculty, and administer departments. A lifelong sportsman, Dr. Dela Cruz's expertise is further enriched by his practical involvement as a former varsity baseball and softball player, a certified basketball coach, and a referee. This multifaceted background informs his holistic approach to physical education, where he champions not only physical fitness but also the enduring values of integrity and sportsmanship. Through his leadership, he is dedicated to cultivating a campus culture that actively promotes health, wellness, and character formation through quality physical education and active engagement.

Hülya Kabakçı Karadeniz is a professor at the Faculty of Law, Pamukkale University. Her academic work focuses on tax law and public finance. Her main research interests include tax policy, tax incentives, wealth taxation, property taxation, and the economic and social effects of tax regulations. She conducts national and international academic research on contemporary issues in tax law and the relationship between taxation policies and public interest.

Abdullah Özdemir is a faculty member in the Department of Economics at Aydın Adnan Menderes University, Faculty of Economics and Administrative Sciences, in Nazilli, Turkey. He earned his undergraduate, master's, and doctoral degrees in Economics from the same university. Throughout his academic career, he has edited several books, including "Globalization" (Ezgi Publishing, 2008), "Socio-Economic Change: The Case of Aydın Province" (Alter Publishing, 2009), and "The Socio-Economic and Political Impacts of the COVID-19 Pandemic" (Nobel Academic Publishing, 2020). Additionally, he has presented papers at numerous national and international academic conferences, contributing significantly to discussions in his field. Dr. Özdemir has published extensively on topics such as economic development, social policies, energy economics, and gender inequality.

His research areas include sustainable development, renewable energy policies, poverty, healthcare expenditures, and gender disparities in labor markets.

Bignya Patnaik is an Assistant Professor at the School of Liberal Studies, KIIT Deemed to be University and holds a doctorate in the area of Diversity, Equity and Inclusivity from NALSAR University of Law in Hyderabad and teaches organizational behaviour, Managing Diversity and Inclusivity etc. Her research interests include sustainable development goals, organizational development etc. She can be reached at bignya.patnaikfhu@kiit.ac.in

Pinaki Nandan Pattnaik, PhD, MBA, heads the School of Leadership at KIIT Deemed to be University in Bhubaneswar, India. He earned his doctoral degree from National Law University in Odisha, India, and holds two masters of business administration degrees, one from the University of Saskatchewan in Saskatoon, Canada, and the other from Maastricht School of Management in the Netherlands. His research interests include services marketing the impact of law on the success and failure of university spinoffs and other businesses, entrepreneurship, smart cities, startups, and technology incubators. He can be reached at pinaki.pattnaikfcm@kiit .ac.in.

Yener Şişman is an academic at Anadolu University, Faculty of Economics and Administrative Sciences. He specializes in labor economics and industrial relations, with a particular focus on social policy, social services, and social security. He completed his undergraduate studies in Labor Economics and Industrial Relations at Uludağ University and earned both his master's and PhD degrees in the same field from Anadolu University's Institute of Social Sciences. Throughout his academic career, he has conducted research on topics such as social policy, employment of people with disabilities, migration, working life, and disadvantaged groups. He has authored numerous academic publications, including books, articles, and conference papers, and has supervised many graduate theses.

Index

T

W

Y

www.ingramcontent.com/pod-product-compliance
Lightning Source LLC
LaVergne TN
LVHW062333300926
849161LV00007B/1679